Computed Tomography of the Head and Neck

Contemporary Issues in Computed Tomography
Volume 5

SERIES EDITOR

Stanley S. Siegelman, M.D.
Professor of Radiology
The Johns Hopkins University School of Medicine
Director of Diagnostic Radiology
The Johns Hopkins Hospital
Baltimore, Maryland

Volumes Already Published

Vol. 1 Computed Tomography of the Pancreas, Stanley S. Siegelman, M.D., Editor

Vol. 2 Computed Tomography of the Spine, Victor M. Haughton, M.D., Editor

Vol. 3 Computed Tomography of the Kidneys and Adrenals, Stanley S. Siegelman, M.D., Olga M. B. Gatewood, M.D., and Stanford M. Goldman, M.D., Editors

Vol. 4 Computed Tomography of the Chest, Stanley S. Siegelman, M.D., Editor

Forthcoming Volumes in the Series

Vol. 6 Computed Tomography of the Pelvis, James W. Walsh, M.D., Editor

Computed Tomography of the Head and Neck

Edited by

Barbara L. Carter, M.D.

Professor of Radiology and Otolaryngology
Tufts University School of Medicine
Chief, CT Body Scanning and ENT Radiology
New England Medical Center
Boston, Massachusetts

CHURCHILL LIVINGSTONE
NEW YORK, EDINBURGH, LONDON, AND MELBOURNE
1985

Acquisitions editor: William R. Schmitt
Copy editor: Ann Ruzycka
Production editor: Michiko Davis
Production supervisor: Sharon Tuder
Compositor: Kingsport Press
Printer/Binder: The Murray Printing Co.

Distributed in the United Kingdom by Churchill Livingstone, Robert Stevenson House, 1-3 Baxter's Place, Leith Walk, Edinburgh EH1 3AF and by associated companies, branches and representatives throughout the world.

First published 1985

Printed in USA

ISBN 0–443–08380–0

7 6 5 4 3 2 1

Library of Congress Cataloging in Publication Data
Main entry under title:

Computed tomography of the head and neck.

  (Contemporary issues in computed tomography; v. 5)
  Includes bibliographies and index.
  1. Head—Radiography. 2. Neck—Radiography.
3. Tomography. I. Carter, Barbara L.
II. Series. [DNLM: 1. Head—radiography. 2. Neck—
radiography. 3. Tomography, X-Ray Computed.
W1 C0769MQK v.5 / WE 700 C737]
RC936.C66 1984   617'.5107'572   84–17565
ISBN 0–443–08380–0

Manufactured in the United States of America

Contributors

Olobunmi K. Abayomi, M.D.
Assistant Professor of Therapeutic Radiology, Tufts University School of Medicine, New England Medical Center, Boston, Massachusetts

Mark S. Bankoff, M.D.
Assistant Professor of Radiology, Tufts University School of Medicine, New England Medical Center, Boston, Massachusetts

Barbara L. Carter, M.D.
Professor of Radiology and Otolaryngology, Tufts University School of Medicine; Chief, CT Body Scanning and ENT Radiology, New England Medical Center, Boston, Massachusetts

Hugh D. Curtin, M.D.
Associate Professor of Radiology, University of Pittsburgh School of Medicine; Director, Department of Radiology, Eye and Ear Hospital, Pittsburgh, Pennsylvania

Harvey S. Glazer, M.D.
Assistant Professor of Radiology, Washington University School of Medicine; Edward Malinckrodt Institute of Radiology, Saint Louis, Missouri

William N. Hanafee, M.D.
Professor of Radiology, University of California, Los Angeles, School of Medicine, UCLA Medical Center, Los Angeles, California

Sven G. Larsson, M.D.
Visiting Assistant Professor, Department of Radiology, University of California, Los Angeles, School of Medicine, UCLA Medical Center, Los Angeles, California

Robert B. Lufkin, M.D.
Assistant Professor in Residence of Radiology, University of California, Los Angeles, School of Medicine, UCLA Medical Center, Los Angeles, California

Roy G. K. McCauley, M.D.
Associate Professor of Radiology, Tufts University School of Medicine; Chief, Pediatric Radiology, New England Medical Center, Boston, Massachusetts

Mahmood F. Mafee, M.D.
Associate Professor of Radiology, University of Illinois College of Medicine; Director, Radiology Section, Eye and Ear Infirmary, University of Illinois Hospital, Chicago, Illinois

Robert Oot, M.D.
Fellow, Department of Radiology, Section of Neuroradiology, Massachusetts General Hospital, Boston, Massachusetts

Deborah L. Reede, M.D.
Assistant Professor of Clinical Radiology, New York University School of Medicine; New York University Medical Center; Bellevue Hospital Center; Manhattan Veterans' Administration Hospital, New York, New York.

Stuart S. Sagel, M.D.
Professor of Radiology, Washington University School of Medicine; Edward Malinckrodt Institute of Radiology, Saint Louis, Missouri

Charles J. Schatz, M.D.
Associate Clinical Professor of Radiology and Otolaryngology, University of Southern California School of Medicine; Director, Ear, Nose, and Throat Radiology, Hollywood Presbyterian Hospital, Los Angeles, California

Lucius F. Sinks, M.D.
Professor of Pediatrics, Tufts University School of Medicine; Chief, Division of Pediatric and Adolescent Oncology/Hematology, New England Medical Center, Boston, Massachusetts

Peter Som, M.D.
Professor of Radiology, Mount Sinai School of Medicine of the City University of New York; Chief, Head and Neck Section, The Mount Sinai Hospital, New York, New York

Galdino E. Valvassori, M.D.
Professor of Radiology and Otolaryngology, Abraham Lincoln School of Medicine, University of Illinois, Chicago, Illinois

Alfred L. Weber, M.D.
Associate Professor of Radiology, Harvard Medical School; Chief of Radiology, Massachusetts Eye and Ear Infirmary; Radiologist, Massachusetts General Hospital, Boston, Massachusetts

Preface

Radiology of the head and neck, until recently a subspeciality practiced by few, has been revitalized by the advent of computed tomography (CT). Pluridirectional tomography made it possible to visualize minute details of the temporal bone and paranasal sinuses, but now with CT, cartilage and soft tissue structures are being imaged with even greater clarity. This has resulted in earlier and more accurate diagnoses and more effective treatment with fewer diagnostic studies.

Laryngography and linear tomography have been completely replaced by computed tomography. CT has proven to be the best way to determine the extension of tumor into the pre-epiglottic space, into the deeper structures of the larynx, and through the cartilage into adjacent tissues. It is also important in assessing trauma to the laryngeal cartilage and the cricoarytenoid joint. Evaluation of tumors of the paranasal sinuses depends heavily on CT to reveal tumor extension into the pterygopalatine fossa, the infratemporal fossa, and other areas. In fact, CT has replaced pluridirectional tomography of the sinuses in the radiographic study of tumor, infection, and congenital anomalies.

CT is of similar importance in the evaluation of patients with apparent abnormality of the nasopharynx, the skull base, and the temporal bone. Imaging of the basal cisterns and epidural space together with the blood vessels, the bone, and the soft tissue structures below the skull is much more informative than plain films or conventional tomograms. Orbital venograms and pneumograms have been relegated to the past by CT scanning of the orbit, which reveals in exquisite detail such fine structures as the optic nerve with its sheath, the orbital muscles, the lacrimal gland, the lens, and choroidal structures of the globe.

Although barium studies are still the procedure of choice for detecting morphologic and functional abnormalities of the pharynx and hypopharynx, CT is needed to identify abnormalities of the deeper structures in the parapharyngeal space, the base of the tongue, and the retromolar trigone. Sialography is still needed for visualization of the major ducts of the salivary glands, but CT with or without sialography is the preferred way to demonstrate benign and malignant tumors, cysts, and abscesses of the salivary glands and their neighboring structures. CT can also reveal unsuspected metastases to neck nodes and benign and malignant lesions of the neck, thyroid, and parathyroid glands.

As described in this book, computed tomography has become an essential tool of modern head and neck radiology. It plays a major role in the evaluation of benign and malignant lesions, congenital defects, and trauma. CT is equally important to the surgeon, the radiotherapist, and the oncologist in planning appropriate initial treatment and follow-up care of patients. Magnetic resonance, now on the horizon, will supplement CT and in some cases may replace it. The evolution of radiographic and other imaging modalities has had as much of an impact on radiology of the head and neck area as on any other area of the body.

Barbara L. Carter, M.D.

Contents

1. The Larynx and Hypopharynx   1
   Harvey S. Glazer and Stuart S. Sagel

2. The Neck—Thyroid and Parathyroid Glands   31
   Deborah L. Reede

3. Nasopharynx, Infratemporal Fossa, and Skull Base   59
   Hugh D. Curtin

4. The Base of the Tongue   85
   Sven G. Larsson

5. Paranasal Sinuses and Pterygopalatine Fossa   101
   Peter Som

6. The Orbit and Globe   131
   Alfred L. Weber and Robert Oot

7. The Temporal Bone   171
   Galdino E. Valvassori and Mahmood F. Mafee

8. The Salivary Glands   207
   Mark S. Bankoff and Barbara L. Carter

9. Head and Neck Lesions in Children   237
   Roy G. K. McCauley, Lucius F. Sinks,
   and Barbara L. Carter

10. Planning Radiotherapy for Head and Neck Tumors   279
    Olobunmi K. Abayomi and Mark S. Bankoff

11. Comparison of CT and MR of the Head and Neck   303
    Robert B. Lufkin and William N. Hanafee

CASE STUDIES

**No. 1. Evaluation of a Young Man for Possible
  Acoustic Neuroma**   329
  Charles J. Schatz
**No. 2. Elderly Male with Decreasing Vision
  of the Left Eye**   331
  Charles J. Schatz
No. 3. Elderly Male with Progressive Hearing Loss   333
  Charles J. Schatz
Index   335

1 The Larynx and Hypopharynx

HARVEY S. GLAZER
STUART S. SAGEL

INTRODUCTION

Computed tomography (CT) has become the most accurate radiological technique for evaluating patients with laryngeal carcinoma or trauma.[1-13] In most cases CT demonstrates more extensive abnormalities than are initially appreciated by other radiological modalities, including laryngography and plain film radiography. The cross-sectional display provided by CT allows evaluation of the entire larynx, including the cartilaginous structures and paralaryngeal soft tissues.

In patients with carcinoma of the larynx, CT supplements the findings detected by indirect or direct laryngoscopy. Although laryngoscopy accurately demonstrates mucosal abnormalities, more extensive spread of tumor is often only suggested by abnormal vocal cord mobility or large tumor bulk. Deep extension of tumor into the paralaryngeal and pre-epiglottic space or adjacent cartilaginous skeleton is not directly visualized and may be difficult to document even with deep biopsy. An accurate demonstration of the extent of tumor is necessary to determine whether conservation laryngeal surgery can be performed.[14-15] CT plays a complementary role to laryngoscopy by assessing the paralaryngeal soft tissues and the supporting cartilaginous structures better than was previously possible using contrast laryngography.[4-8]

TECHNIQUE

The most accurate demonstration of laryngeal anatomy is obtained with CT scanners that provide thinly collimated sections at rapid scanning times (<5 sec). The patient is examined supine with the neck slightly hyperextended to make the larynx perpendicular to the scanning plane. Contiguous 4- or 5-mm thick sections are obtained during slow inspiration, starting at the base

1

of the tongue and extending to the subglottic region. If the scans are obtained during suspended inspiration, the airway may appear falsely narrowed because of adduction of the true vocal cords. In selected instances very thin (1.5-mm) collimated contiguous scans with multiplanar reconstruction may have some merit in evaluating carcinoma of the larynx.[16]

Additional scans may be performed during phonation ("e") to distend the pyriform sinuses and improve visualization of the aryepiglottic folds.[17] A modified Valsalva maneuver is also helpful in distending the pyriform sinus.

Intravenous administration of iodinated contrast media is used in selected cases to separate vascular structures from adjacent neoplasm or to assess possible cervical lymphadenopathy more definitively.

NORMAL ANATOMY

Although symmetry of the normal laryngeal structures is helpful in evaluating laryngeal abnormalities, some normal degree of asymmetry must be appreciated in order to avoid misinterpretation. The normal anatomy of the larynx and surrounding structures can best be approached by a discussion of the laryngeal skeleton, superficial and deep soft tissue, the laryngeal airway, and the vascular anatomy of the neck.

Laryngeal Skeleton

The laryngeal skeleton, which protects the airway and supports the soft tissue structures (true and false vocal cords, aryepiglottic folds) within the larynx, consists of the hyoid bone and the epiglottic, thyroid, arytenoid, and cricoid cartilages (Figs. 1.1 and 1.2). The unique appearance of these individual bony and cartilaginous structures allows for easy orientation of the CT sections. The degree of cartilage mineralization varies widely and is generally most extensive in older men.[18]

The *hyoid bone* is a tripartite (body and two greater cornua) structure that surrounds the upper free portion of the epiglottis (Fig. 1.3). The paired greater cornua extend posteriorly from the more anterior body. The normal separation between the components of the hyoid bone may be visible and should not be confused with a fracture.

The air-containing valleculae, which are commonly asymmetrical in size, lie posterior to the hyoid bone and anterior to the free margin of the epiglottis. They are separated by the median glossoepiglottic fold.

The *epiglottis* appears on CT as a thin curved band of soft tissue density anterior to the air-containing laryngeal vestibule and posterior to the valleculae (Fig. 1.3). It is broadest at its superior extent just above the hyoid bone. It quickly tapers below the level of the hyoid bone to a point at its inferior margin, the petiole. Here, in the midline just below the thyroid notch, it attaches to the thyroid lamina via the thyroepiglottic ligament. Since the epiglottis consists of elastic cartilage, it rarely calcifies (Fig. 1.4).

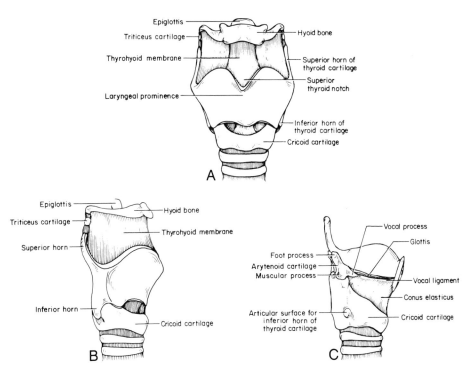

FIG. 1.1. Laryngeal skeleton. (A) Anterior. (B) Lateral. (C) Lateral view with removal of right lamina of thyroid cartilage. (Sagel SS: Larynx. pp. 37–53. In Lee JKT, Sagel SS, Stanley RJ (eds): Computed Body Tomography. Raven Press, New York, 1983. With permission.)

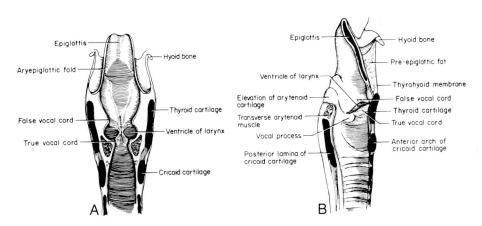

FIG. 1.2. Sections through larynx and surrounding tissues. (A) Coronal. (B) Sagittal. (Sagel SS: Larynx. pp. 37–53. In Lee JKT, Sagel SS, Stanley RJ (eds): Computed Body Tomograpy. Raven Press, New York, 1983. With permission.)

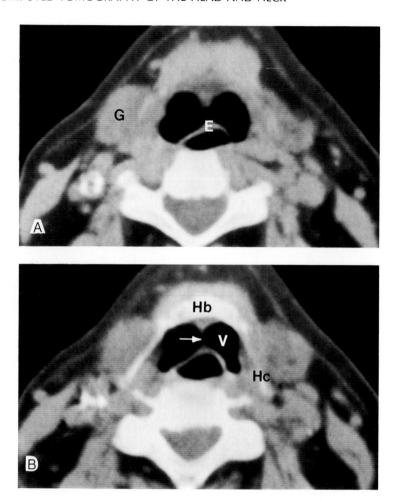

FIG. 1.3. Normal anatomy: high supraglottic larynx (serial scans at 5-mm intervals). (A) The suprahyoid portion of the epiglottis (E) lies posterior to the valleculae and anterior to the laryngeal vestibule. Normal asymmetry in the size of the submandibular glands (G) should not be confused with enlarged lymph nodes. (B) Inferiorly, the body (Hb) and greater cornua (Hc) of the hyoid bone are seen. The two valleculae (V), which can normally be asymmetric, are separated by the median glossoepiglottic fold (arrow).

The *thyroid cartilage,* which is open posteriorly, consists of two laminae that fuse anteriorly in the midline at the laryngeal prominence (Fig. 1.5). The superior thyroid notch, a normal separation where the two laminae do not meet, lies just above the glottis. This should not be confused with cartilaginous destruction. Normal paramedian thinning may be seen anteriorly. At the true vocal cord level the thyroid cartilage is V-shaped, whereas infraglottically it appears more U-shaped. The infrahyoid strap muscles are seen as a soft tissue density band anterior and parallel to the thyroid lamina. The superior and inferior cornua are calcified projections off the posterior bodies of the lamina. The

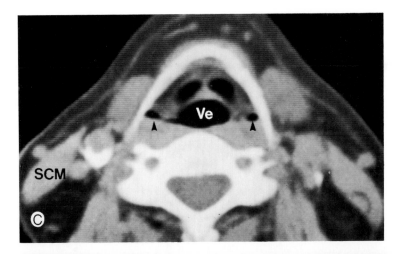

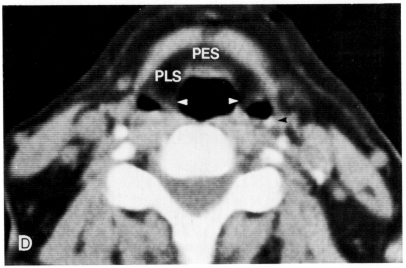

FIG. 1.3 (*Cont.*). (C) At the next inferior level, the valleculae have decreased in size. The top of the air-filled pyriform sinuses (arrowheads) are seen lateral to the laryngeal vestibule (Ve). (SCM) sternocleidomastoid muscle. (D) The fat-containing pre-epiglottic space (PES) is seen anterior to the soft tissue density epiglottis. The fat in the pre-epiglottic space extends laterally into the paralaryngeal space (PLS) and then postero-laterally into each aryepiglottic fold (white arrowheads). Black arrowhead, triticeus cartilage. (Sagel SS: Larynx. pp. 37–53. In Lee JKT, Sagel SS, Stanley RJ (eds): Computed Body Tomography. Raven Press, New York, 1983. With permission.)

superior cornua attach to the hyoid bone via the thyrohyoid ligament; these contain the small triticeus cartilages, which may calcify. The inferior cornua articulate with the cricoid cartilage posteriorly, forming the cricothyroid joint.

There is considerable variation in the degree of calcification and ossification of the thyroid cartilage. In general, there is a rim of cortical calcification with

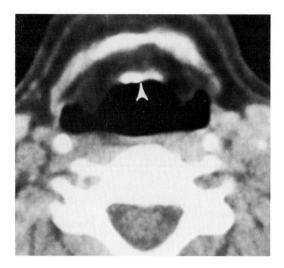

FIG. 1.4. Calcification in epiglottic cartilage (arrowhead).

a more lucent medullary space. However, the pattern may be irregular and incomplete, simulating neoplastic invasion. The laminae tend to be relatively symmetrical in appearance in each individual.

The *arytenoid cartilages* are paired densely calcified triangular structures that lie laterally on top of the cricoid cartilage (Fig. 1.5). The small tapering vocal processes, projecting anteriorly from the base of the arytenoids to attach to the vocalis muscles, define the level of the true vocal cords. The foot processes project superiorly at the level of the false vocal cords, whereas the muscular processes of the arytenoid project posterolaterally toward the thyroid lamina. The muscular processes are separated from the thyroid cartilage by 2 mm or less.

The corniculate cartilages, which sit atop the arytenoids, are usually inseparable from the foot processes of the arytenoids. The paired cuneiform cartilages, when calcified, can occasionally be seen anterior to the foot processes within the aryepiglottic folds.

During phonation the arytenoid cartilages adduct and rotate symmetrically toward the midline to oppose each other (Fig. 1.6).

The *cricoid cartilage,* the most inferior portion of the laryngeal skeleton, is the only circumferential cartilaginous ring in the airway (Fig. 1.7). It sits on the first tracheal ring and, thus, provides the major foundation for the larynx. It is a signet-ring-shaped structure, with a wide posterior lamina that measures 2 to 3 cm vertically and a narrower anterior arch. The cricoid cartilage usually has a well-defined outer cortical rim with a lower-density central medullary space.

At the cricothyroid joint, the thyroid and cricoid cartilages are in close apposition, with approximately 1.5-mm separation between the two. More importantly, the two joints should be symmetrical in appearance.

The cricoid ring defines the level of the subglottic space. Normally, no soft

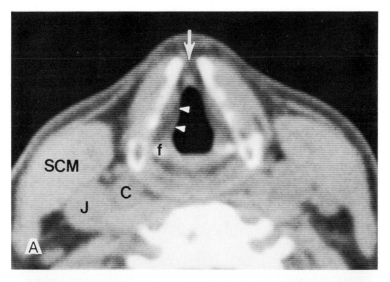

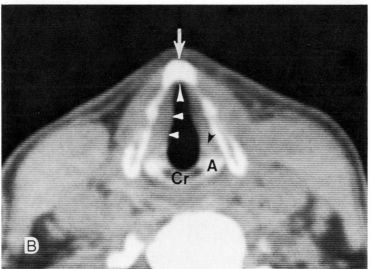

FIG. 1.5. Normal anatomy: false and true vocal cords. (A) The false vocal cords (arrow-heads) lie medial to the fat-containing paralaryngeal space. The foot processes (f) of the arytenoid cartilages are seen posteriorly. The superior thyroid notch (arrow) is seen anteriorly between the thyroid laminae. The thyroid alae are incompletely calcified, a normal variation that should not be confused with cartilage destruction. C, Carotid artery; J, jugular vein; SCM, sternocleidomastoid muscle. (B) The true vocal cords (small white arrowheads) are located at the level of the vocal processes (black arrowhead) of the arytenoid cartilages (A), which articulate with the cricoid cartilage (Cr). The thyroid laminae fuse anteriorly to form the laryngeal prominence (arrow). The soft tissues at the anterior commissure (large white arrowhead) should be less than 2 mm in thickness. The laryngeal airway, which closely abuts the cartilage posteriorly, is elliptical in shape with a long anteroposterior axis.

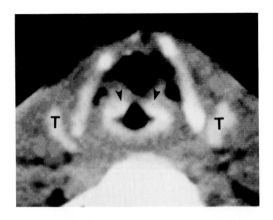

FIG. 1.6. Scan performed during phonation demonstrates adduction of the vocal process (arrowheads) of the arytenoid cartilages. (T) thyroid gland.

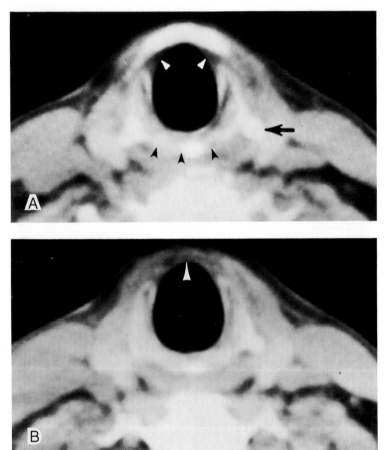

FIG. 1.7. Normal anatomy: subglottic level. (A) The cricoid cartilage (black arrowheads) articulates with the inferior cornua (arrow) of the thyroid cartilage. The undersurfaces of the true vocal cords (white arrowheads) are seen anterolaterally. (B) 1 cm inferiorly, the cricoid ring is almost complete, except at the cricothyroid membrane (arrowhead) anteriorly. The circular subglottic airway is closely apposed to the cricoid cartilage.

tissue density between the airway and the inner surface of the cricoid ring should be detectable.

Laryngeal Soft Tissues

The intrinsic soft tissue structures of the larynx include the aryepiglottic folds, true vocal cords, and false vocal cords.

The *aryepiglottic folds* are obliquely oriented, paired soft tissue structures that separate the laryngeal vestibule and pyriform sinus (Fig. 1.3). They extend first laterally and then medially from the top of the epiglottis caudally toward the false vocal cords. Although the aryepiglottic folds may normally be asymmetrical during inspiration, distension of the pyriform sinuses during phonation or a modified Valsalva maneuver results in a more symmetrical appearance (Fig. 1.8).

The pyriform sinuses are bilateral air-containing structures that lie lateral to the aryepiglottic folds. The two pyriform sinuses join behind the cricoid cartilage to form the cervical esophagus. They are partially collapsed during quiet breathing but distend during a modified Valsalva maneuver or phonation (Fig. 1.8). They are frequently asymmetrical in both their size and their caudal extent.

The *true vocal cords* are visualized during slow inspiration in an abducted position (Fig. 1.5). They are triangularly shaped, soft tissue density structures that are wider posteriorly (approximately 9 mm) than anteriorly (about 2 mm). The anterior commissure is seen anteriorly between the points of attachment of the true vocal cords to the thyroid cartilage, just behind the laryngeal promi-

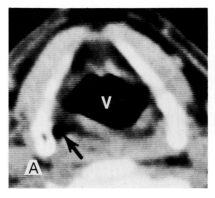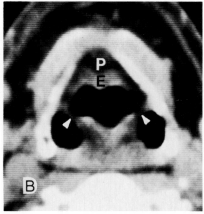

FIG. 1.8.   (A) The pyriform sinuses (arrow) are not well visualized during slow inspiration. (V) laryngeal vestibule. (B) Scan performed during a modified Valsalva maneuver distends the pyriform sinuses. The aryepiglottic folds (arrowheads), which separate the pyriform sinuses from the laryngeal vestibule, are also better visualized. E, epiglottis; P, pre-epiglottic space.

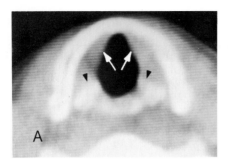
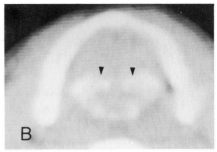

FIG. 1.9. (A) The true vocal cords (arrows) and vocal processes (arrowheads) of the arytenoid cartilages are abducted during slow inspiration. (B) During expiration, the glottis is obliterated and the laryngeal soft tissues appear falsely thickened. The vocal processes (arrowheads) are adducted. (Sagel SS: Larynx. pp. 37–53. In Lee JKT, Sagel SS, Stanley RJ (eds): Computed Body Tomography. Raven Press, New York, 1983.)

nence. When the vocal cords are abducted, no soft tissue thickening of greater than 1–2 mm should be visible at the anterior commissure. The posterior commissure lies between the vocal processes of the arytenoids on the anterior surface of the cricoid lamina. Again, only minimal soft tissue density is seen here when the cords are abducted. If the cords are adducted, the soft tissues in the region of both the anterior and the posterior commissures may appear falsely thickened (Fig. 1.9).

The *false vocal cords* appear as a band of soft tissue, thicker than the true cords, both laterally and anteriorly (Fig. 1.5). The foot processes of the arytenoids are usually visible posteriorly. The false vocal cords are slightly less dense than the true vocal cords because of their higher fat content. At the level of the false vocal cords, normally the soft tissue is appreciably thickened anteriorly behind the thyroid lamina, secondary in part to insertion of the thyroepiglottic ligament.

The laryngeal ventricle separating the true and false vocal cords is visualized

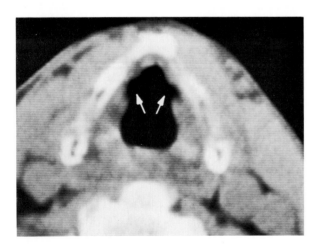

FIG. 1.10. Laryngeal ventricle. Scan performed during reverse "e" maneuver demonstrates the laryngeal ventricle (arrows). Note the irregular ossification of the thyroid cartilage, a normal variation.

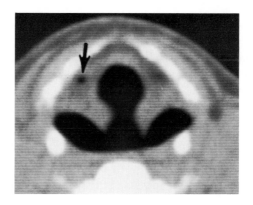

FIG. 1.11.   Saccule of laryngeal ventricle. Scan performed   during   modified Valsalva maneuver demonstrates   air   in   the   saccule of the laryngeal ventricle (arrow).

in only 10 percent of patients, because of partial volume averaging. A reverse "e" maneuver may help fill out the ventricles (Fig. 1.10) but is difficult for most patients to accomplish in the supine scanning position.

A small collection of air may occasionally be seen on CT anterolateral to the false vocal cord (Fig. 1.11). This represents the normal saccule of the laryngeal ventricle. This structure has been reported to be visualized in 40 percent of laryngograms;[19] it is seen less frequently on CT because specific maneuvers to distend the saccule by increasing intralaryngeal pressure are not usually performed.

Deep Soft Tissue Spaces of the Larynx

The soft tissue deep to the endolarynx is composed primarily of fat and consequently is of lower density than the true vocal cords or neoplasm. The preepiglottic space is a triangularly shaped region that is bordered superiorly by the valleculae, posteriorly by the epiglottis, and anteriorly by the thyrohyoid membrane (Fig. 1.3). It extends inferiorly from the hyoid bone caudally to the anterior commissure. It is usually composed of homogeneous fat density. However, an area of higher density may be seen superiorly at the level of the hyoid bone because of the presence of the hyoepiglottic ligament, which should not be confused with an infiltrating tumor.

The pre-epiglottic space is contiguous laterally with the paralaryngeal space (Figs. 1.3, 1.8). On CT the paralaryngeal space also appears as a low density zone bounded laterally by the thyroid cartilage, medially by the aryepiglottic folds, and posteriorly by the pyriform sinus. The paralaryngeal space narrows caudally as scans proceed toward the level of the true vocal cord.

Laryngeal Airway

The *laryngeal airway* has different configurations at different CT levels (Figs. 1.3, 1.5, 1.7). The supraglottic portion of the airway, the laryngeal vestibule, is elliptical in shape. The anteroposterior axis of the airway increases at the

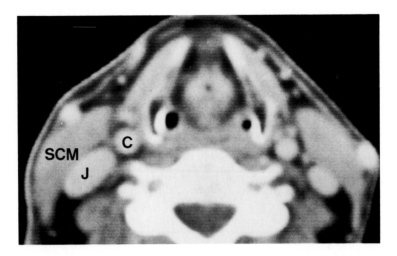

FIG. 1.12.   Normal vascular anatomy. Scan performed after administration of intravenous contrast demonstrates the common carotid artery (C) and internal jugular vein (J) posteromedial to the sternocleidomastoid muscle (SCM). The laryngeal vestibule is obliterated because the patient performed a Valsalva maneuver during the injection of contrast.

level of the true vocal cords. The subglottic region is more circular, with a flat posterior border at the level of the trachea.

Vascular Anatomy

The jugular vein and carotid artery lie posterolateral to the thyroid laminae (Fig. 1.12). The jugular vein lies posterolateral to the carotid artery and can be quite variable in size. The right jugular vein, which is usually larger than the left, can be confused both on CT and on physical examination with lymph node enlargement (Fig. 1.13). In difficult cases, scanning after intravenous contrast administration improves depiction of the normal vascular structure.

LARYNGEAL NEOPLASMS

Laryngoscopy is the best method to examine the laryngeal mucosa and glottic function. Although CT may demonstrate mucosal abnormalities secondary to small tumors, subtle asymmetries of the laryngeal soft tissues may fall within the normal range. CT scans may also appear entirely normal when laryngoscopy discloses a small laryngeal carcinoma. However, these findings are indicative of a localized tumor.

In deciding between radiation therapy, conservation surgery, and total laryngectomy an accurate demonstration of tumor extent is necessary.[14-15] The major role of CT is to examine those areas of the larynx that are not well visualized by laryngoscopy. Laryngeal tumors may be bulky, making examination of much

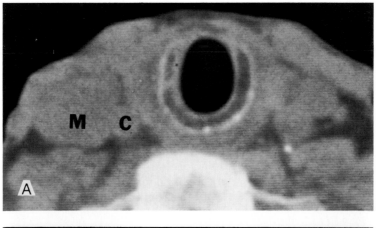

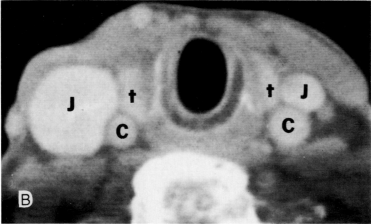

FIG. 1.13.   Dilatation of right internal jugular vein. (A) Scans performed because of palpable right neck mass demonstrate a soft tissue density mass (M) lateral to the common carotid artery (C) in the expected position of the internal jugular vein. (B) Scan performed after intravenous contrast administration shows that the apparent soft tissue mass is an enlarged right internal jugular vein (J). More caudal scans confirmed the absence of a mass obstructing the jugular vein. C, carotid artery; J, left internal jugular vein; t, enhancing thyroid gland.

of the larynx difficult by laryngoscopy. In addition, CT may demonstrate deep (submucosal) extension of the tumor and invasion of cartilage that are not suspected clinically.

Neoplasm appears on CT as an area of increased soft tissue density that alters the normal symmetrical laryngeal anatomy. Such CT findings are not histologically specific and may also be caused by edema, hemorrhage, inflammation, or fibrosis. The CT examination must be correlated with the clinical history and should be performed prior to laryngeal biopsy to prevent confusion of post-biopsy hemorrhage and edema with neoplasm.

Glottic Tumors

If a vocal cord carcinoma is confined to a normally mobile true vocal cord, it may be treated with radiation therapy or partial laryngectomy.[14] CT scans may be normal in these cases or may show focal or diffuse cord thickening (Fig. 1.14). Although a paralyzed true vocal cord can simulate a thickened cord secondary to neoplasm on CT, distinction between the two conditions should have been made by previous laryngoscopy.

The major role of CT in patients with true vocal cord neoplasms is in evaluating involvement of the anterior commissure, the thyroid and cricoid cartilages, and the paralaryngeal and subglottic spaces. Involvement of greater than 30 percent of the contralateral true vocal cord, invasion of thyroid cartilage, or subglottic extension of tumor precludes successful conservation surgery.[14]

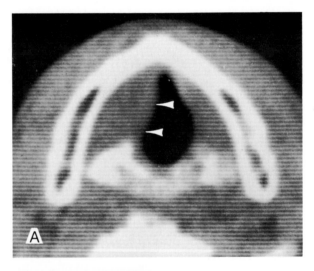

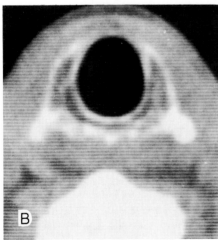

FIG. 1.14. Localized true vocal cord carcinoma. (A) Neoplasm diffusely thickens the right true vocal cord (arrowheads). (B) No subglottic extension is seen as evidence by close apposition of the airway to the cricoid cartilage. Right hemilaryngectomy was performed.

Soft tissue is normally less than 2 mm thick at the anterior commissure. An increase in thickness should be considered abnormal, whether it is secondary to tumor, to hemorrhage, or to edema (Fig. 1.15). If true vocal cord carcinomas reach the anterior commissure, they can extend infraglottically to the contralateral vocal cord or invade the thyroid cartilage.[20] Large true vocal cord neoplasms may bulge across the midline and appear to extend to the contralateral cord. In these cases, CT may demonstrate a clear tissue plane between the anterior commissure and the contralateral true vocal cord. Neoplasms may also extend posteriorly, resulting in soft tissue thickening over the arytenoid cartilages (Fig. 1.16); concomitant rotation or displacement of the arytenoid cartilages may occur. When the bulk of tumor is in close proximity to the arytenoid cartilages, cartilage involvement is very likely, especially if the arytenoid cartilages are fixed or limited in motion.[12]

Although CT is helpful in demonstrating cartilaginous invasion, certain pitfalls and limitations exist (Figs. 1.17–1.19).[2,5] Since the thyroid cartilage may normally have an irregular pattern of calcification and ossification, only moderately or far advanced neoplastic involvement can be confidently diagnosed. Extensive cartilage destruction may appear as fragmentation of the normal cartilage, with tumor spread outside the confines of the thyroid cartilage. Cartilage involvement may also be suggested by the presence of distortion without obvious destruction (e.g., bowing of the thyroid cartilage). When CT findings are equivocal, biopsy of the cartilage after the initial surgical incision should be recommended to confirm the need for possible radical surgery.

The paralaryngeal space provides access for vertical extension of laryngeal carcinoma. At the level of the true vocal cords a thin line of fat density may be seen medial to the thyroid cartilage.[10] Bilateral absence of this line may be a normal finding. However, absence only on the side of the neoplasm is

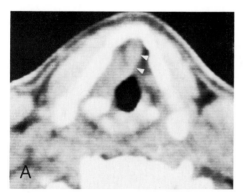 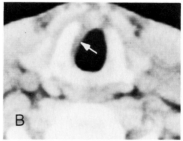

FIG. 1.15. True vocal cord carcinoma with involvement of anterior commissure and subglottic extension. (A) Neoplasm of the right true vocal cord spreads anteriorly to involve the anterior commissure (arrowheads). (B) Inferior extension of tumor is seen in the subglottic region, producing soft tissue (arrow) thickening between the airway and the cricoid arch. Total laryngectomy was performed.

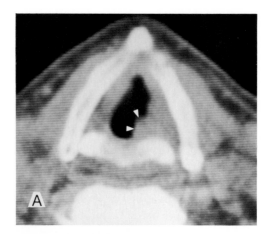

FIG. 1.16. True vocal cord carcinoma with involvement of posterior commissure and subglottic extenstion. (A) Left true vocal cord tumor extends posteromedially over arytenoid cartilage (arrowheads) toward the posterior commissure. (B) Subglottic extension (arrowheads) is noted inferiorly. Total laryngectomy was performed. (Sagel SS: Larynx. pp. 37–53. In Lee JKT, Sagel SS, Stanley RJ (eds): Computed Body Tomography. Raven Press, New York, 1983.)

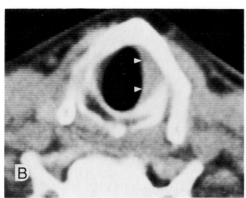

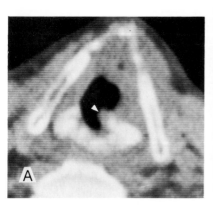
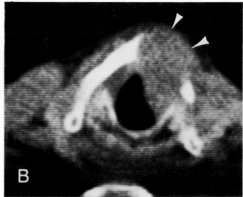

FIG. 1.17. True vocal cord carcinoma with thyroid cartilage destruction. (A) Left true vocal cord neoplasm extends over vocal process of arytenoid (arrowhead) and anteriorly across anterior commissure. (Sagel SS: Larynx. pp. 37–53. In Lee JKT, Sagel SS, Stanley RJ (eds): Computed Body Tomography. Raven Press, New York, 1983.) (B) Tumor extends inferiorly into the subglottic space and through the left thyroid ala into the adjacent subcutaneous tissue (arrowheads). Total laryngectomy was performed.

16

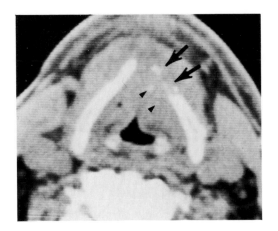

FIG. 1.18. Thyroid cartilage destruction. A large carcinoma involves the anterior commissure and destroys the anterior portion of the left thyroid ala (arrows). Several small bony fragments can be seen within the tumor (arrowheads).

highly suggestive of tumor invasion of the paralaryngeal space. Extension into the paralaryngeal space at the false vocal cord level is easier to demonstrate, because the space is wider. CT, however, is somewhat limited in its ability to define extension into the false vocal cord itself; such assessment generally is more easily defined by laryngoscopy.

Subglottic extension of a true vocal cord carcinoma greater than 1 cm anteriorly and 6 mm posteriorly is an indication for total laryngectomy.[14,20] However, the relationship between the tumor and the cricoid ring, which is easily demonstrated by CT, is more important than any arbitrary measurement (Figs. 1.15–1.17). Below the undersurface of the true vocal cords the soft tissue is not normally thickened between the cricoid cartilage and the airway, although a small degree of thickening may be seen anteriorly just beneath the bottom of the true vocal cords (Fig. 1.7).

Laryngoscopic demonstration of vocal cord fixation is thought to be a sign

FIG. 1.19. True vocal cord carcinoma without cartilage invasion. Irregularity of the right thyroid ala (arrowheads) is seen adjacent to a tumor of the right true vocal cord. A total laryngectomy was performed because of anterior commissure involvement and subglottic extension demonstrated on more inferior scans. Pathological examination of the surgical specimen demonstrated no evidence of cartilage invasion.

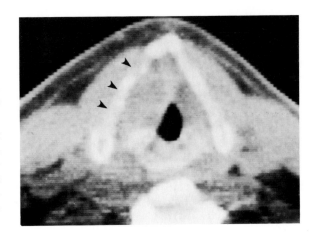

suggesting deep infiltration by tumor.[20] Although phonation scans may demonstrate vocal cord fixation, CT is most helpful in separating the variety of causes of cord fixation preoperatively as well as in demonstrating deep infiltration in those patients with mobile true vocal cords.[6] Causes of vocal cord fixation include subglottic extension of tumor, thyroid cartilage invasion, and invasion

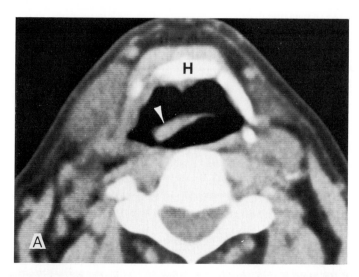

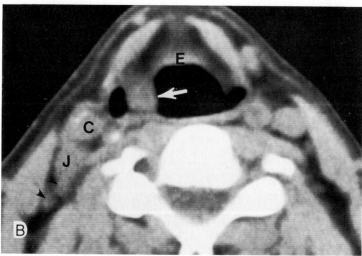

FIG. 1.20.   Epiglottic carcinoma. (A) Tumor produces thickening of right side of the epiglottis (arrowhead) at the level of the hyoid bone (H). (Sagel SS: Larynx. pp. 37–53. In Lee JKT, Sagel SS, Stanley RJ (eds): Computed Body Tomography. Raven Press, New York, 1983.) (B) 2 cm inferiorly the tumor extends into the right aryepiglottic fold (arrow). The epiglottis (E) at this level and pre-epiglottic space are normal. A few mildly enlarged lymph nodes (arrowheads) are seen posterior to the right jugular vein (J). Supraglottic laryngectomy and right radical neck dissection performed. (C) carotid artery.

of the cricoarytenoid joint. CT cannot distinguish between a paramedian cord secondary to paresis and direct tumor involvement of the vocalis muscle. Occasionally, CT will demonstrate that the cord fixation is secondary to prior trauma and the laryngeal neoplasm is less extensive than predicted by laryngoscopy.

Supraglottic Tumors

Supraglottic tumors include those that arise at or above the false vocal cord level. Carcinoma of the epiglottis may appear on CT as thickening of one of the margins of the epiglottis or as a bulky mass (Fig. 1.20). Early carcinoma of the epiglottis may be treated with radiation therapy or with supraglottic laryngectomy.[21] However, if the pre-epiglottic space is invaded, radiation therapy alone is inadequate treatment.[22] Extension of epiglottic carcinoma to the pre-epiglottic space is usually difficult or impossible to demonstrate clinically or with contrast laryngography. The pre-epiglottic and paralaryngeal spaces serve as pathways for spread of supraglottic neoplasms. In particular, those lesions that involve the infrahyoid epiglottis have an increased tendency to invade the pre-epiglottic space. CT is helpful in evaluating these spaces, with their normal fat density, for infiltration by higher attenuation value neoplasm (Fig. 1.21). Attention should also be drawn to the region of the anterior commissure, since a 3- to 5-mm free margin is needed above the level of the anterior commissure for a supraglottic laryngectomy.[14] Tumors that extend deep into the pre-epiglottic space may also extend inferiorly to invade the thyroid cartilage.

Lesions of the aryepiglottic fold, which result in thickening of the fold, often are better demonstrated on scans performed during phonation or a modified Valsalva maneuver (Fig. 1.22). The tumor may spread into the paralaryngeal space as well as posteroinferiorly to the arytenoid. If the tumor extends anteriorly across the midline, it may be difficult on CT to determine whether the lesion arose in the aryepiglottic fold or the epiglottis.

Neoplasms of the pyriform sinus are more aggressive than lesions arising in the endolarynx. They may invade the aryepiglottic fold and mimic primary

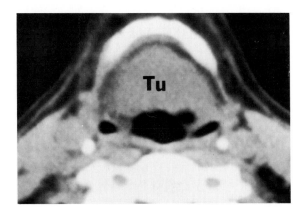

FIG. 1.21. Epiglottic carcinoma. A large epiglottic tumor (Tu) extends into the pre-epiglottic space. No neoplasm was visible at the level of the false cords or below. Supraglottic laryngectomy performed.

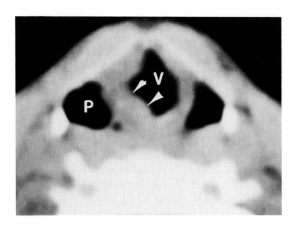

FIG. 1.22. Aryepiglottic fold carcinoma. CT scan performed during phonation demonstrates a tumor involving the right aryepiglottic fold (arrowheads). P, pyriform sinus; V, vestibule.

tumors of the aryepiglottic fold. Pyriform sinus carcinomas are associated with a high incidence of thyroid cartilage invasion. In these patients tumor spread outside of the larynx between the thyroid and cricoid cartilages, is frequently evident, a finding usually seen only with pyriform sinus lesions (Fig. 1.23).[23]

Transglottic Tumors

Transglottic tumors include those that extend across the laryngeal ventricle to involve the supraglottic, glottic, and often the subglottic compartments. The transglottic extension of tumor may be mucosal, submucosal, or both.[24] Transglottic tumors are associated with a very high incidence of thyroid cartilage destruction and extralaryngeal spread (Fig. 1.24) and are treated by total laryngectomy, with or without radiation therapy.

Lymph Nodes

In general, enlarged lymph nodes identified on CT can be palpated clinically. Occasionally, CT may detect enlarged lymph nodes that are not palpable on physical examination (Fig. 1.25).[25] CT can also show the relationship of enlarged lymph nodes to adjacent vascular structures (Fig. 1.26). Encasement or invasion of the carotid artery makes successful surgical resection and cure less likely.

Postoperative Larynx

Physical examination may be difficult in patients who have undergone prior radiation therapy, conservation surgery, or total laryngectomy because of edema of the soft tissues or alteration of the normal laryngeal anatomy. CT can define the anatomy of the normal postoperative larynx and may be invaluable in detecting recurrent neoplasm.[26]

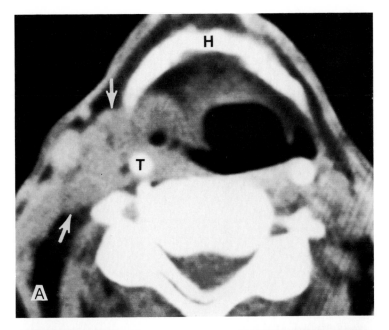

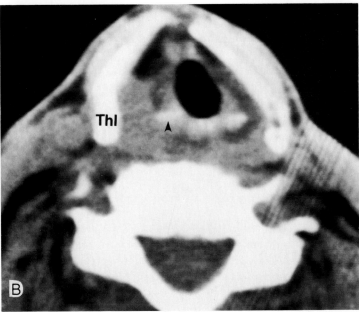

FIG. 1.23. Pyriform sinus carcinoma. (A) Tumor arises in the right pyriform sinus and extends through the thyrohyoid membrane into the soft tissues of the neck (arrows) surrounding the carotid and jugular vessels. (H) hyoid bone, (T) superior cornu of thyroid cartilage. (B) Tumor extends inferiorly to infiltrate normal low-density paralaryngeal space and widen the distance between the right thyroid lamina (Thl) and the arytenoid cartilage (arrowhead). ((A), (B) from Sagel SS: Larynx. pp. 37–53. In Lee JKT, Sagel SS, Stanley RJ (eds): Computed Body Tomography. Raven Press, New York, 1983.)

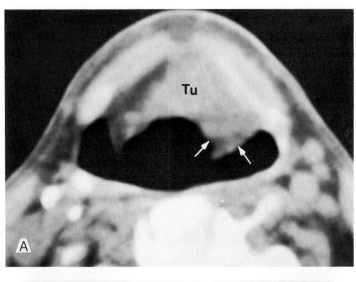

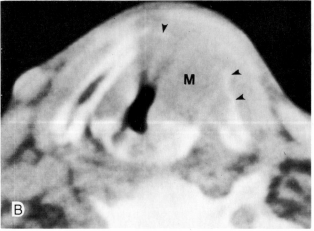

FIG. 1.24. Transglottic carcinoma. (A) A large tumor of the epiglottis (Tu) infiltrates the pre-epiglottic space and extends into the left aryepiglottic fold (arrows). (B) Inferiorly the mass (M) involves the left true vocal cord and destroys the left thyroid ala (arrowheads) with extension into the subcutaneous tissues.

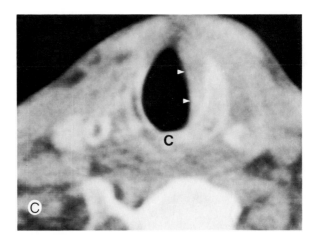

FIG. 1.24 (*Cont.*). (C) At level of the cricoid cartilage (C) extension is seen into the subglottic space (arrowheads).

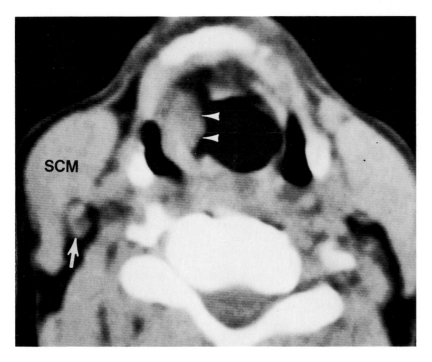

FIG. 1.25. Aryepiglottic fold carcinoma without palpable neck masses. Neoplasm is seen thickening the right aryepiglottic fold (arrowheads). A few mildly enlarged lymph nodes (arrow) are seen posteromedial to the sternocleidomastoid muscle (SCM). These were felt on repeat physical examination and confirmed as metastatic lymph nodes at surgery.

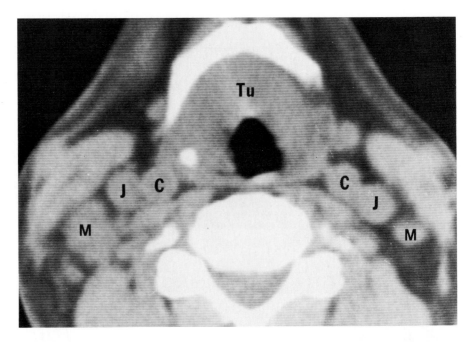

FIG. 1.26. Epiglottic carcinoma with lymph node metastases. A large epiglottic tumor (Tu) is seen infiltrating the pre-epiglottic space. Lymph node metastases (M) are seen bilaterally posterolateral to the internal jugular veins (J) and internal carotid arteries (C).

BENIGN LARYNGEAL MASSES

Most benign laryngeal tumors have a nonspecific but typically smooth appearance on CT. Small vocal cord polyps and retention cysts frequently are not detected by CT or may cause only minimal bulging of the true vocal cord. A lipoma arising from an aryepiglottic fold has been diagnosed on CT by its negative CT numbers.[10]

CT is accurate in establishing the definitive diagnosis of a laryngocele and mapping its total extent.[11,27] A laryngocele is an abnormal dilatation of the saccule of the laryngeal ventricle and occasionally may mimic a submucosal neoplasm on laryngoscopy. Laryngoceles may be confined to the paralaryngeal space or extend through the thyrohyoid membrane into the neck. When the CT appearance of a laryngocele is that of a well-defined structure of air or near water density, the diagnosis is easily established (Figs. 1.27, 1.28). When the mass is of soft tissue density because it contains mucoid or purulent material, its location and smooth surface in the absence of a mucosal abnormality on laryngoscopy should suggest a laryngocele (Fig. 1.29).

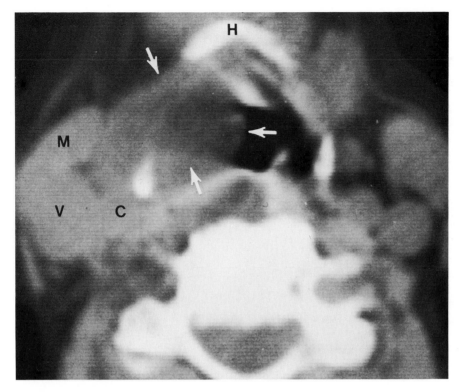

FIG. 1.27. Fluid-filled mixed laryngocele. CT scan at inferior border of hyoid bone (H) demonstrates a water-density mass (arrows) in the right paralaryngeal space extending through the thyrohyoid membrane medial to the sternocleidomastoid muscle (M) and anterior to jugular vein (V) and carotid artery (C). (Glazer HS, Mauro MA, Aronberg DJ, et al.: Computed tomography of laryngoceles. AJR 140: 549–552, 1983.)

TRAUMA

The cross-sectional display of CT allows easy evaluation of the extent of injury to the cartilaginous structures of the larynx and adjacent soft tissues.[5] CT is particularly helpful in those patients in whom supraglottic swelling prevents adequate airway evaluation by laryngoscopy. If laryngeal abnormalities are not appreciated and treatment is delayed, laryngeal stenosis may result.[28,29]

Blood and edema spread through the deep soft tissues of the larynx in a manner similar to neoplasm. CT can demonstrate the extent of hematoma and edema through the paralaryngeal and pre-epiglottic space as well as their effect on the airway (Fig. 1.30). In contrast to conventional radiography, CT gives the true cross-sectional dimensions of the airway.[30]

Trauma to the laryngeal cartilage may be manifested by fracture, displace-

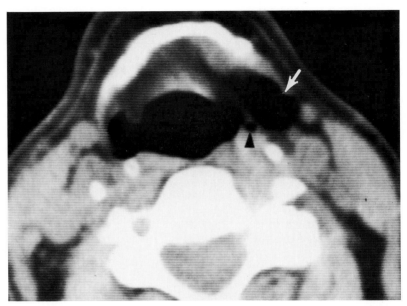

FIG. 1.28.   Air-filled mixed laryngocele. The communication between the air-filled internal and external components of the laryngocele (arrow) is seen. The left pyriform sinus (arrowhead) is compressed by the internal component of the laryngocele. (Glazer HS, Mauro MA, Aronberg DJ, et al.: Computed tomography of laryngoceles. AJR 140: 549–552, 1983.)

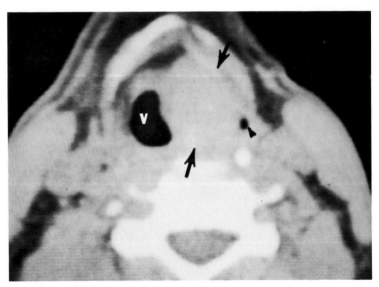

FIG. 1.29.   Infected internal laryngocele. A soft-tissue density mass with smooth borders in the left paralaryngeal space (arrows) compresses the laryngeal vestibule (V) and left pyriform sinus (arrowhead). (Glazer HS, Mauro MA, Aronberg DJ, et al.: Computed tomography of laryngoceles. AJR 140: 549–552, 1983.)

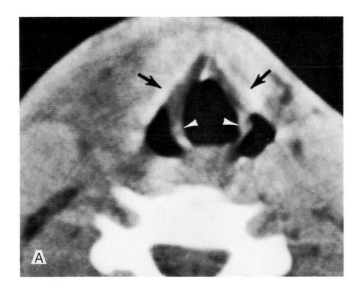

FIG. 1.30. Soft tissue swelling with intact cartilage. (A) Marked swelling of the soft tissues of the neck is seen with obliteration of the normal perivascular planes, especially on the right. The thyroid cartilage (arrows) and aryepiglottic folds (arrowheads) appear normal. (B) In another patient, marked swelling of the left true vocal cord (arrowheads) is seen with narrowing of the airway. The thyroid ala and top of the cricoid cartilage are intact. Extensive subcutaneous emphysema is secondary to a mucosal tear resulting from an emergency tracheostomy.

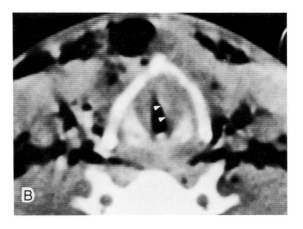

ment, or dislocation of the individual cartilages (Figs. 1.31, 1.32). In blunt trauma to the larynx, the force is usually directed from anterior to posterior in a compressive manner against the cervical spine. Injuries include transverse or vertical fractures of the thyroid or cricoid cartilage, dislocation of the arytenoid cartilages at the cricoarytenoid joint, avulsion of the base of the epiglottis, and disruption of the cricothyroid joint. The normal cleft of the thyroid lamina

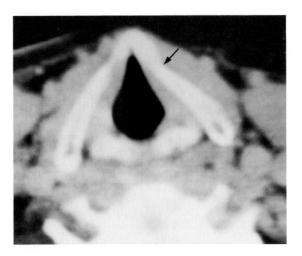

FIG. 1.31. Fractured thyroid cartilage. A minimally depressed fracture of the left thyroid lamina (arrow) is seen with associated swelling of the adjacent thyrohyoid muscle. The vocal cords and cricoid cartilage are normal.

anteriorly should not be confused with a fracture (Fig. 1.5). If a fracture is present, there usually is associated soft tissue swelling.

Occasionally CT will disclose an unsuspected old occult fracture that distorts the laryngeal skeleton and results in the false impression of a laryngeal mass on laryngoscopy (Fig. 1.33).

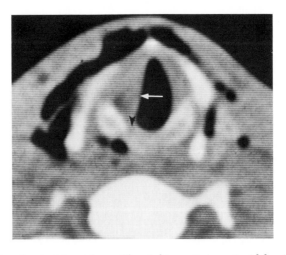

FIG. 1.32. Fractured cricoid cartilage. The right posterior cricoid lamina (arrowhead) is fractured. Swelling of the right true vocal cord (arrow) is also seen. Air is present in the surrounding soft tissue secondary to recent tracheostomy and probable mucosal tear.

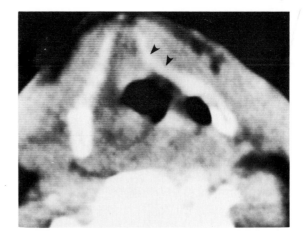

FIG. 1.33. Old "occult" fracture of left thyroid ala (arrowheads) resulted in the erroneous impression of a left false vocal cord mass at laryngoscopy.

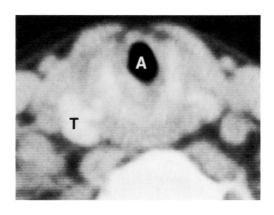

FIG. 1.34. Subglottic stenosis secondary to previous intubation. (A) airway, (T) thyroid gland.

CHRONIC LARYNGEAL STENOSIS

CT may be helpful in evaluating laryngeal stenosis secondary to prior trauma or intubation (Fig. 1.34). CT depicts airway size more accurately than conventional radiography, particularly when the airway is irregular.

REFERENCES

1. Mancuso AA, Calcaterra TC, Hanafee WN: Computed tomography of the larynx. Radiol Clin North Am 16:195–208, 1978.
2. Archer CR, Yeager VL, Friedman WH, Katsantonis GP: Computed tomography of the larynx. J Comput Assist Tomogr 2:404–411, 1978.
3. Archer CR, Friedman WH, Yeager VL, Katsantonis GP: Evaluation of laryngeal cancer by computed tomography. J Comput Assist Tomogr 2:618–624, 1978.
4. Mancuso AA, Hanafee WN: A comparative evaluation of computed tomography and laryngography. Radiology 133:131–138, 1979.
5. Mancuso AA, Hanafee WN: Computed tomography of the injured larynx. Radiology 133:139–144, 1979.

6. Mancuso AA, Tamakawa Y, Hanafee WN: CT of the fixed vocal cord. Am J Roentgenol 135:529–534, 1980.

7. Sagel SS, Aufderheide JF, Aronberg DJ, Stanley RJ, Archer CR: High resolution computed tomography in the staging of carcinoma of the larynx. Laryngoscope 91:292–300, 1981.

8. Archer CR, Sagel SS, Yeager VL, Martin S, Friedman WH: Staging of carcinoma of the larynx: comparative accuracy of computed tomography and laryngoraphy. Am J Roentgenol 136:571–575, 1981.

9. Scott M, Forsted DH, Rominger CJ, Brennan M: Computed tomographic evaluation of laryngeal neoplasms. Radiology 140:141–144, 1981.

10. Shulman HS, Noyek AM, Steinhardt MJ: CT of the larynx. J Otolaryngol 11:395–406, 1982.

11. Mancuso AA, Hanafee WN: Computed Tomography of the Head and Neck. Williams & Wilkins, Baltimore, 1982.

12. Mafee MF, Schild JA, Valvassori GE, Capek V: Computed tomography of the larynx: correlation with anatomic and pathologic studies in cases of laryngeal carcinoma. Radiology 147:123–128, 1983.

13. Sagel SS: Larynx. pp. 37–53. In Lee JKT, Sagel SS, Stanley RJ (eds): Computed Body Tomography. Raven Press, New York, 1983.

14. Ogura JH, Heeneman H; Conservation surgery of the larynx and hypopharynx—Selection of patients and results. Can J Otolaryngol 2:11–16, 1973.

15. Lesinski SG, Bauer WC, Ogura JH: Hemilaryngectomy for T_3 (fixed cord) epidermoid carcinoma of the larynx. Laryngoscope 10:1563–1571, 1976.

16. Silverman PM, Korobkin M, Thompson WM, et al.: Work in progress: high resolution, thin-section computed tomography of the larynx. Radiology 145:723–725, 1982.

17. Gamsu G, Mark AS, Webb WR: Computed tomography of the normal larynx during quiet breathing and phonation. J Comput Assist Tomogr 5:353–360, 1981.

18. Archer CR, Yeager VL: Evaluation of laryngeal cartilages by computed tomography. J Comput Assist Tomogr 3:604–611, 1979.

19. Bassett LW, Hanafee WN, Canalis RF: The appendix of the ventricle of the larynx. Radiology 120:571–574, 1976.

20. Kirchner JA: Two hundred laryngeal cancers: patterns of growth and spread as seen in serial section. Laryngoscope 87:474–482, 1977.

21. Cocke EW, Wang CC: Part 1. Cancer of the larynx: selecting optimum treatment. CA 26:194–200, 1976.

22. Klein R, Fletcher GH: Evaluation of the clinical usefulness of roentgenologic findings in squamous cell carcinomas of the larynx. AJR 92:43–54, 1964.

23. Larrson S, Mancuso A, Hoover L, Hanafee W: Differentiation of pyriform sinus cancer from supraglottic laryngeal cancer by computed tomography. Radiology 141:427–432, 1981.

24. Tucker GF: The anatomy of laryngeal cancer. Can J Otolaryngol 3:417–431, 1974.

25. Mancuso AA, Maceri D, Rice D, Hanafee WN: CT of cervical lymph node cancer. AJR 136:381–385, 1981.

26. Disantis DJ, Balfe DM, Hayden R, et al: The neck after vertical hemilaryngectomy: Computed tomographic study. Radiology 151:683–687, 1984.

27. Glazer HS, Mauro MA, Aronberg DJ, et al.: Computed tomography of laryngoceles. AJR 140:549–552, 1983.

28. Ogura JH, Biller HF: Reconstruction of the larynx following blunt trauma. Ann Otolaryngol 80:492–506, 1971.

29. Ogura JH, Powers WF: Functional restitution of traumatic stenosis of the larynx and pharynx. Laryngoscope 74:1081–1110, 1964.

30. Brown BM, Oshita AK, Castellino RA: CT assessment of the adult extrathoracic trachea. J Comput Assist Tomogr 7:415–418, 1983.

2 The Neck—Thyroid and Parathyroid Glands

DEBORAH L. REEDE

INTRODUCTION

High-resolution CT has greatly enhanced evaluation of soft tissue and bony structures of the neck. With this imaging technique, examination of tissue volumes that once necessitated the use of several imaging modalities (plain films, tomograms, angiograms, and/or laryngography) can now be evaluated using a single one. CT allows determination of both the precise location of a lesion and its effect on adjacent structures without body invasion. Although an exact tissue diagnosis probably cannot be made purely on the basis of the CT, correlation of the history and the clinical and CT findings will provide a reasonable working differential diagnosis in every circumstance.

As with other derived images, informed analysis of CT images requires that one have a working knowledge of the normal anatomy. The normal gross and CT anatomy, therefore, will be reviewed prior to the presentation of pathology.

GROSS ANATOMY

The neck spans the distance between the head and the chest. Its superior limits are the occiput posteriorly and the tip of the chin anteriorly. The mylohyoid muscle, which forms a sling between the horizontal rami of the mandible, serves as the boundary between the floor of the mouth (above) and the neck (below) (Fig. 2.1). All the structures located above the mylohyoid muscle are located within the floor of the mouth or tongue, whereas those below the mylohyoid are in the neck.[1]

Inferiorly, the neck occupies a plane that parallels the first rib and, therefore, tilts downward anteriorly at the level of the thoracic inlet.

The neck may be divided into two paired triangles, anterior and posterior (Fig. 2.2).

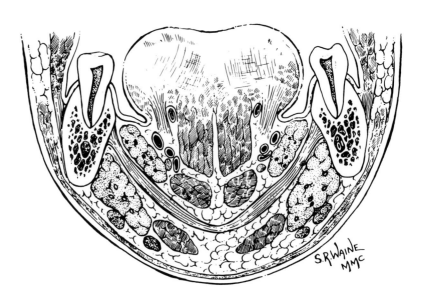

FIG. 2.1. Coronal section of the suprahyoid neck, tongue, and floor of mouth. The mylohyoid muscle is depicted as a sling between the horizontal rami of the mandible.

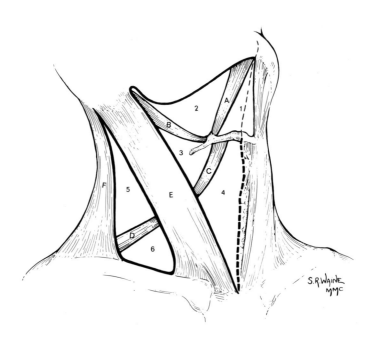

FIG. 2.2. Triangles of the neck: A, anterior belly of the digastric muscle; B, posterior belly of the digastric muscle; C, superior belly of the omohyoid muscle; D, inferior belly of the omohyoid muscle; E, sternocleidomastoid muscle; F, trapezius muscle; 1, submental triangle; 2, submandibular triangle; 3, carotid triangle; 4, muscular triangle; 5, occipital triangle; 6, subclavian triangle.

Anterior Triangle

The anterior triangles abut one another in the midline and, therefore, share a common side (medial border). The boundaries are the sternocleidomastoid posterolaterally, the mandible superiorly, and the midline medially. The hyoid bone divides this triangle into supra- and infrahyoid portions, each of which has two subdivisions.

Suprahyoid Portion

The submental and submandibular triangles are located above the level of the hyoid bone. These triangles are limited superiorly by the mylohyoid muscle, separating them from the floor of the mouth.

Submental triangle: The sides of the submental triangle are formed by the opposing anterior bellies of the two digastric muscles. These muscles attach to the anteroinferior aspect of the mandible anteriorly and the hyoid bone posteriorly. The hyoid bone forms the base of this triangle. Only a few lymph nodes and small branches of the facial artery and vein are located in this triangle.

Submandibular triangle: This is an inverted triangle. Its sides are formed by the two bellies of the digastric muscle: its medial border is formed by the anterior belly and the lateral border is formed by the posterior belly. The mandibular ramus forms its base. The major structures contained within this space are the submandibular salivary glands and numerous small lymph nodes.

Infrahyoid Division

Below the level of the hyoid bone the anterior triangle is divided by the superior belly of the omohyoid muscle into the carotid triangle superolaterally and the muscular triangle inferomedially.

All the major visceral structures in the neck (larynx, trachea, hypopharynx, esophagus, thyroid, and parathyroid glands) are located in the anterior triangle. The carotid sheath structures traverse the entire length of the anterior triangle, delimiting its posterior border, lying deep to the anterior margin of the sternocleidomastoid muscle.

Portions of all the layers of the deep cervical fascial layers contribute to the formation of the carotid sheath. Superiorly it begins at the base of the skull where it attaches to the periosteum around the periphery of the jugular foramen and carotid canal. Inferiorly it terminates at the level of the thoracic inlet. Within this sheath, the common carotid artery lies medially, the internal jugular vein laterally, and the vagus nerve posteriorly, situated between the two vessels. The external carotid artery exits from the carotid sheath in the upper neck; the internal carotid artery remains within it. Located posterior to, and sometimes embedded within, the carotid sheath is the cervical sympathetic plexus.

Posterior Triangle

The boundaries of the posterior triangle are formed by the sternocleidomastoid muscle anteriorly, the trapezius muscle posteriorly, and the clavicle, which forms the base. This triangle is divided by the inferior belly of the omohyoid muscle into two unequal parts. The larger subdivision is the occipital triangle, which is located superiorly. The subclavian triangle is located inferiorly.

The major structures located within the posterior triangle are the lymph nodes, nutrient vessels, and nerves (cutaneous branches of the cervical plexus and spinal accessory nerve).

Thoracic Inlet

The thoracic inlet is located at the junction between the root of the neck and the superior mediastinum. It occupies an oblique plane, paralleling the first rib.

One should be aware of the major neural–vascular relationships at this level. If the anterior scalenus muscle is used as a reference point, it is easy to remember these relationships: The anterior scalenus muscle attaches to the superior border of the first rib; the subclavian vein lies *anterior* to it and the subclavian artery *posterior* to it.

Three major neural structures cross the thoracic inlet: the inferior trunk of the brachial plexus, the phrenic nerve, and the vagus nerve. The phrenic and vagus nerves cross the thoracic inlet side by side (phrenic nerve laterally and vagus medially) between the anterior scalenus muscle and the subclavian artery. Posterior to the subclavian artery is the inferior trunk of the brachial plexus.

NORMAL CT ANATOMY

The review of normal anatomy below will begin at the level of the mylohyoid muscle, since it serves as the dividing line between the neck and the floor of the mouth. The mylohyoid muscle is readily identified as a soft tissue density located between the mandible anteriorly and the hyoid bone posteriorly (Fig. 2.3). Lateral to the mylohyoid muscle are the submandibular glands. Superficial to it are the anterior bellies of the digastric muscles (Fig. 2.4). These muscles attach anteriorly to the mandible and posteriorly to the hyoid bone. Occasionally the mylohyoid muscle can be seen between these two muscles.

The hyoid bone is a semicircular calcified structure located anteriorly in the neck. If the chin is sufficiently extended at the time of the scan, the submandibular glands will not be seen at the level of the hyoid bone, since these are suprahyoid structures. Posterior to the hyoid bone are seen portions of the upper airway: the valleculae, base of the tongue, epiglottis, and superior portion of the pyriform sinuses (Figs. 2.3, 2.4). The major vascular structures are located posterolaterally to the hyoid bone: the internal carotid artery medially, the external carotid artery and its branches anterolaterally, and the internal

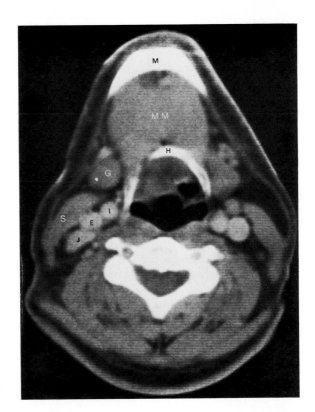

FIG. 2.3. G, submandibular gland; M, mandible; H, hyoid bone; MM, mylohyoid muscle; S, sternocleidomastoid muscle; I, internal carotid artery; E, external carotid artery; J, internal jugular vein.

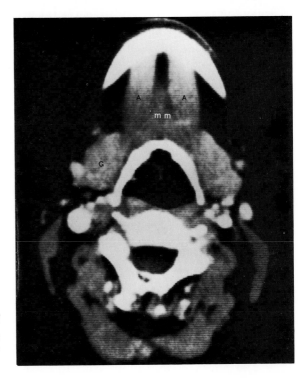

FIG. 2.4. A, anterior belly of the digastric muscle; MM, mylohyoid muscle; G, submandibular gland.

jugular vein posterolaterally. The external jugular vein may be seen on the superficial surface of the sternocleidomastoid muscle.

A constant landmark seen on all CT scans obtained through the neck is the sternocleidomastoid muscle. Superiorly it occupies a lateral position; inferiorly it moves to an anterior position so that it can attach to the sternum and clavicle. This muscle can be used to identify the anterior and posterior triangles of the neck on CT. Structures that are located deep to the sternocleidomastoid muscle, superficial to the scalenes, and posterior to the carotid sheath, are in the posterior triangle. On CT the posterior triangle appears as a fat-filled cleft except for a few structures with positive attenuation values caused by the presence of lymph nodes, small nutrient vessels, and nerves. Carotid sheath structures, as well as the major visceral structures in the anterior aspect of the neck (larynx, hypopharynx, thyroid, parathyroid, and esophagus), lie within the anterior triangle.

Scans obtained just below the level of the hyoid bone will demonstrate the superior cornua of the thyroid cartilage. They are readily identified as paired calcified structures located lateral to the longus coli muscle (Fig. 2.5). The major vascular structures lie lateral to this cartilage. The strap muscles (sternohyoid, sternothyroid, thyrohyoid, and superior belly of the omohyoid muscle) are the most anteriorly placed structures at this level.

The body of the thyroid cartilage resembles a triangle without a base. Located at the superior aspect of this cartilage is the thyroid notch (Fig. 2.6). At the level of the thyroid notch the two halves of the cartilage do not meet anteriorly. Anterior to the thyroid cartilage are the strap muscles; lateral to it are the carotid sheath structures. Between the two laminae of this cartilage are the

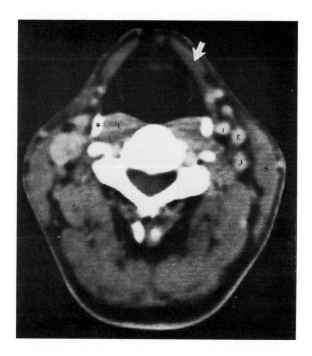

FIG. 2.5. *, superior cornu of the thyroid cartilage; arrow, strap muscles; E, external carotid artery; I, internal carotid artery; J, internal jugular vein; S, sternocleidomastoid muscle; L, longus colli muscle.

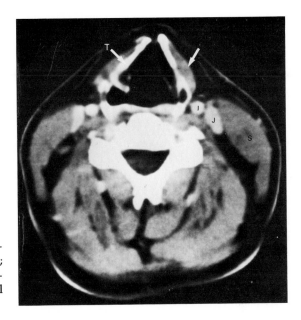

FIG. 2.6. S, sternocleidomastoid muscle; T, thyroid cartilage; open arrow, strap muscles; I, internal carotid artery; J, internal jugular vein.

vestibule of the larynx, lying centrally, and the pyriform sinuses, laterally. Occasionally a soft tissue density is visualized on the undersurface of the sternocleidomastoid muscle (Fig. 2.7). This is the inferior belly of the omohyoid muscle. It should not be mistaken for a lymph node or some other soft tissue mass.

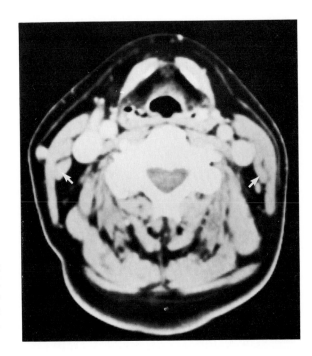

FIG. 2.7. Contrast scan at the level of the thyroid cartilage demonstrating the omohyoid muscle (arrow) deep to the sternocleidomastoid muscle.

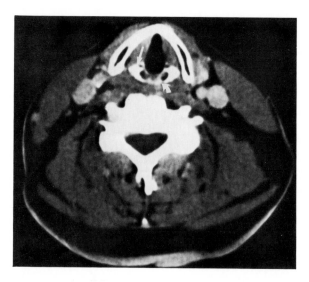

FIG. 2.8. Scan at the level of the superior aspect of the cricoid cartilage (small arrow) where it articulates with the arytenoid cartilages (large arrows).

The cricoid cartilage forms the base of the larynx. It is the only cartilaginous structure of the airway that forms a complete circle. It has a lucent medullary center with a peripheral rim of calcification. The posterior portion of the cricoid cartilage has greater vertical dimension than the anterior portion; cuts obtained through the superior portion of the cartilage only will demonstrate this characteristic pattern of calcification posteriorly (Fig. 2.8), with a "deficiency" anteriorly.

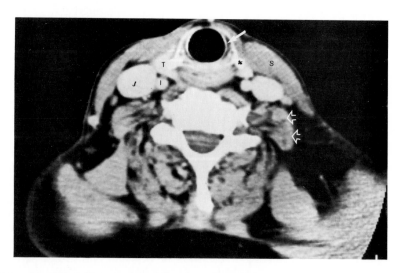

FIG. 2.9. Asterisk, inferior cornu of the thyroid cartilage; closed arrow, cricoid cartilage; open arrows, scalene muscles; S, sternocleidomastoid muscle; T, thyroid gland; I, internal carotid artery; J, internal jugular vein.

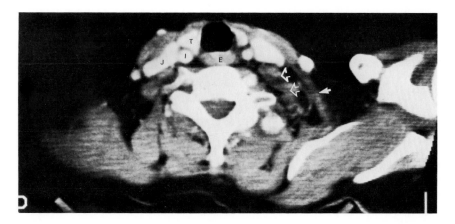

FIG. 2.10.   I, internal carotid artery; J, internal jugular vein; T, thyroid gland; E, esophagus; open arrows, scalene muscles; closed arrow, inferior belly of the omohyoid muscle.

The inferior cornua of the thyroid cartilage articulate with the posterolateral aspects of the cricoid cartilage (Fig. 2.9). Usually at about the level of the cricoid cartilage the superior poles of the thyroid gland come into view, located between the cricoid cartilage medially and the common carotid artery posterolaterally. The strap muscles lie anteriorly, with the anterior jugular veins superficial to them. One should note that at this level the sternocleidomastoid muscle

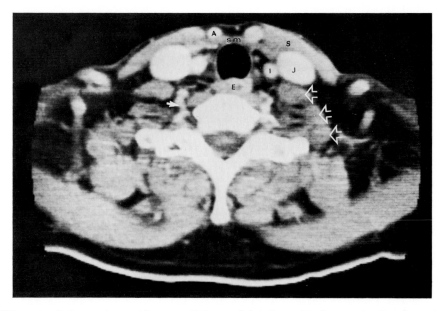

FIG. 2.11.   I, internal carotid artery; J, internal jugular vein; A, anterior jugular vein; S, sternocleidomastoid muscle; E, esophagus; open arrows, scalene muscles; closed arrow, vertebral artery.

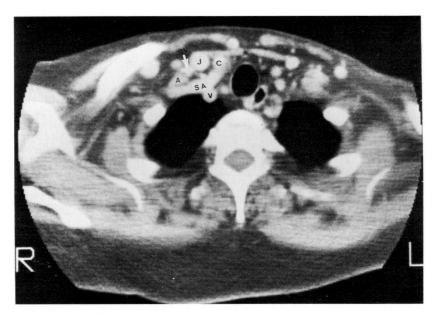

FIG. 2.12. Scan at the level of the thoracic inlet. C, internal carotid artery; J, internal jugular vein; SA, subclavian artery; SV, subclavian vein; V, vertebral artery; A, anterior scalenus muscle.

is at a more anterior position in the neck than seen on scans obtained at higher levels, where it is more lateral.

Images at the level of the body of the thyroid gland may show both lobes of the gland connected anteriorly by the thyroid isthmus. At this level the scalenus muscles and inferior belly of the omohyoid muscle are often visualized (Fig. 2.10).

Below the level of the thyroid gland the carotid sheath structures move medially to occupy the space occupied at a higher level by the thyroid gland (Fig. 2.11). The strap muscles are seen anterior to the trachea with the anterior jugular veins superficial to them. Between the scalenus muscles the vertebral arteries are seen lying outside of the foramina transversaria. The esophagus is situated between the trachea anteriorly and the vertebral body posteriorly.

Only rarely will any *one* CT image visualize both the subclavian artery and the subclavian vein with the anterior scalenus muscle situated between them (Fig. 2.12). Careful analysis of sequential scans, however, often make it possible to visualize these structures.

TECHNIQUE

All neck scans should be performed with intravenous contrast unless it is contraindicated. Use of contrast permits differentiation of normal vascular structures from lymph nodes and other structures with positive attenuation values.

A 300-cc sample of Reno-M-Dip is infused over a 15-min period. Scanning starts after approximately 150 cc are infused. The patient is placed in the supine position, with the chin extended so that the horizontal ramus of the mandible is parallel to the x-ray beam. All scans are performed at a gantry angle of 0°. This prevents distortion of the anatomy. Contiguous cuts of 5 mm each are obtained through the area of interest.

THYROID GLAND

A number of imaging modalities, including radionuclide scans and ultrasound, are available for the evaluation of the thyroid gland. The use of CT in evaluating thyroid disease is somewhat limited. However, it may provide clinical information such as the degree of airway compression, presence of nodal involvement, and the precise caudal extent of a substernal goiter, that cannot be obtained by any other means.

Normal Thyroid

Normal thyroid tissue is seen as an "enhanced" soft tissue structure on a noncontrast CT scan. This is a result of its (physiologically normal) high iodine content (Fig. 2.13). Its CT numbers range between 70 and 100 Hounsfield units (HU).[2,3] Hounsfield measurements taken after contrast administration will increase (by approximately 25 HU) because of the rich blood supply of the gland. In patients who are hypothyroid, or on thyroid replacement or suppression, the thyroid glands may show less "enhanced" thyroid tissue on a noncontrast scan (Fig. 2.14). The thyroid glands in older patients tend to have an nonhomogeneous pattern of enhancement on both the pre- and postcontrast scans.

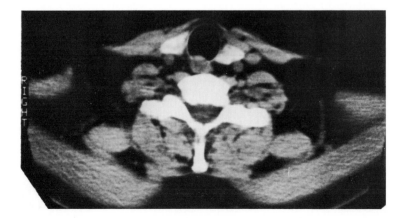

FIG. 2.13. Noncontrast scan demonstrating normal thyroid tissue, which is "enhanced" prior to contrast administration.

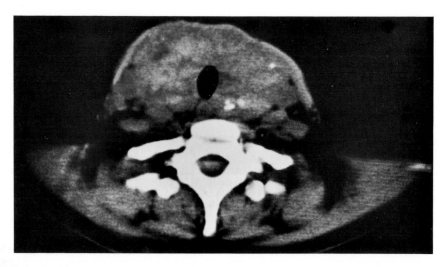

FIG. 2.14. Noncontrast scan of a hypothyroid patient with a multinodular goiter. The gland is markedly enlarged and nonhomogeneous in appearance. Multiple areas of amorphous calcification are seen. Note the tracheal deviation.

Pathology

Thyroglossal duct cyst, lingual thyroid tissue, and aberrant thyroid tissue may be diagnosed on CT. A knowledge of the embryology of the thyroid gland is helpful in explaining the locations of these various conditions.

The thyroid gland arises as a midline outgrowth from the floor of the pharynx at a level between the first and second branchial pouches. The site of origin is termed the *foramen cecum*. It is located behind the apex of the V-shaped row of circumvallate papillae. Once the thyroid gland develops, it penetrates the underlying mesoderm, enlarges, and descends in front of the pharynx as a bilobed diverticulum. During this migration the diverticulum remains patent and is known as the *thyroglossal duct*. Once the thyroid gland reaches its final position in front of the trachea, the duct normally undergoes atrophy and dissolution, and disappears. If any portion of the duct persists, a cyst will develop secondary to the secretions of the epithelial lining of the duct.[4,5] These cysts can occur anywhere along the course of the duct as well as within the hyoid bone, since the embryological development of the hyoid bone is intimately associated with that of the thyroglossal duct. Therefore, these cysts may be located anterior to, posterior to, or within the hyoid bone. About 65 percent of these cysts are located below the level of the hyoid bone, in the region of the thyrohyoid membrane. Another 20 percent are located above and 15 percent at the level of the hyoid bone.[6] Fistulas are not commonly seen in association with these lesions unless the cyst has become infected and/or the patient has had previous surgery.

Thyroglossal duct cysts usually present clinically as an asymptomatic neck mass, in the midline or slightly off midline in location. Most of these cysts appear before the age of 10 years; however, it is not uncommon to see them in older patients.

On CT these lesions appear as a smooth, well-circumscribed mass anywhere along the course of the thyroglossal duct. The density of these cysts is quite variable, but it is usually less than that of surrounding muscle (Fig. 2.15). If the cyst is located in the region of the hyoid bone, it may produce bone erosion secondary to pressure effect.

Fragments of thyroid tissue may be found anywhere along the course of the thyroglossal duct. A lingual thyroid results when there has been an arrest in the migration of the thyroid from the region of the foramen cecum.

Lingual thyroids are more common in females, presenting clinically as a lobulated mass in the midline at the base of the tongue. Frequently, they may go undetected until normal physiological enlargement of the gland occurs, which usually takes place at puberty or during pregnancy. Approximately 70 to 80 percent of patients with lingual thyroids have no other thyroid tissue.[6] There is approximately a 4 to 6 percent incidence of carcinoma in these glands.[7] This relatively high incidence of carcinoma may be related to excessive TSH stimulation.[8]

Plain film examination of this area may demonstrate a soft tissue mass in the region of the base of the tongue. This is a nonspecific finding, since a number of conditions, such as carcinoma, lymphoma, and enlarged lingual tonsils, may produce similar findings. Aberrant thyroid tissue is most often identified with certainty on radionuclide scans (Fig. 2.16).

The CT findings are also fairly specific. On a noncontrast scan the tissue appears as a high-attenuation mass at the base of the tongue. This is a reflection of the high iodine content of the thyroid tissue. After intravenous contrast it will enhance to a greater degree because of the rich blood supply of the gland (Fig. 2.17). Nonthyroid lesions that occur in this area tend to be of the same

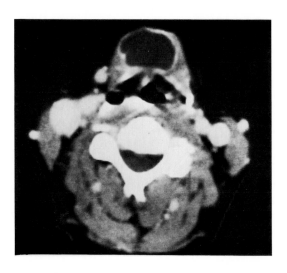

FIG. 2.15. Thyroglossal duct cyst. Contrast scan demonstrating a well-circumscribed low-density anterior midline mass.

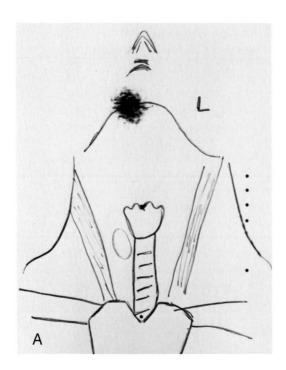

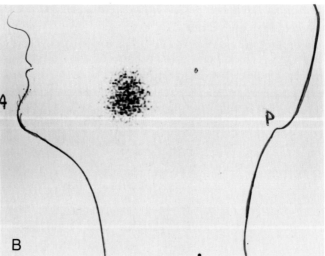

FIG. 2.16. Lingual thyroid. [123]I radionuclide scan. Frontal (A) and lateral (B) views demonstrating uptake of radionuclide at the base of the tongue.

density as muscle (Fig. 2.18). Occasionally, lymphoid tissue at the base of the tongue may be less dense than the adjacent muscle.[9] It should be noted that the use of contrast with inorganic iodine may precipitate thyroid storm in patients with autonomous thyroid nodules and multinodular goiters.[11-13]

Residual thyroid tissue located along the course of the thyroglossal duct

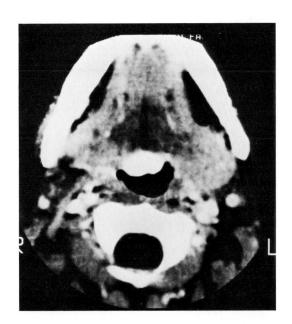

FIG. 2.17. Lingual thyroid. An enhancing midline mass is seen at the base of the tongue on this contrast scan.

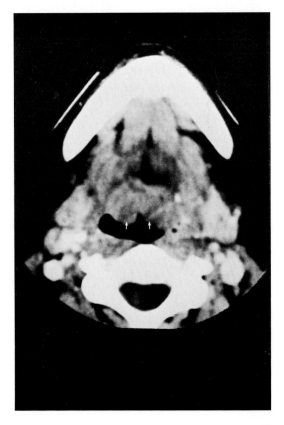

FIG. 2.18. Hypertrophied lingual tonsils. Lobulated soft-tissue masses (arrows) are seen at the base of the tongue.

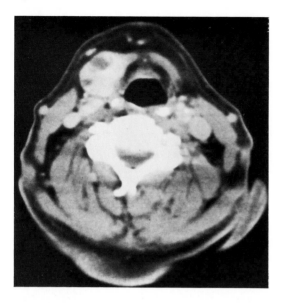

FIG. 2.19. Adenoma in ectopic thyroid tissue. Contrast scan shows a nonhomogeneous enhancing mass intimately associated with the strap muscles on the right side. This mass was separate from the thyroid gland but located along the course of the thyroglossal duct.

other than the base of the tongue may also escape detection until it becomes pathologically enlarged. The CT appearance of this tissue may resemble normal thyroid tissue or show evidence of an nonhomogeneous enhancement pattern with low density areas within it (Fig. 2.19).

It is not possible to differentiate benign from malignant disease in the thyroid

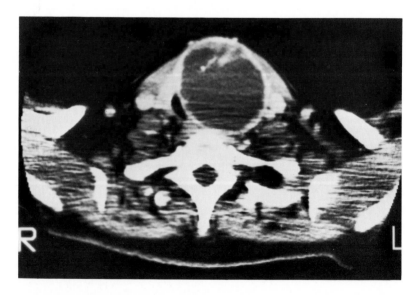

FIG. 2.20. Multinodular goiter. Contrast scan at the level of the thoracic inlet demonstrating a cystic mass involving the left lobe and isthmus of thyroid. The trachea is deviated to the left and the left carotid sheath structures are displaced laterally.

based on the CT characteristics of the lesion. This is contrary to early reports on the CT characteristics of thyroid lesions.[13] Ancillary findings such as lymph node enlargement and bone and/or cartilage destruction in association with a thyroid lesion would suggest a diagnosis of malignancy. Recurrent laryngeal nerve palsy in the presence of a thyroid mass is also highly suggestive of malignancy, since this rarely occurs with benign thyroid lesions. Only 10 percent of patients with goiters develop vocal cord paralysis secondary to pressure on the recurrent laryngeal nerve.[14]

CT can provide valuable information in the assessment of patients with goiters. Often this information may not be obtained by any other noninvasive means. CT makes it possible to identify the precise location of a lesion and the degree of airway compression and vascular displacement (Fig. 2.20, 2.21).

FIG. 2.21. Multinodular goiter. (A) Scan at the level of the hyoid shows bilateral nonhomogeneous enhancing masses medial to the carotid sheath structure. The lesion extends into the prevertebral area and is causing posterolateral displacement of the carotid sheath structures. It is retrotracheal. (B) At level of the thyroid cartilage. The shape of the lesions resembles that of normal thyroid tissue, but the gland is massively enlarged and demonstrates retrotracheal extension.

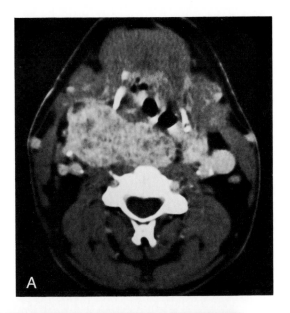

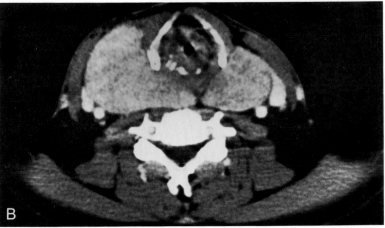

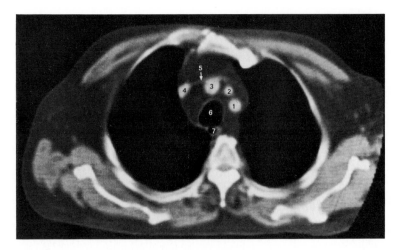

FIG. 2.22. Contrast scan at the level where the right and left innominate veins join. Note the following normal vascular structures at this level: 1, left subclavian artery; 2, left carotid artery; 3, right innominate artery; 4, right innominate vein; 5, left innominate vein; 6, trachea; 7, esophagus.

In the case of malignant disease, nodal metastasis may also be detected.[15-21]

Intrathoracic goiters can be divided into two groups based on their relationship to the great vessels at the level of the thoracic inlet. Anterior goiters lie in front of the arteries and innominate veins; posterior goiters lie posterior to these vessels. Goiters arising from the inferior poles of the thyroid gland or isthmus tend to lie anterior to the carotid and subclavian arteries. Those arising from the posterior and lateral portions of the gland are usually situated posterior to the trachea, esophagus, and vascular structures.[22] Goiters descend into the thoracic cavity along the perivisceral fascia, which is located around the trachea and esophagus. Most goiters descend inferiorly to the level of the left innominate vein, as it crosses the anterior mediastinum (Fig. 2.22) at the cervicothoracic junction. This vessel prevents caudal progression of these lesions. Occasionally, however, a goiter may cascade anterior to the great vessels, presenting as an anterior mediastinal mass (Fig. 2.23) or posterior to the great vessels to present as a posterior or middle mediastinal mass (Fig. 2.24, 2.25). If a goiter is located on the left and extends below the level of the innominate vein, it is usually posterior in location. Its extension to the right of the midline is delineated anteriorly by the innominate vein and the aortic arch. The aorta prevents its extension to the left of the midline. The caudal descent of a right-sided goiter is usually limited by the azygos arch or right hilum.[23]

The CT findings of intrathoracic goiters have been described.[24-26] Bashist et al. report six common CT findings:[26]

1. Continuity with the cervical gland
2. Well-defined borders
3. Punctate coarse or ring-like calcification

4. Nonhomogeneous enhancement, with well-defined, low density areas

5. Precontrast attenuation values usually at minimum 15 HU greater than adjacent musculature, with at least a 25 HU enhancement after intravenous administration of contrast

6. Patterns of extension

   a. Cradling of the goiter by the innominate vessels high in the mediastinum

   b. Retrovascular extension in the paratracheal and retrotracheal area

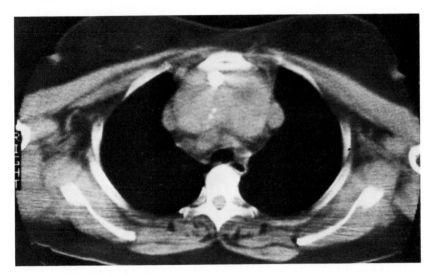

FIG. 2.23. Substernal goiter—anterior extension. A goiter extending into the mediastinum anterior to the great vessels. Note the amorphous calcification within the lesion.

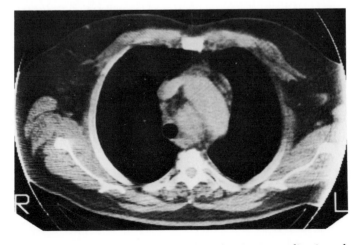

FIG. 2.24. Substernal goiter—posterior extension. A goiter extending into the mediastinum delimited laterally by the trachea on the right and anterolaterally by the aortic arch on the left.

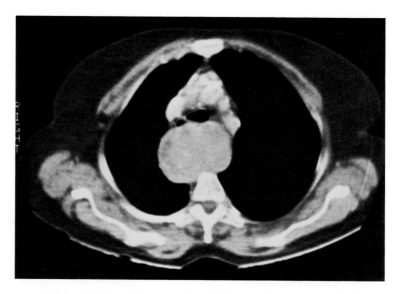

FIG. 2.25. Substernal goiter—posterior extension. Goiter extending into the mediastinum in a retrotracheal location.

Postoperative scans obtained on patients who have had a partial or total thyroidectomy often demonstrate medial displacement of the carotid sheath structures (Fig. 2.26). This may be confused clinically with recurrent disease or residual thyroid tissue. If the anterior scalene muscle is mistaken for the jugular vein on CT (a not uncommon interpretative error), the displaced jugular

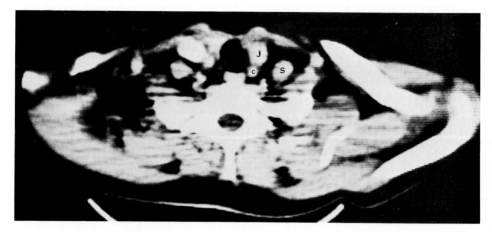

FIG. 2.26. Postoperative thyroid with anteromedial migration of carotid sheath structures. A contrast scan on a patient who has had the left lobe of the thyroid gland removed. Note the medial displacement of the left carotid sheath structures. C, common carotid artery; J, internal jugular vein; S, anterior scalenus muscle.

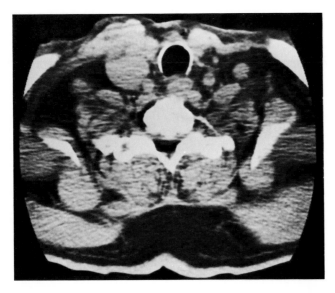

FIG. 2.27.   Recurrent papillary carcinoma of the thyroid. A nonhomogeneous mass is seen involving the thyroid bed with invasion into the medial aspect of the right sternocleidomastoid muscle.

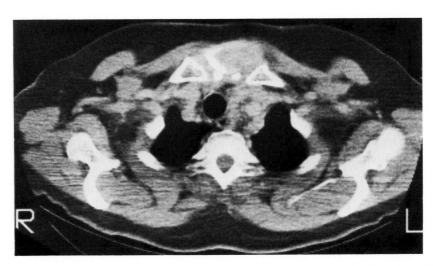

FIG. 2.28.   Metastatic papillary carcinoma of the thyroid gland. A vascular, expansile, lytic lesion is seen involving the manubrium in this patient with a history of thyroid carcinoma 10 years previously.

vein may similarly be confused with recurrent disease. CT is also capable of demonstrating the precise location of recurrent disease and its effect on adjacent structures (Figs. 2.27, 2.28).

PARATHYROID GLANDS

The parathyroid glands arise from the third and fourth pharyngeal pouches. Along with the thymus, the inferior parathyroid glands arise from the third pharyngeal pouch; they are sometimes referred to as the "parathyroids III" or "parathymic glands." The superior parathyroid glands arise from the fourth pharyngeal pouch and they are often referred to as "parathyroids IV."[27,28]

Wong,[29] in his study of 645 normal adult parathyroid glands in 160 cadavers, demonstrated a definite pattern of anatomic distribution based on the embryological development of the parathyroid, thyroid, and thymus glands. Seventy-seven percent of the upper parathyroid glands were located posteriorly, at the level of the cricothyroid junction. Twenty-two percent were found embedded in the thyroid, behind the upper pole; these glands were subcapsular in location, that is, lying deep to the surgical capsule of the thyroid gland. Less than one percent were found behind the lower pharyngeal and upper esophageal junction in the midline. The lower pole parathyroid glands have a more widespread distribution. Forty-two percent were found on the anterior or lateral surface of the lower pole of the thyroid gland. Thirty-nine percent were located in the lower neck within a tongue of thymic tissue. Two percent were found inside the mediastinal thymic tissue. Fifteen percent were located lateral to the lower pole of the thyroid gland and two percent were ectopic in location. Even though the lower pole glands are widely distributed, they are almost always in the immediate vicinity of the lower pole of the thyroid.[30] In brief, it may be said that the *majority* of the superior parathyroid glands are found posteriorly, outside the thyroid capsule at the cricothyroid junction and that the inferior parathyroids are usually found either in the lower poles of the thyroid, superficial to the capsule, or within a tongue of cervical thymic tissue in the neck.

When the parathyroid glands enlarge, they are usually displaced caudally. An enlarged (posteriorly) situated upper pole gland will be displaced inferiorly from the tracheo-esophageal sulcus into the posterior mediastinum. The lower glands, when enlarged, may be displaced into either the anterior or the posterior mediastinum, depending on the site of origin.[30] A study of 84 patients with mediastinal adenomas showed that the majority of the lesions (67 cases) occurred in the anterior mediastinum.[28] Parathyroid glands originating within the surgical capsule of the thyroid tend to remain stationary in position even when they are enlarged.[29]

There is almost equal right/left distribution of parathyroid adenomas. However, there is a distinct preference for involvement of the inferior glands.[31]

The radiographic evaluation of parathyroid adenoma suspects has traditionally consisted of angiography, venous sampling for PTH levels, and barium swallow. Recently, ultrasound and CT have been added to this diagnostic regimen.

High-resolution CT has greatly improved detection of enlarged parathyroid glands;[32-39] however, the ultimate value of routine preoperative localization of parathyroid adenomas remains questionable at best. Preoperative localization does not appreciably decrease operation time, since most surgeons will attempt to identify all the parathyroid glands, not necessarily only the "one" identified as enlarged on CT or ultrasound. In addition, 90 percent of parathyroid adenomas may be identified at the time of surgery without any preoperative attempts at localization whatsoever.[39]

Ultrasound is capable of detecting enlarged parathyroid glands in the cervical

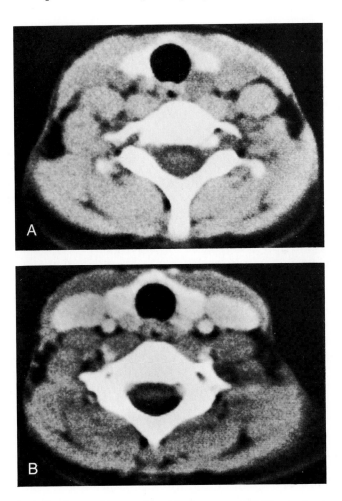

FIG. 2.29. Bilateral subcapsular parathyroid adenomas. (A) Noncontrast scan demonstrating low density areas in the posterior aspect of both lobes of the thyroid. (B) After contrast administration these areas are enhanced.

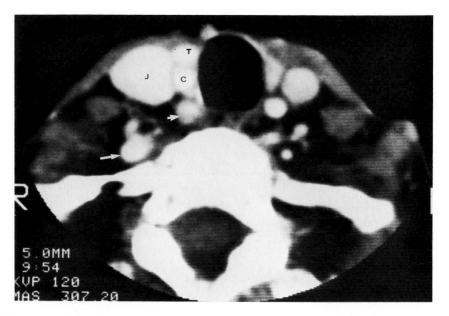

FIG. 2.30. Right parathyroid adenoma. A contrast scan demonstrates an enhancing mass in the right tracheal esophageal sulcus (small arrow). C, common carotid artery; J, internal jugular vein; T, thyroid gland; large arrow, vertebral artery.

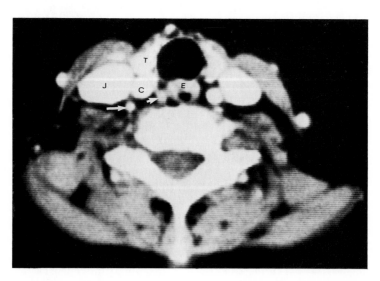

FIG. 2.31. Right parathyroid adenoma. An enhancing mass is seen adjacent to the right side of the esophagus in the tracheoesophageal sulcus (small arrow). E, esophagus; T, thyroid; C, common carotid artery; J, internal jugular vein; large arrow, vertebral artery.

region. However, if the lesion is small (less than 5 mm in size)[40] or located in the mediastinum, ultrasound is often incapable of detecting the lesion. CT is often helpful in evaluating patients with negative or equivocal ultrasound findings or previous unsuccessful neck surgery.

CT scans should be performed both with and without intravenous contrast for assessment of the thyroid region. Superior mediastinal evaluation may be carried out with the contrast portion of the study alone. Enlarged glands located within the thyroid capsule will be seen on the non-contrast scan as a low density area embedded within the posterior aspect of the normally "enhanced" thyroid gland (Fig. 2.29A). After contrast administration, the degree of enhancement of the adenoma is variable. At times it will enhance to the same degree as the surrounding thyroid tissue (Fig. 2.29B). For this reason, there must be a non-contrast study for comparison so that these lesions do not escape detection. Extracapsular adenomas are more common. They appear as a homogeneous enhancing mass in the tracheoesophageal groove or lying against the posterolateral wall of the trachea (Figs. 2.30, 2.31).[35] Normal, enlarged, or tortuous vessels may be mistaken for an adenoma in these areas.

REFERENCES

1. Last RJ: Anatomy: Regional and Applied. Churchill Livingstone, New York, 1978.
2. Machida K, Yoshikawa K: Aberrant thyroid gland demonstrated by computed tomography. J Comput Assist Tomogr 3:689–690, 1979.
3. Wolf BS, Nakagawa H, Cjeh HC: Visualization of the thyroid gland with computed tomography. Radiology 123:368, 1977.
4. Davies J: Embryology and anatomy of the head, neck, face, palate, nose, and paranasal sinuses. pp. 63–123. In Paparrella MM and Shumrick DA (eds): Otolaryngology. Vol. 1. WB Saunders, Philadelphia, 1980.
5. Hollinshead WH: Anatomy for Surgeons. Vol. 1: The Head and Neck. Harper and Row, New York, 1968.
6. Batsakis JG: Tumors of the Head and Neck. Clinical and Pathological Considerations. Williams and Wilkins, Baltimore, 1979.
7. Fish J, Moore RM: Ectopic thyroid tissue and extopic thyroid carcinoma: a review of the literature and report of a case. Ann Surg, 157:212–222, 1963.
8. Wertz ML: Management of undescended lingual and subhyoid thyroid glands. Laryngoscope 84:507–521, 1974.
9. Larsson SG, Mancuso AA, Hanafee WN: Computed tomography of the tongue and floor of the mouth. Radiology 144:493–499, May 1972.
10. Vagenakis AG, Wang C, Barger A: Iodine-induced thyrotoxicosis in Boston. N Engl J Med 287:523–527, 1972.
11. Blum M, Weinberg U, Shenkman L, Hollander CS: Hyperthyroidism after iodinated contrast medium. N Engl J Med 291:24–25, 1974.
12. Blum M, Kranjac T, Park CM, Engleman RM: Thyroid storm after cardiac angiography with iodinated contrast medium: occurrence in a patient with a previously euthyroid autonomous nodule of the thyroid. JAMA 235:2324–2325, 1976.
13. Sekiya T, Toda S, Kanakami K, et al.: Clinical application of computed tomography of thyroid disease. Comput Tomogr 3:185–193, 1979.
14. Waugh JM: Relation between disease of the thyroid gland and laryngal function. pp.

55–64. In Roland AF (ed): The Thyroid Gland. Clinics of George W. Crile and Associates. 2nd Ed. WB Saunders, Philadelphia, 1922.

15. Mancuso AA, Maceri D, Rice D, Hanafee WN: CT of cervical lymph node cancer. AJR 136:381–385, 1981.

16. Reede DL, Whelan MA, Bergeron RT: Computed tomography of the infrahyoid neck, Part I: Normal anatomy. Radiology 145:389–395, 1982.

17. Reede DL, Whelan MA, Bergeron RT: Computed tomography of the infrahyoid neck, Part II: Pathology. Radiology 145:397–402, 1982.

18. Reede DL, Bergeron RT: CT of cervical lymph nodes. J Otolaryngol 11:411–418, 1982.

19. Reede DL, Bergeron RT, Whelan MA, et al.: Computed tomography of cervical lymph nodes. RadioGraphics, 3:339–351, 1983.

20. Mancuso AA, Harnsberger HR, Muraki AS, Stevens MH: Computed tomography of cervical and retropharyngeal lymph nodes. Normal anatomy, variants of normal, and applications in staging head and neck cancer. Part I: Normal anatomy. Radiology 148:709–714, 1983.

21. Mancuso AA, Harnsberger HR, Muraki AS, Stevens MH: Computed tomography of cervical and retropharyngeal lymph nodes: normal anatomy, variants of normal, and applications in staging head and neck cancer. Part II: Pathology. Radiology 148:715–723, 1983.

22. McCort JJ: Intrathoracic goiter: its incidence, symptomatology, and roentgen diagnosis. Radiology 53:227–236, 1949.

23. Heitzman ER: The Mediastinum. Radiologic Correlation with Anatomy and Pathology. CV Mosby, St. Louis, 1977.

24. Glazer GM, Axel L, Moss AA: CT diagnosis of mediastinal thyroid. AJR 138:495–498, 1982.

25. Morris UL, Colletti PM, Rolls PW, et al.: Case report: CT demonstration of intrathoracic thyroid tissue. J Comput Assist Tomogr 6:821–824, 1982.

26. Bashist B, Ellis K, Gold RP: Computed Tomography of Intrathoracic Goiters. AJR 140:450–460, 1983.

27. Warwick R, Williams RL: Gray's Anatomy, WB Saunders, Philadelphia, 1973.

28. Nathaniels EK, Nathaniels AM, Wang C: Mediastinal parathyroid tumors: a clinical and pathological study of 84 cases. Ann Surg 171:165–170, 1970.

29. Wang C, The Anatomic Basis of Parathyroid Surgery. Ann Surg 183:271–275, 1976.

30. Edis AS: Surgical anatomy and technique of neck exploration for primary hyperparathyroidism. Surg Clin N Am 57:495–504, 1977.

31. Norris EH: The parathyroid adenomas: a study of 322 cases. Int Abstr Surg, 84:1–41, 1947.

32. Doppman JL, Brennan MF, Koehler JO, Marx SJ: Computed tomography for parathyroid localization. J Comput Assist Tomogr 1:30–36, 1977.

33. Krudy AG, Doppman JL, Brannan MF, et al.: The detection of mediastinal parathyroid glands by computed tomography, selective angiography, and venous sampling: an analysis of 17 cases. Radiology 140:739–744, 1981.

34. Wolverson MK, Sundaram M, Eddelston B, Prendergast J: Diagnosis of parathyroid adenoma by computed tomography. J Comput Assist Tomogr 5:818–821, 1981.

35. Doppman JL, Krudy AG, Brennan MF, et al.: CT appearance of enlarged parathyroid glands in the posterior superior mediastinum. J Comput Assist Tomogr 6:1099–1102, 1982.

36. Sommer B, Welter HF, Spelsberg F, et al.: Computed tomography for localizing enlarged parathyroid glands in primary hyperparathyroidism. J Comput Assist Tomogr 6:521–526, 1982.

37. Whitley NO, Bohlman M, Connor TB, et al.: Computed tomography for localization of parathyroid adenomas. J Comput Assist Tomogr 5:812–817, 1981.

38. Editor's Note: CT localization of cervical parathyroid glands: it deserves a second look. J Comput Assist Tomogr 6:519–520, 1982.

39. Satava RM, Beahrs OH, Scholz DA: Success rate of cervical exploration for hyperparathyroidism. Arch Surg, 110:625–628, 1975.

40. Sample WF, Mitchell SP, Bledsoe RC: Parathyroid ultrasonography. Radiology 127:485–490, 1978.

3 Nasopharynx, Infratemporal Fossa, and Skull Base

HUGH D. CURTIN

INTRODUCTION

The focal point of this chapter is the nasopharynx. The infratemporal fossa, parapharyngeal space, and skull base are so integrally related to the nasopharynx that the entire area can be discussed as one region. Prior to the advent of the CT scanner, the radiologist played a very limited role here, seeking to detect pathology by identifying subtle bone erosions or even more subtle airway displacement. The fat planes around the muscles in the region are very distinct and are constant enough that CT now serves a key role in the evaluation of the region. CT can miss small lesions of the mucosa of the nasopharynx and so is not a substitute for direct visualization by mirror or nasopharyngoscope. Rather, CT assumes its importance in evaluation of deeper structures.[1-8]

ANATOMY

The nasopharynx extends from the choana to the level of the soft palate (Fig. 3.1). The roof and posterior wall are made up of the inferior surface of the sphenoid and the anterior surface of the basiocciput. The rectus and longus capitis muscles separate the posterior mucosa of the nasopharynx from the bone of the basiocciput. Anterior to the insertion of the rectus and longus capitis (anterior basilar portion of the occipital bone), the mucosa and submucosa of the roof of the nasopharynx are closely applied to the bone with no intervening musculature. The roof and posterior wall of the nasopharynx may form either a right angle or a smooth curve.

On the lateral wall of the nasopharynx is an inverted hook-like prominence made up of the torus tubarius and the salpingopharyngeal fold. This prominence partially surrounds the nasopharyngeal opening of the Eustachian tube. Along the outer circumference of the hook is a small indentation called the pharyngeal recess or fossa of Rosenmuller.

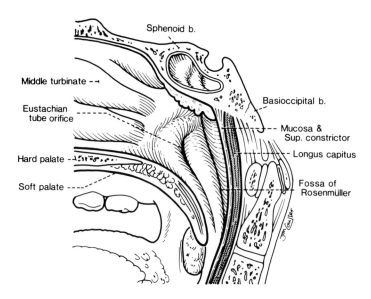

FIG. 3.1.   View of the lateral surface of the nasopharynx. Specimen has been sagittally sectioned. Note the junction of the longus capitis with the base of the skull. The fossa of Rosenmuller, or pharyngeal recess, follows the posterior margin of the salpingopharyngeal fold and curves over the torus tubarius.

The pharyngeal tonsil arises in the midline of the roof and posterior wall. Lymphoid tissue (adenoid) can fill the fossa of Rosenmuller and extend onto the wall of the torus tubarius. The lymphoid tissue usually atrophies significantly by late adolescence but may persist to some extent to the second and third decades.

Excluding the prevertebral muscles, the musculature of the region can be separated into the muscles of mastication and those of deglutition. The muscles of deglutition form an inner ring around the nasopharynx and the muscles of mastication are found more laterally in the infratemporal fossa (Fig. 3.2). They are separated for the most part by the parapharyngeal space, a fat plane that plays a key role in interpretation of the CT scan.

The muscles of deglutition are made up of the palatal musculature and the superior pharyngeal constrictors. The pharyngeal constrictors become very thin above the level of the soft palate and are incomplete along the lateral aspect of the upper nasopharynx. The space between the upper margin of the superior constrictors and the skull base is closed by the pharyngobasilar fascia, a tough fibrous sheet that attaches to the base of the skull. Inferiorly, the pharyngobasilar fascia fuses with the fascia of the superior constrictors and continues through the nasopharynx. The pharyngobasilar fascia, though strong, is quite thin and, therefore, the levator and tensor veli palatini are responsible for the muscle density along the lateral border of the nasopharynx at the upper levels of the nasopharynx on CT scan. The levator veli palatini and the Eustachian tube pass through the pharyngobasilar fascia and are thus medial to it. The

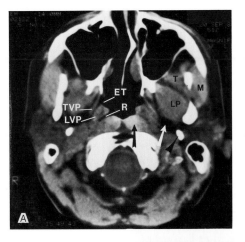
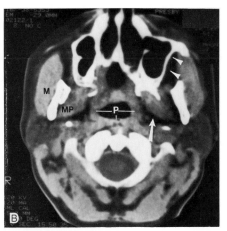
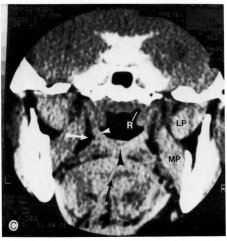

FIG. 3.2. (A) Axial slice through nasopharynx. ET, nasopharyngeal orifice of the Eustachian tube; R, fossa of Rosenmuller. The torus (unlabeled) is the prominence between ET and R. Deglutitional muscles: TVP, tensor veli palatini; LVP, levator veli palatini. Masticator muscles: LP, lateral pterygoid; M, masseter; T, temporalis. Black arrow, prevertebral musculature; white arrow, parapharyngeal space; black arrowhead, styloid process. Note how the tensor veli palatini extends toward the hamulus of the medial pterygoid. (B) Axial slice inferior to (A) at the level of Passavant's ring and the hard palate. P, Passavant's ring encircling the nasopharynx at the level of the soft palate; M, masseter; MP, medial pterygoid; arrow, parapharyngeal space; arrowheads demonstrate the fat planes just posterior to the maxillary sinus. (C) Coronal slice through the nasopharynx taken during a metrizamide cisternogram for unrelated abnormality. The deglutitional muscles, in this case the levator veli palatini (white arrowhead), extend from the base of the skull into the soft palate (black arrowhead). The fossa of Rosenmuller (R) is seen just superior to the torus. The masticator muscles are seen laterally. LP, lateral pterygoid; MP, medial pterygoid. The deglutitional and masticator muscles are separated by the parapharyngeal space (white arrow). Black arrow, musculature of the tongue.

tensor veli palatini is a thin muscle that passes outside the fascia from the base of the skull to the hamulus of the medial pterygoid and then curves into the soft palate. The Eustachian tube, tensor veli palatini, and levator veli palatini seem to merge into one image on CT scan but can be partly separated on high-resolution machines. At the level of the hard palate, according to some authors, fibers of the superior constrictor merge with fibers of the various palatal muscles to form a ring encircling the pharynx and making up Passavant's muscle. This can be seen on axial CT scan as a continuous ring if the palate is not elevated during the scan (Fig. 3.2B). If the scan is performed with the palate raised, the palate meets the ring to close off the nasopharynx and on CT appears to merge with the ring.

The muscles of mastication include medial and lateral pterygoid, masseter, and temporal muscles. All pass through or are located in the infratemporal fossa, which is defined as the area medial to the zygomatic arch, inferior to the middle cranial fossa, and lateral to the inner surface of the pterygoid muscle and pterygoid plates. Perhaps a better term is the masticator space, as discussed below. The anterior wall of the fossa is the posterior wall of the maxilla. The roof is for the most part made up of the sphenoid and a small part of the temporal bone. The infratemporal fossa communicates with the pterygo-palatine fossa medially via the pterygomaxillary fissure and with the orbit superiorly via the inferior orbital fissure. These communications represent potential routes of spread of disease.

The deglutition and mastication muscles are separated for the most part by the parapharyngeal space. Some authors include the parapharyngeal space as part of the infratemporal fossa; others treat them separately. This fat-filled space extends from the skull base to the hyoid, roughly forming an inverted pyramid. Most authors separate the parapharyngeal space into anterior and posterior parts, which are separated by an extension of the fascia surrounding the styloid musculature. This fascia passes anteriorly and medially toward the tensor veli palatini.[8] The separation is useful from a diagnostic viewpoint, as the posterior space contains the carotid sheath.

The parapharyngeal space is wider posteriorly than anteriorly, and superiorly than inferiorly. Thus obliquity of scan slice must be taken into account when symmetry of the spaces is judged.

The retropharyngeal area is made up of the prevertebral musculature—the longus capitis and colli—and the retropharyngeal space, a potential space between the pharyngobasilar fascia and the prevertebral musculature.

The discussion of the skull base will be limited to those structures intimately related to the nasopharynx and its related structures. This limits the discussion to the sphenoid, basiocciput, and temporal bones. The sphenoid and basiocciput are fused together and, along with the prevertebral muscles, form the roof and the posterior wall of the nasopharynx. These bones are most likely to be eroded by nasopharyngeal tumors. The temporal bone is separated from the basiocciput by the foramen lacerum and more posteriorly by the petro-occipital suture. The temporal bone contains the carotid canal and the anterior wall of the jugular foramen, which are key structures in the posterior parapharyngeal lesions.

The vomer forms the posterior margin of the nasal septum and meets the rostrum of the sphenoid. This junction can often be identified in the roof of the nasopharynx on CT and indeed the alae of the vomer make up a small portion of the roof of the nasopharynx.

Fascial Planes[9-12]

The potential fascial spaces of the neck and face are formed by fascia covering certain muscles (Fig. 3.3). These fascia bind to the periosteum, thus compartmentalizing the area to some extent. Detailed description of the fascial spaces is beyond the scope of this volume, but since the compartments may direct the spread of pathology, some familiarity is useful to the radiologist. The important fascial compartments in this area include the masticator space, temporal space, buccal space, parapharyngeal space, and retropharyngeal space. The ca-

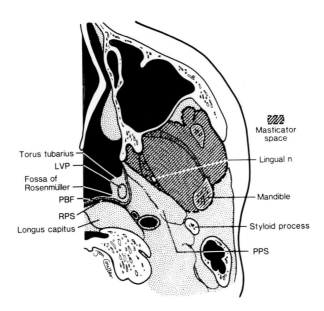

FIG. 3.3. Horizontal section showing one-half of the nasopharynx and infratemporal fossa. The masticator space is shaded. The parapharyngeal space is between the pharyngobasilar fascia and the masticator space. The carotid artery and jugular vein are seen in the poststyloid space. The line extending through the parapharyngeal space is an approximation of the separation between pre- and poststyloid compartments. LVP, levator veli palatini; PBF, pharyngobasilar fascia; RPS, retropharyngeal space; PPS, parapharyngeal space.

rotid sheath is located in the posterior parapharyngeal space and communicates partially with the retropharyngeal space.

The masticator space contains the pterygoid muscles, masseter, and insertion of the temporalis muscle, as well as a portion of the angle and ramus of the mandible. The space continues anterosuperiorly as the temporal space passing medially to the zygomatic arch on either side of the temporalis muscle.

The buccal space is anterior to the masticator space and superficial (lateral) to the buccinator muscle.

The parapharyngeal space has been described above. The fascial covering of the parotid gland is considered by some authors to separate the deep portion of the parotid from the parapharyngeal space. The deep portion of the parotid extends through the gap or tunnel between the styloid and the mandible and abuts on the parapharyngeal space just posterior to the pterygoid musculature.

The space separating the pharyngeal mucosa from the skull base and vertebral arches is made up of the prevertebral muscular space and the retropharyngeal space. The prevertebral muscular space contains the prevertebral muscles, the longus capitis, and the colli. The retropharyngeal space is a potential space between the fascia of the prevertebral muscles and the pharyngobasilar fascia. According to some authors, this retropharyngeal space is separated into two compartments by an extra fascial layer called the alar fascia.[12] The retropharyngeal spaces are important as pathways for extension of infection into the mediastinum. The retropharyngeal space contains small chains of lymph nodes that are medial to the carotid artery.[13]

The fascial boundaries are not always complete and may communicate with each other. Indeed, there is considerable disagreement about the integrity of some of the fascial layers and, therefore, the definition of some of the compartments.

CT TECHNIQUE

Axial scans are taken from the sphenoid to a point well below the hard palate. In cases of possible malignancy, the nodes most likely to be involved are included. Scans are taken 5 mm apart while intravenous contrast is administered with rapid flow during the actual scanning. The scan angle is approximately at Reid's baseline or parallel to the hard palate. Coronal sections may be helpful in further defining the lesion (Fig. 3.2C).

Maneuvers, such as blowing out against pinched nostrils (Valsalva maneuver), tend to open the Eustachian tube orifice and fossa of Rosenmuller (lateral pharyngeal recess).

PATHOLOGY

Nasopharynx

Tumors in the nasopharynx can cause airway obstruction, Eustachian tube malfunction, or cranial nerve palsies. Middle ear effusion, presenting for the first time in an older person, suggests the possibility of a carcinoma of the nasopharynx. One difficulty in evaluating the nasopharynx is differentiating lymphoid tissue in the nasopharynx from tumor. The pharyngeal tonsils or adenoids attach to the roof and posterior wall of the nasopharynx and are intraluminal, showing masses in the nasopharynx on CT. They are often but not always symmetrical and may have a midline sulcus. At times the pharyngeal mucosa blushes slightly with intravenous contrast and the adenoids can then be defined, but this is not always the case. The pharyngeal tonsils or any intraluminal soft tissue mass such as a choanal polyp may appear to blend into the deglutitional muscles but should not affect the appearance of the parapharyngeal fat, which should retain bilateral symmetry. Thus the symmetry of the parapharyngeal fat assumes its importance.

Squamous Cell Carcinoma[14,15]

Squamous cell carcinoma accounts for 90 percent of nasopharyngeal malignancies. Small tumors may cause apparent thickening of the deglutitional muscles or may appear to flatten or efface the fossa of Rosenmuller and the Eustachian tube (Figs. 3.4–3.6). Small asymmetries of the airway may be normal and should be confirmed by direct visualization and biopsy.

As a larger nasopharyngeal tumor extends laterally, it pushes into the medial aspect of the parapharyngeal fat, which then outlines the lateral margin of the tumor (Fig. 3.7). The parapharyngeal spaces lose their symmetry. Extension posteriorly involves the prevertebral musculature and eventually the base of the skull (Fig. 3.5, 3.8). The tumor can finally erode into the intracranial area, appearing as a "bulge" in the dura or impinging on the cerebellospinal fluid cistern anterior to the brainstem. A tumor can also grow through the foramen lacerum to reach the dura (Fig. 3.6) of the middle cranial fossa. Anteriorly the lesion may grow into the nasal cavity or up into the sphenoethmoid recess,

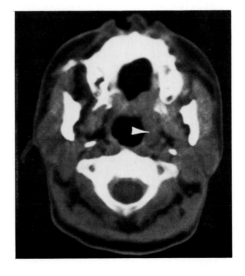

FIG. 3.4. Carcinoma of the oro- and nasopharyngeal wall extending into the margin of the soft palate. Note the thickening of the nasopharyngeal wall (arrowhead). The inner ring of the deglutitional muscles appears to be enlarged on the involved side.

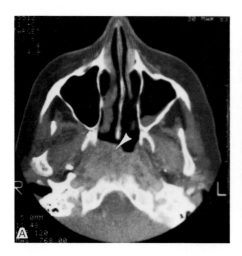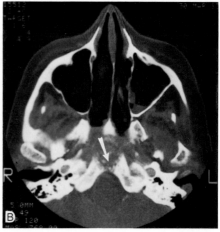

FIG. 3.5. (A) Carcinoma of the nasopharynx with effacement of the fossa of Rosenmuller and orifice of the Eustachian tube. The mass is asymmetric (arrowhead). (B) At a slightly higher level, the base of the skull is eroded (arrow). Erosion does not extend intracranially.

ethmoid sinuses, pterygopalatine fossa, and orbital apex. The precise limits of extension are very important in planning treatment, which in the case of carcinoma of the nasopharynx is usually radiotherapy.

In cases where the Eustachian tube is involved, the middle ear and mastoid will often be filled with fluid but may be normal in the degree of mastoid

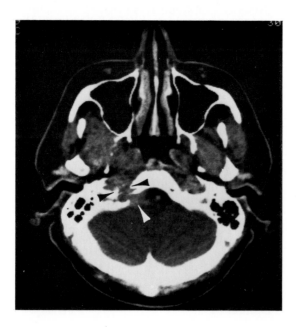

FIG. 3.6. Tumor extending through the petro-occipital suture (between black arrowheads) and extending into the dura with a characteristic enhancing bulge seen in the posterior fossa (white arrowhead).

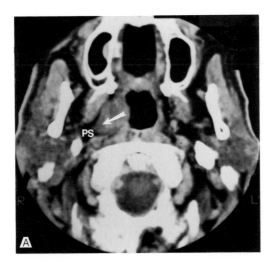

FIG. 3.7. (A) Tumor involving the nasopharyngeal wall (neurilemmoma). The tumor extends beyond the wall of the nasopharynx into the parapharyngeal space (arrow). PS, parapharyngeal space. This 60-year-old patient presented with middle ear effusion because of an obstructed Eustachian tube. (B) Coronal view showing tumor (T) extending from the nasopharyngeal wall and impinging on the parapharyngeal space (white arrowhead). Note the relationship of the tumor to the lower part of the bony Eustachian tube (black arrow). The tumor partly effaces the fossa of Rosenmuller.

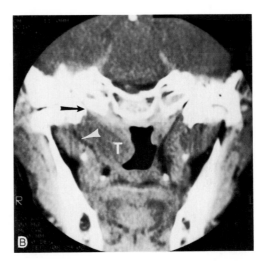

air cell formation. In a patient with chronic ear infection since childhood, the mastoid air cells are usually underdeveloped.

Lymph Node Involvement

Lymphatic spread from the nasopharynx may be to the jugular digastric nodes or to the retropharyngeal nodes. Of special interest are the nodes high in the posterior triangle of the neck (spinal accessory nodes) (Fig. 3.9). Enlargement of these nodes is strongly suggestive of nasopharyngeal carcinoma. The nodes involved with squamous cell carcinoma often show necrotic centers that appear as low densities with peripheral enhancement.

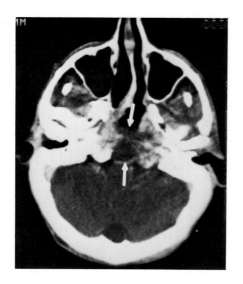

FIG. 3.8. Nasopharyngeal carcinoma (between arrows) arising in the nasopharynx. The tumor extended through the basiocciput and impinges on the dura and subarachnoid cistern.

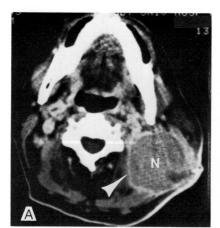

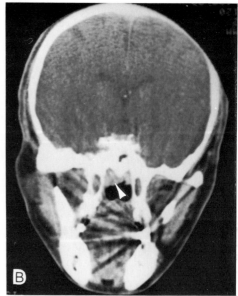

FIG. 3.9. (A) Patient presents with a large mass in the posterior triangle. CT scan demonstrates an enlarged lymph node (N) with characteristic peripheral enhancement (arrowhead). (B) Coronal section through the nasopharynx shows asymmetry of the soft tissue, which was biopsied and was a nasopharyngeal squamous cell carcinoma. Without bone erosion small asymmetries of the nasopharynx can be normal, and biopsy is required for diagnosis.

Other Malignancies

Rhabdomyosarcoma is the most common malignancy involving the nasopharyngeal area in a child. By the time of presentation, the tumor may have progressed into the ear or the skull base and the precise point of origin may not be clear. Extension into and through the skull base is best detected by CT.

Adenoid cystic carcinoma, melanoma, lymphoma, plasmacytoma, and a number of other tumors including metastases may occasionally arise in the nasopharynx but are much less common than squamous cell carcinoma.[14]

Secondary Involvement

Tumors may impinge on the nasopharynx from any side. Of importance is superior extension from carcinoma of the tonsillar pillar and soft palate. Submucosal spread may efface the fossa of Rosenmuller without involving the mucosa and thus may be missed by direct visualization by the clinician (Fig. 3.10). Tumors of the sella turcica, sphenoid sinus, sphenoid bone, foramen ovale, jugular fossa, temporal bone, and even the foramen magnum may encroach on the nasopharynx from above.

Benign Lesions of the Nasopharynx

Juvenile angiofibromas present with nosebleeds and nasal obstruction, usually in an adolescent male. These tumors arise in the upper anterior nasopharynx. The most common origin is along the lateral wall. The tumor characteristically widens the pterygopalatine fossa and enhances intensely when intravenous contrast is administered (Fig. 3.11). Rarely, the lesion may extend laterally through the pterygopalatine fossa into the infratemporal fossa or may erode into or through the sphenoid.[16,17]

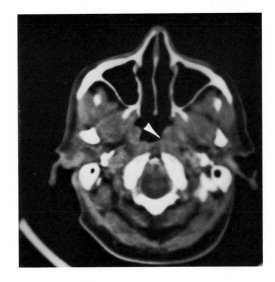

FIG. 3.10. Carcinoma of the tonsillar pillar extending superiorly into the nasopharynx. The tumor is submucosal and, therefore, not visible to the clinical examiner at this level. The fossa of Rosenmuller is effaced (white arrowhead) suggesting the submucosal spread.

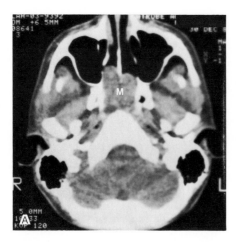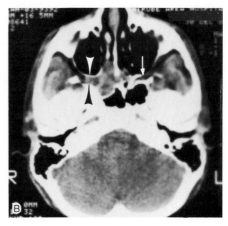

FIG. 3.11. (A) Juvenile angiofibroma mass (M) is seen filling the airway and bulging into the nasal cavity. (B) Slightly higher cut at the level of the pterygopalatine fossa shows a soft tissue mass in the upper nasopharynx and posterior nasal cavity. The parapharyngeal space is involved (between arrowheads). Note that the fat, normally seen in the pterygopalatine fossa, is obliterated. Compare with the normal pterygopalatine fossa on the opposite side. (Case courtesy of Dr. William Stilley, Latrobe Hospital, Latrobe, Pennsylvania).

The appearance of these tumors is usually characteristic and, coupled with a clinical history, is almost diagnostic, but angiography is done to demonstrate blood supply and to evaluate the possibility of embolization.

Tornwaldt's cyst can form in the pharyngeal bursa and present in the second and third decades as a submucosal mass or cyst high in the midline of the posterior wall of the nasopharynx. It originates from remnants of the notochord.

Antral choanal polyps protrude into the nasopharynx. The parapharyngeal fascia remains symmetrical. The nasal cavity is partly filled with soft tissue and the maxillary sinus as the site of origin is usually opacified (Fig. 3.12).

Encephalocele may extend through a defect in the sphenoid bone to the nasopharynx.

The Parapharyngeal Space

Lesions of the parapharyngeal space are infrequent and usually benign.[18,19] Those in the anterior or prestyloid space are predominantly of salivary gland origin, whereas those in the posterior or poststyloid space are more commonly of neurogenic origin (neurilemmoma, paraganglioma).[8,19] Again, the effect of the tumor on the fat in the parapharyngeal space helps to define tumor origin.

Prestyloid lesions are usually extensions from either the pharyngeal area or the deep portion of the parotid. Those arising from the parotid are often dumbbell shaped, being constricted as the tumor "squeezes" through the stylo-

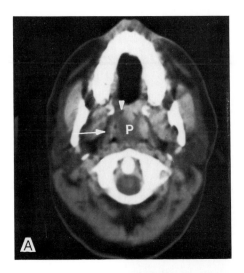

FIG. 3.12. (A) Antral choanal polyp. The polyp is seen as a mass (P) in the lumen of the nasopharynx. The polyp appears to merge partially with the deglutitional muscles along the left side. The small amount of air (arrowhead) separates the polyp from the soft palate. The parapharyngeal spaces are symmetrical. Parapharyngeal space (arrow). (B) Higher cuts shows soft tissue obliterating the nasal cavity (N) and the maxillary sinus (M). No bone destruction is defined. It is difficult to tell how much of the maxillary sinus represents the mass and how much represents obstruction.

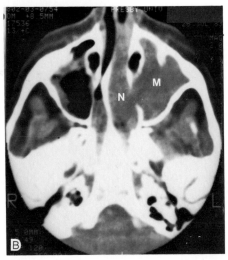

mandibular gap or tunnel (Fig. 3.13). The fat in the parapharyngeal space is pushed medially. Parotid sialography can be used to determine the precise relationship of the lesion to the parotid gland (Fig. 3.14).[20] Contrast injected into the parotid duct opacifies the "finger" of the parotid passing through the stylomandibular tunnel in those lesions that are entirely within the parapharyngeal space. This is of considerable importance when determining the surgical approach.[19]

A salivary gland tumor in the parapharyngeal space can also arise from ectopic or minor salivary glands. These may be differentiated from neuromas (neurilemmomas) of the fifth cranial nerve, which usually enhance with intravenous contrast, and from parapharyngeal cysts, which tend to have a lower attenuation.

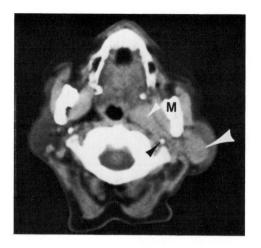

FIG. 3.13. Benign tumor (cystic Warthin's tumor). Typical "dumbbell" lesion arising in the parotid (large white arrowhead) and extending through the stylomandibular tunnel into the parapharyngeal space (small white arrowhead). The fat planes of the parapharyngeal space are displaced but not obscured. The fat plane just posterior to the parapharyngeal component of the tumor indicates that this is in the prestyloid space. Small black arrowhead, styloid M, mandible.

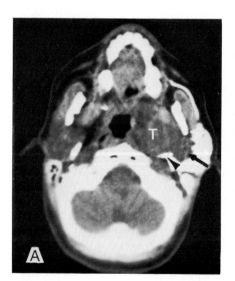

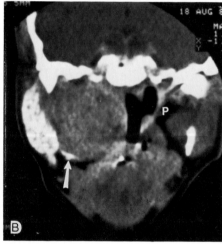

FIG. 3.14. (A) Pleomorphic adenoma. CT sialogram shows tumor (T) extending into the parapharyngeal space. The tumor "squeezes" through the stylomandibular tunnel to involve the parotid (black arrow). Small amount of contrast (small arrowhead) extends as far as the styloid process. The typical dumbbell or bilobed shape suggests a parotid origin. (B) Coronal of the same patient shows the relationship of the tumor to the base of the skull. A small amount of contrast (arrow) is seen at the lower margin of the tumor, again indicating a parotid origin. The airway and parapharyngeal space are effaced and displaced. Note the normal parapharyngeal space (P) on the opposite side.

Tumors of the poststyloid parapharyngeal space are usually related to the neural elements associated with the carotid and jugular. Cranial nerves IX, X, XI, and XII, as well as the sympathetic chain, are close to these vessels just beneath the skull base. Lesions of the space push the parapharyngeal space fat anteriorly and slightly laterally.

Neuromas may arise in the poststyloid parapharyngeal space, usually enhance, and are at least partially posterior and medial to the styloid (Fig. 3.15).

Paragangliomas or chemodectomas involve the poststyloid parapharyngeal space. An intensely enhancing lesion may be the inferior extension of a glomus jugulare arising in the jugular bulb or may be a glomus intravagale arising beneath the base of the skull in the region of the ganglion of the vagus nerve.

Glomus jugulare tumors exhibit destruction of the jugular fossa and usually extend into the middle ear or intracranially through the jugular canal. The lower margin may be estimated by the rapid tapering in size of the enhancing lesion in the poststyloid compartment, as seen on axial slices. Coronal images can better demonstrate the lower margin of the tumor.

The glomus intravagale arises beneath the jugular foramen and pushes the carotid forward on angiography. Paragangliomas may be multiple and bilateral but are rarely malignant.

Meningiomas may involve either the pre- or poststyloid space as well as the infratemporal fossa. They are vascular and blush on intravenous enhancement. They cause hyperostosis of bone and may calcify. (See also infratemporal fossa).

Lateral retropharyngeal nodes behave as poststyloid parapharyngeal masses displacing the parapharyngeal fat anteriorly (Fig. 3.16). When infiltrated with squamous cell carcinoma, they often exhibit a central necrotic area.

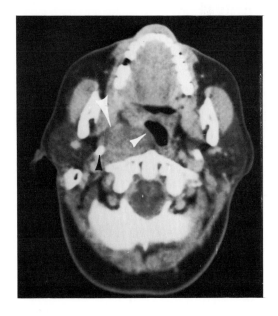

FIG. 3.15. Neuroma arising in the poststyloid parapharyngeal space. A fine fat plane (small white arrowhead) separates the tumor from the pharyngeal mucosa. The parapharyngeal space fat (large white arrowhead) is displaced anteriorly and laterally, indicating the poststyloid origin of the tumor. Styloid process (small black arrowhead).

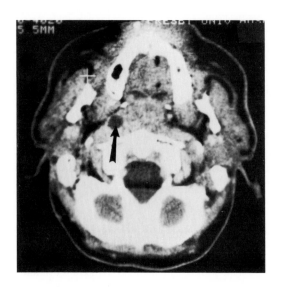

FIG. 3.16. Patient with carcinoma of the hypopharynx with nodal involvement. The node has central lucency (arrow) and behaves as a poststyloid parapharyngeal mass. This would represent the node of Rouviere and is just medial to the carotid.

Other types of tumors, such as hemangiomas and various sarcomas, are very rare. Skull base tumors extend into the parapharyngeal space and will be discussed below.

When a lesion is localized in the poststyloid parapharyngeal space, angiography is performed. This technique can help to differentiate neurilemmomas from paragangliomas; more importantly it defines the blood supply and the relation of the tumor to the great vessels.

Infratemporal Fossa

Most tumors involving the infratemporal fossa do so secondarily, extending into the fossa from the maxillary sinus, nasopharynx, sphenoid bone, or other surrounding structures. Less commonly, a primary tumor may arise in the mandible or the soft tissues of the fossa (Fig. 3.17). At times, the point of origin can be predicted fairly accurately, but biopsy is necessary as in other areas for precise histological definition before therapy is planned. Tumors may erode bone as they progress, or they may extend through natural ostia or along soft tissue planes.[21] Medially, they can pass into or through the pterygopalatine fossa or extend toward the parapharyngeal space. Superiorly, the inferior orbital fissure gives access to the orbit and the foramen ovale leads to the middle cranial fossa. Each of these exits from the infratemporal fossa can be evaluated by CT. Usually the routes of exit contain fat, which is obliterated as the tumor encroaches on the area. Tumor extending through into the middle cranial fossa enhances more than does the brain, so the tumor margin can be detected (Fig. 3.17C).

As tumor pushes anteriorly against the posterior wall of the maxillary sinus, the bone may be destroyed with the tumor breaking into the maxillary antrum.

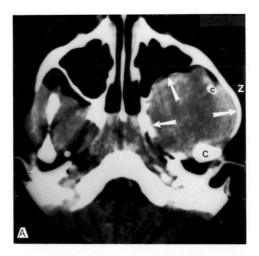

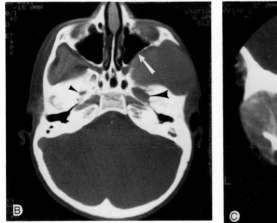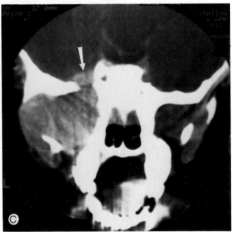

FIG. 3.17. (A) Synovial sarcoma. Large mass bows the zygoma (Z) laterally, bows the posterior wall of the maxillary sinus anteriorly, and flattens the pterygoid plate. Remodeling of the mandible is present, separating the coronoid process (c) from the condyle (C). (B) Slightly higher cut. Again, the posterior wall of the maxillary sinus is shown bowed forward but not destroyed (white arrow). The foramen ovale is enlarged on the ipsilateral side (black arrowhead). (C) Coronal view shows the tumor extending through the foramen ovale. The margin of the tumor (arrow) can be seen because the enhancing tumor has a different density from that of the brain.

The tumor may bow a thin bone forward without actually breaking through. This finding does not necessarily mean that the lesion is benign but has been described in malignancy as well.[22] Again, biopsy is necessary for diagnosis.

Meningiomas can involve the infratemporal fossa (Fig. 3.18). They enhance and often cause sclerosis of the bone surrounding them, in this case the ptery-

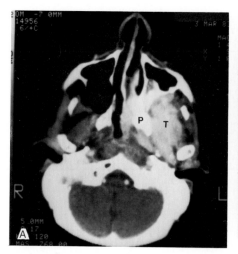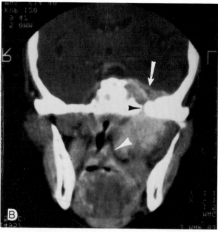

FIG. 3.18. (A) Meningioma. Tumor (T) in the infratemporal fossa with bowing of the maxillary sinus, posterior wall. Hyperostosis involving the pterygoid plates (P) is present. (B) Coronal view shows the tumor that deviates the parapharyngeal fat (large white arrowhead). The tumor extends through the foramen ovale (small black arrowhead) and has a large intracranial component (white arrow) in the floor of the middle cranial fossa.

goids, sphenoid, and maxilla. When they are detected in the infratemporal fossa, the usual routes of spread are evaluated, with special attention given to the floor of the middle cranial fossa. Coronal scans are often necessary.

Tumors may grow along a nerve to spread more centrally. Perineural spread is usually associated with adenocystic carcinoma but can be seen in other cell types, including squamous cell carcinoma.[23,24] The trigeminal nerve is susceptible because it courses through areas prone to adenocystic carcinoma, i.e., the area of the major and minor salivary glands. Several nerves may be affected in the infratemporal fossa. The segment of the second division of the trigeminal nerve between the posterior end of the infraorbital canal and the pterygopalatine fossa passes along the posterior wall of the maxillary sinus and is in the fat plane of the infratemporal fossa. The nerve parallels the inferior orbital fissure into the pterygopalatine fossa. If the lesion can be seen in the infratemporal fossa, the fat in the pterygopalatine fossa is usually obliterated.

Similarly, the superior alveolar nerves pass along the posterior wall of the maxilla and are then in the margin of the infratemporal fossa (see Fig. 3.23).

The lingual nerve passes very close to the submandibular gland. More superiorly the nerve passes lateral to the medial pterygoid muscle and medial to the lateral pterygoid muscle. Tumor can follow this nerve through the foramen ovale to the gasserian ganglion. Defining the enlargement of the nerve itself would be very unusual. If an irregularity is seen at the margin of the pterygoid muscle, the foramen ovale and middle cranial fossa should be examined (Fig. 3.19).

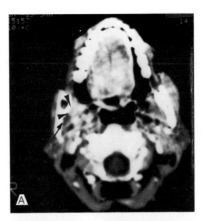

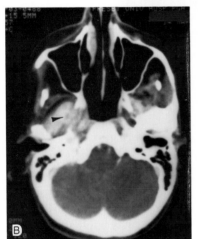
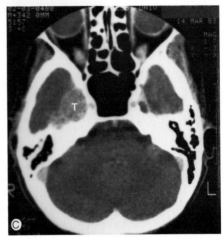

FIG. 3.19. (A) Patient with adenoid cystic carcinoma of the submandibular gland. CT scan shows peculiar ring-like density (black arrowheads) along the inner margin of the mandible just anterior to the entrance to the mandibular canal (black arrow). This would correspond to the position of the lingual nerve just lateral to the medial pterygoid muscle. (B) Slightly higher cut shows ring-like density (small black arrowhead) along the inner margin of the lateral pterygoid. (C) The tumor (T) resurfaced in the region of the gesserian ganglion and middle cranial fossa. There was destruction of the foramen ovale. At surgery perineural invasion was demonstrated along the lingual nerve, which was grossly enlarged. Although it would be very difficult to say preoperatively that the irregularity associated with the pterygoid muscles represented an enlarged lingual nerve, the region of the foramen ovale and middle cranial fossa should be carefully evaluated.

Tumor may spread along a nerve without necessarily enlarging it, in which case no abnormality would be seen. In this case, a tumor may "resurface" more centrally after following a nerve through its basilar foramen. More experience is needed before definitive statements can be made in this regard.

Hematogenous metastasis may affect the mandible, usually in the region

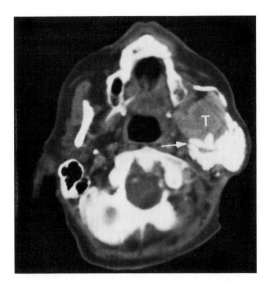

FIG. 3.20. Metastatic carcinoma of the lung to the mandible. Tumor (T) destroys the anterior portion of the ramus of the mandible and although it displaces the parotid duct, it does not involve the parotid itself. A small finger of the parotid extends through the stylomandibular tunnel towards the parapharyngeal space (arrow).

of the molars (Fig. 3.20). Primaries are usually breast, kidney, lung, colon, or prostate.[25]

Skull Base

A brief discussion of the skull base is warranted because of the close relationship between it and the nasopharyngeal and parapharyngeal structures. Tumors extend into the base of the skull from the nasopharynx and the parapharyngeal space as described above, or tumors of the base may grow down into the soft tissues beneath the base of the skull and thus impinge on the area under discussion.

The tumors of the base of the skull are quite varied, but some order can be achieved by defining their points of origin. If the discussion is limited to the sphenoid, basiocciput, and temporal bone, the differential diagnosis is usually limited to a few entities.

The temporal bone is covered elsewhere in this volume but is briefly mentioned here. Carcinoma of the external canal, glomus jugulare tumor, and more medially neuromas all arise in the temporal bone and may extend into the parapharyngeal spaces. Epidermoids (primary cholesteatomas) are of low density. They involve the petrous apex but usually do not extend inferiorly.

A chondromatous lesion can arise in many areas of the skull base but has a definite predilection for the petro-occipital suture or posterior foramen lacerum.[2] This lesion may be difficult to differentiate from a lesion of the jugular foramen. Chondromatous lesion may calcify and thus mimic meningiomas but would not show the hyperostosis (Fig. 3.21).

The clivus is the characteristic location of a chordoma arising from notochord remnants. These midline remnants are most frequent in the basiocciput itself

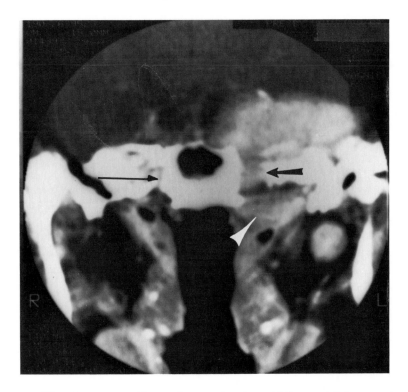

FIG. 3.21. Chondrosarcoma. Tumor is seen in the middle cranial fossa, extending through the petro-occipital suture (large black arrow) into the parapharyngeal area (white arrowhead). Note the normal petro-occipital suture on the opposite side (small black arrow). Tumor arising in the petro-occipital suture suggests a chondromatous lesion. It may be difficult to differentiate this from tumor arising in the jugular area. This tumor showed a small amount of calcification indicating the chondromatous nature.

or along the intracranial surface of the clivus.[26] Chordomas can destroy enough bone to reach the nasopharynx. They can arise in the posterior nasopharyngeal wall itself, but this would be very unusual.

Rathke's pouch tumors, such as craniopharyngiomas, would be more likely to affect the nasopharynx higher in the vault close to the nasal septum.[27] They are much more likely to be intracranial than extracranial. They calcify and arise in the midline.

Pituitary tumors rarely erode inferiorly all the way through the sphenoid sinus. Teratomas may affect the basiocciput and sphenoid, as can plasmacytomas.

Hematogenous metastatic disease can cause osteoblastic changes or a lytic destruction of the base of the skull. There are many diseases that may mimic malignant destruction. In the temporal bone Paget's disease, petrositis, and histiocytosis can look much like tumoral destruction, whereas fibrous dysplasia can mimic hyperostotic changes of meningioma.

Infection

Infections can extend into the compartments deep to the nasopharynx and the parapharyngeal area from an abscessed tooth, a peritonsillar abscess, sinusitis (especially sphenoid), or a more distant site with bacteremia. Infection can drain to the nodes in the retropharyngeal space, thus giving rise to an abscess in that region.[9] Once the infection is established, the various fascial planes may partially contain the spread and direct it preferentially to certain areas. For instance, infections of the masticator space (mandible, pterygoids, and masseter) can easily spread superiorly beneath the zygoma into the temporal space (Fig. 3.22). Infection reaching the parapharyngeal space can spread inferiorly toward the hyoid. Retropharyngeal infections may spread down into the mediastinum. Osteomyelitis of the skull base can develop from sinusitis. Parapharyngeal space infections may be a direct extension from the parotid gland.

The fascial planes are not to be considered impervious to spread of infection. There are often gaps in the fascia, or infection can follow the nerves or blood vessels that perforate the fascia, thus entering bordering compartments. For instance, infection of the buccal space may spread to the masticator space or, less commonly, the parapharyngeal space.[11]

Malignant external otitis is a *Pseudomonas* infection seen predominantly in elderly diabetics. It can extend from the external auditory canal down into the soft tissues beneath the skull base. Usually the spread is quite lateral,

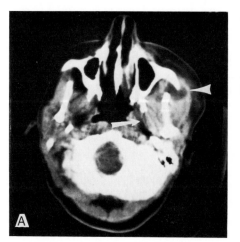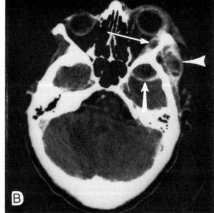

FIG. 3.22. (A) Infection of the masticator space secondary to dental extraction. The abscess obliterates the fat plane with an area of necrosis. The lateral margin approximates the position of the masseter muscle (arrowhead). The medial margin involves the pterygoid musculature but not the parapharyngeal space (arrow). (B) Infection extends superiorly in the temporal space (arrowhead). Infection also extended through the infraorbital fissure and presented as a subperiosteal abscess in the orbit (small white arrow), and unsuspected epidural abscess was also identified on the CT (large white arrow). The precise route to the epidural space was not clear.

but infection can also extend medially into the pharyngeal region.[28] Again, involvement is detected because the infection obliterates the normal fat planes.

Miscellaneous

Atrophy of the muscles in the elderly accentuates the fat planes in the nasopharynx and related areas.

The muscles of mastication are all innervated by cranial nerve V. Any pathological process involving the central connections of cranial nerve V may lead to unilateral atrophy (Fig. 3.23). These changes can be detected on CT and may reflect disease more central to a clinically obvious lesion.

The palatal muscles are innervated through the pharyngeal plexus by cranial nerve X with the exception of the tensor veli palatini, which is cranial nerve V. The tensor veli palatini attaches to the lateral wall of the Eustachian tube and is partly responsible for its normal function.[29] Involvement of the innervation of the tensor veli palatini, therefore, causes Eustachian tube malfunction and middle ear effusion without extension of the tumor directly into the tube itself. Atrophy of the tongue is indicative of hypoglossal nerve involvement.

Pseudoenlargement of the pterygoid muscles has been seen after hemimandibulectomy (Fig. 3.24). If the body of the mandible is removed, the pterygoids

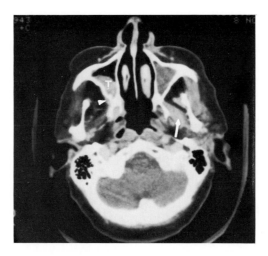

FIG. 3.23. Patient with adenoid cystic carcinoma (T) of the maxillary antrum. There was extensive perineural involvement. The small density (small arrowhead) seen in the fat just posterior to the wall of the maxillary sinus most likely represents tumor following the alveolar nerves. The pterygopalatine fat was obliterated on a more superior cut. Note the atrophy of the lateral pterygoid muscle compared with the normal thickness on the opposite side (arrow). The fossa of Rosenmuller and Eustachian tube orifice appear to be more prominent on the involved side. The opposite maxillary sinus is opacified by retained secretions.

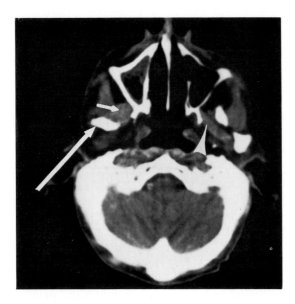

FIG. 3.24. Patient with hemimandibular resection because of carcinoma of the mandibular alveolar ridge. Because of the absence of the mandible and teeth on the right side, the mandibular condyle (large white arrow) has been pulled forward out of the glenoid fossa. The lateral pterygoid muscle (small white arrow) appears to be much thicker than the normal lateral pterygoid (white arrowhead) on the opposite side. This should not be mistaken for tumor.

and masseters (if present) pull the remnant of the ramus anteriorly and superiorly. This shortens the lateral pterygoid muscle and may cause it to appear larger than the muscle on the opposite side, which remains in normal position. This effect should not be mistaken for tumor involvement.

SUMMARY

The nasopharynx and related soft tissues lend themselves to evaluation by CT because of the presence of distinct symmetrical fat planes, which are distorted by pathology. Displacement of the fat-filled parapharyngeal space is particularly useful in localizing the origin of a tumor. Knowledge of the anatomy and the behavior of various tumors is essential if the limits of a neoplasm are to be accurately defined. Although the cell type of a tumor can occasionally be predicted, the radiologist's primary role is to define precisely the extent of the disease process.

REFERENCES

1. Silver AJ, Mawad ME, Hilal SK, et al.: Computed tomography of the nasopharynx and related spaces. Part I. Anatomy. Radiology 147:725–731, 1983.
2. Silver AJ, Mawad ME, Hilal SK, et al.: Computed tomography of the nasopharynx and related spaces. Part II. Pathology. Radiology 147:733–738, 1983.
3. Bohman L, Mancuso A, Thompson J, Hanafee WN: CT approach to benign nasopharyngeal masses. AJR 136:173–180, 1981.
4. Mancuso A, Bohman L, Hanafee W, Maxwell D: Computed tomography of the nasopharynx: normal and variants of normal. *Radiology 137:113–121, 1980.*
5. Doubleday LC, Jing B, Wallace S: Computed tomography of the infratemporal fossa. Radiology 138:619–624, 1981.

6. Mancuso A, Hanafee WN: Computed Tomography of the Head and Neck. Williams & Wilkins, Baltimore, 1982.

7. Carter B: Computed Tomography. pp. 212–240. In Valvassori GE, Potter GD, Hanafee WN, et al. (eds): Radiology of the Ear, Nose and Throat. WB Saunders, Philadelphia 1982.

8. Som PM, Biller HF, Lawson W: Tumors of the parapharyngeal space (preoperative evaluation, diagnosis, and surgical approaches). Ann Otol Rhinol Laryngol 90:3–15, 1981.

9. Wong YK, Novotny GM: Retropharyngeal space—a review of anatomy, pathology, and clinical presentation. J Otolaryngol 7:528–536, 1978.

10. Coller FA, Yglesias L: Infections of the lip and face. Surg Gynecol Obstet 60:277–290, 1935.

11. Kostrubala JG: Potential anatomical spaces in the face. Am J Surg 68:28–37, 1945.

12. Grodinsky M, Holyoke EA: The fascia and fascial spaces of the head, neck, and adjacent regions. Am J Anat 63:367–408, 1938.

13. Mancuso AA, Harnsberger HR, Muraki AS, Stevens MH: Computed tomography of cervical and retropharyngeal lymph nodes: normal anatomy, variants of normal, and applications in staging head and neck cancer. Part I: normal anatomy. Radiology 148:709–714, 1983.

14. Goldstein JC, Sisson GA: Tumors of the nose, paranasal sinuses, and nasopharynx. pp. 2078–2114. In Paparella MM, Shumrick DA (eds): Otolaryngology, Vol. III (Head and Neck), WB Saunders, Philadelphia 1980.

15. Choa G: Cancer of the Nasopharynx. pp. 372–414. In Suen JY, Myers EN (eds): Cancer of the Head and Neck. Churchill Livingstone, New York, 1981.

16. Weinstein MA, Levine H, Duchesneau PM, Tucker HM: Diagnosis of juvenile angiofibroma by computed tomography. Radiology 126:703–705, 1978.

17. Bryan RN, Sessions RB, Horowitz BL: Radiologic management of juvenile angiofibroma. AJNR 2:157–166, 1981.

18. Lawson VG, LeLiever WC, Makerewich LA, et al.: Unusual parapharyngeal lesions. J Otolaryngol 8:241–249, 1979.

19. Bass R: Approaches to the diagnosis and treatment of tumors of the parapharyngeal space. Head Neck Surg 4:281–289, 1982.

20. Som PM, Biller HF: The combined CT-sialogram. Radiology 135:387–390, 1980.

21. Hesselink JR, Weber AL: Pathways of orbital extension of extra-orbital neoplasms. J Comput Assist Tomogr 613:593–597, 1982.

22. Som PM, Shugar JM, Cohen BA, Biller HF: The nonspecificity of the antral bowing sign in maxillary sinus pathology. J Comput Assist Tomogr 5:350–352, 1981.

23. Dodd GD, Dolan PA, Ballantyne AJ, et al.: The dissemination of tumors of the head and neck via the cranial nerves. Radiol Clin N Am 8:445–461, 1970.

24. Conley J, Dingman D: Adenoid cystic carcinoma in the head and neck (cylindroma). Arch Otolaryngol 100:81–90, 1974.

25. Batsakis JG: Tumors of the Head and Neck, Clinical and Pathological Considerations, 2nd Ed. Williams & Wilkins, Baltimore, 1979.

26. Bonneville J, Belloir A, Mawazini H, et al.: Calcified remnants of the notochord in the roof of the nasopharynx. Radiology 137:373–377, 1980.

27. Caffey J: Pediatric X-ray Diagnosis. p. 149. Year Book Medical Publishers, Chicago, 1945.

28. Curtin HD, Wolfe P, May M: Malignant external otitis: CT evaluation. Radiology 145:383–388, 1982.

29. Cantekin EI, Doyle WJ, Bluestone CD: Effect of levator veli palatini muscle excision on eustachian tube function. Arch Otolaryngol 109:281–284, 1983.

4 The Base of the Tongue

SVEN G. LARSSON

INTRODUCTION

The oropharynx forms a relatively passive crossroad between the airway and the digestive tract. It extends from a plane through the soft palate superiorly down to a plane through the hyoid bone. The base of the tongue is separated from the oral tongue by the circumvallate papillae and forms the anterior portion of the oropharynx together with the vallecula and the free margin of the epiglottis. The lateral borders are made up of the anterior and posterior tonsillar pillars, with the palatine tonsil in between, and the lateral pharyngeal wall. The posterior pharyngeal wall forms the remaining boundary.

Although parts of the oropharynx are available for inspection, evaluation of its deeper structures, particularly the base of the tongue, is difficult because of usually well-developed gagging reflexes. Clinical assessment of the base of the tongue can therefore be accomplished only after application of topical anesthesia; sometimes even general anesthesia is needed to evaluate the deeper portions.

Studies using computed tomography have shown that the technique can clearly and with ease outline the base of the tongue and its accompanying deep fascial planes and structures.[1-3] With that in mind CT can be of value in the work-up of any base-of-tongue lesion.

TECHNIQUE

For scanning in the axial plane, the patient is placed supine with the neck and chin slightly hyperextended in order to immobilize and stretch the suprahyoid and extrinsic tongue muscles. The body of the mandible is thereby positioned parallel to the x-ray beam.

An intravenous drip infusion containing approximately 40 g of iodine is started as soon as the patient is positioned. The study is begun when two-thirds of the infusion has been administered in order to obtain good arterial and venous visualization. The contrast enhancement will also help in identifying pathological lymph nodes. A double-dose technique can be of value, if the patient is well hydrated, in identifying a base-of-tongue carcinoma.[2] The examination is then begun halfway through the second contrast bottle.

Continous scans are obtained from the level of the hyoid bone to the hard palate at 5-mm intervals with 5-mm collimation. With the chin hyperextended most of the tongue base is covered without interference from dental fillings. The patient should be instructed not to swallow during the actual scanning sequence.

Coronal views can be of value in outlining certain lesions. Unless the patient either has no dental fillings or is edentulous, good quality scans can be difficult to obtain because of artifacts from dental fillings. With a tilting gantry some of these problems can be avoided.

NORMAL ANATOMY

Muscle Anatomy

The anatomy of the floor of the mouth and of the tongue has to be reviewed together in order to fully understand the topography of the base of the tongue. The floor of the mouth is comprised of three muscle groups. The supporting structure of the floor of the mouth is the V-shaped mylohyoid muscle, which takes its origin from the mylohyoid line on the inside of the mandible. It converges in the midline into a fibrous midline raphé and inserts posteriorly onto the body of the hyoid bone. The anterior bellies of the digastric muscle run in a characteristic parallel fashion underneath the mylohyoid muscles. After swinging around the intermediate tendon of the hyoid bone, these muscles run forward just off the midline to insert on the inferior border of the mandible (Fig. 4.1). Opposite these two muscle bundles and on the oral side of the mylohyoid muscles are the paired geniohyoid muscles. These last take their origin from the inferior genial tubercles behind the symphysis of the mandible and run in a slightly diverging fashion in the midline back to the body of the hyoid bone (Fig. 4.2).[4,5]

The tongue itself consists of both extrinsic and intrinsic musculature. The tongue is attached to the surrounding structures by the extrinsic musculature, which is responsible for the tongue's position. The extrinsic muscles consist of three paired muscle groups; the genioglossus, hyoglossus, and styloglossus muscles. The genioglossus muscles take their origin from the superior genial tubercle. They run just above the geniohyoid muscles before spreading out into the base of the tongue in a fanlike fashion (Figs. 4.2A, 4.3). The hyoglossus muscle runs lateral to the genioglossus muscle, rising like a palisade from the greater cornu of the hyoid bone. In its superior posterior aspect this muscle interdigitates with the styloglossus muscle as it comes down from the styloid process to insert along the lateral border of the tongue (Figs. 4.2A, 4.3).[4,5]

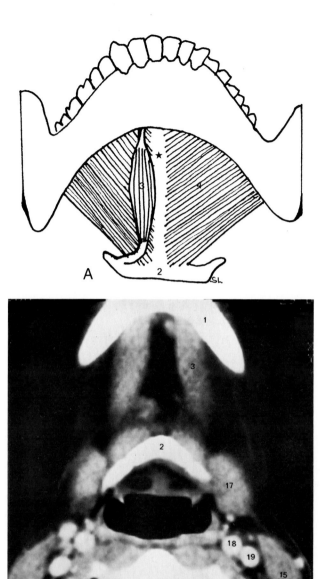

FIG. 4.1. Normal anatomy. (A) Schematic drawing of the floor of the mouth viewed from below. One digastric muscle has been removed. The mylohyoid muscles (4) can be seen converging down into the midline raphé (★), with the anterior belly of the digastric muscle (3) running just off the midline. (B) Axial scan through the level of the hyoid bone with contrast enhancement. The paired anterior bellies of the digastric muscles run parallel toward the mandible. Note the characteristic shape of the submandibular glands (17) lateral to the hyoid bone (2).

Key to Figures 4.1–4.3: 1, mandible; 2, hyoid bone; 3, anterior belly of the digastric muscle; 4, mylohyoid muscle; 5, geniohyoid muscle; 6, genioglossus muscle; 7, hyoglossus muscle; 8, styloglossus muscle; 9, inferior longitudinal muscle; 10, oblique and transverse intrinsic muscles; 11, superior longitudinal muscle; 12, fibrous lingual septum; 13, anterior tonsillar pillar; 14, posterior tonsillar pillar; 15, sternocleidomastoid muscle; 16, posterior belly of the digastric muscle; 17, submandibular gland; 18, internal carotid artery; 19, internal jugular vein; 20, lingual artery and vein; 21, arteria et vena profunda linguae; 22, sublingual artery and vein; 23, vena comitans nervi hypoglossi.

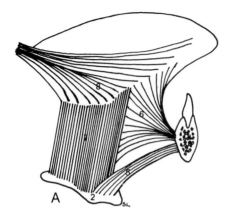

FIG. 4.2. Normal anatomy. (A) Schematic drawing of the extrinsic muscles of the tongue viewed from the side. The genio-hyoid muscle (5) running on the inside of the mylohyoid muscle is part of the floor of the mouth. The genioglossus muscle (6) is attached to the mandible, whereas the hyoglossus muscle (7) and the styloglossus muscle (8) are attached to the hyoid bone and the styloid process, respectively. (B) Axial scan through the low base of tongue with contrast enhancement. The genio-hyoid muscle (5) can be seen tapering off in a characteristic smooth fashion before inserting onto the mandible (1). The hyo-glossus muscle (7) is outlined by the lin-gual vasculature, with the vena comitans nervi hypoglossi (23) accompanying the hypoglossal nerve. (See Fig. 4.1 for abbre-viations.)

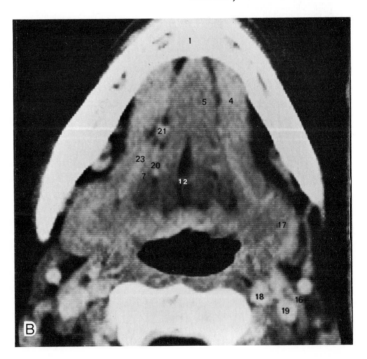

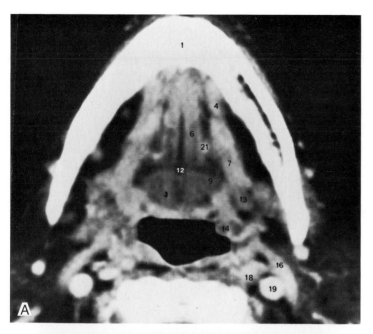

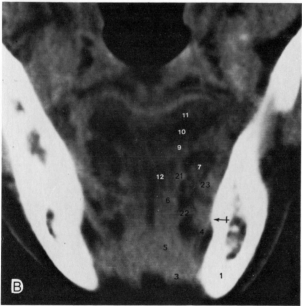

FIG. 4.3.   Normal anatomy. (A) Axial scan through the midbase of tongue with contrast
enhancement. The paired genioglossus muscle (6) can be seen separated by the fibrous
lingual septum (12) and fat. The inferior longitudinal muscle (9) can be seen having a
well-demarcated anterior border. (B) Coronal scan through the mid-tongue. The tongue
can be seen separated into two halves by the fibrous lingual septum (12). The mylohyoid
muscles (4) are shown to a great advantage as they come down from the mylohyoid
line on the mandible (⊢—+). (See Fig. 4.1 for abbreviations.)

The intrinsic muscles, which make up the body of the tongue, are responsible for shaping the tongue during the speech process. The intrinsic muscles consist of one superior longitudinal group and one inferior longitudinal group separated by the transverse and oblique muscles, which are woven together.

One has to remember that the base of the tongue, because of its embryological origin, is made up of two halves, which are fused together along the fibrous lingual septum. This septum can be seen dividing the intrinsic musculature into two halves and it also extends down in between the genioglossus muscles (Fig. 4.2B).[6] The superior longitudinal muscles are fused together along the lingual septum. They run like a broad sheet from the root of the tongue toward the tip, just beneath the mucosal layer. Underneath this muscle layer the transverse and oblique muscles are interwoven. They take their origin from the lingual septum, with the transverse muscles running out toward the lateral borders of the tongue. The inferior longitudinal muscles can often be seen as two distinct muscle bundles deep in the tongue running medial to the hyoglossus muscles (Fig. 4.3).[4,5]

Arteries and Veins

The blood supply of the tongue is mainly from the lingual artery, a branch of the external carotid artery. The lingual artery leaves the external carotid artery at the level of the hyoid bone and runs in the carotid triangle. The second part passes deep to the hyoglossus muscle where it gives off dorsal branches to the dorsum of the tongue. At the inferior border of the hyoglossus muscle it branches into the sublingual artery and arteria profunda linguae. The arteria profunda linguae first takes a vertical course up between the genioglossus and the inferior longitudinal muscle (Fig. 4.2B, 4.3B) and then branches out toward the tip of the tongue. Venous return is through the vena profunda linguae, also sometimes called the ranine vein. This is the vein one can see in the submucosal layer lateral to the frenulum on the undersurface of the tongue. This vein joins the sublingual vein and forms the vena comitans nervi hypoglossi as it runs lateral to the hyoglossus muscle, following the course of the hypoglossal nerve (Fig. 4.2B). The lingual artery itself also has an accompanying vein. Both these veins empty directly or indirectly into the internal jugular vein.[4-6]

Lymphatic Drainage

The lymphatic drainage of the base of the tongue is independent from that of the oral tongue. The collecting trunks from the deep central portion descend down in between the two genioglossus muscles. Some lymphatic trunks cross the median plane, thereby draining the contralateral side. The main trunks pass through the lateral pharyngeal wall below the palatine tonsil and empty into the jugulodigastric node.[4,5]

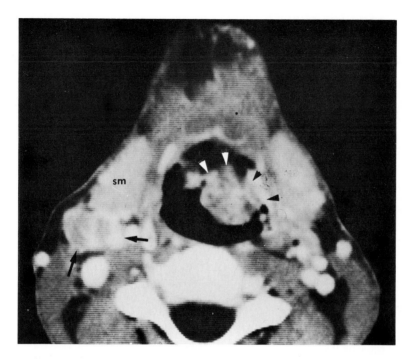

FIG. 4.4.   Lingual tonsil. Axial scan through the low base of tongue. Lobulated superficial mass made up of normal hyperplastic lymphoid tissue (▶) can be seen in this patient with a metastatic lymph node (⟶) behind the submandibular gland (sm).

The lingual tonsil is an aggregation of lymphoid tissue found in the submucosa of the base of the tongue. It can be responsible for nodular asymmetries of the tongue surface, because it bulges out into the vallecula.[7] Characteristically on CT the tonsils show a multilobulated border without any evidence of extension deep into the tongue (Fig. 4.4). Still, they should be evaluated with care, since they show the same amount of contrast enhancement as the surrounding mucosal layer and should not be mistaken for a carcinoma of the base of the tongue.[3]

CONGENITAL LESIONS

The congenital lesions of the base of the tongue are related to the development of the thyroid gland. The thyroid anlage descends from the region of the foramen cecum at the midline angle of the circumvallate papillae. In its descent it passes through the middle of the base of the tongue and continues in close relationship to the body of the hyoid bone.[8] This tract is obliterated under normal circumstances but otherwise can give rise to either cysts or aberrant thyroid tissue.[5]

Thyroglossal Duct Cyst

Thyroglossal duct cysts can be found in all age groups, but they are often discovered before the age of 10. The history is that of a gradually increasing mass in the midline that may fluctuate on palpation. Ultrasound examination usually reveals a cystic mass. If CT studies are done in the preoperative work-up, care should be taken to demonstrate the full length of the thyroglossal tract from the foramen cecum to the thyroid isthmus.[9] In particular, its relationship to the body of the hyoid bone should be delineated. This is because

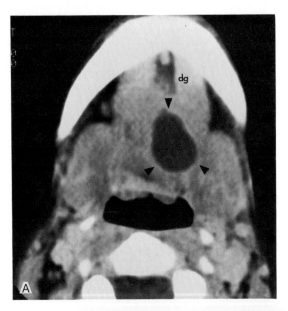

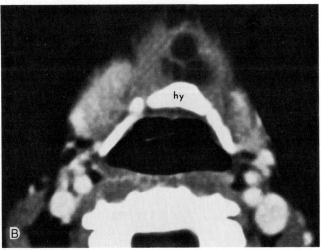

FIG. 4.5. Thyroglossal duct cyst. (A) Axial scan through the low base of tongue. A cystic mass (▶) can be seen in the midline separating the two anterior bellies of the digastric muscle (dg). (B) Same patient. Scan through the level of the hyoid bone. The septated cystic mass can here be seen in close relationship to the body of the hyoid bone (hy).

the treatment is surgery, with removal of all tissue along the tract including the body of the hyoid bone in order to avoid a recurrence of the cyst (Fig. 4.5).

Lingual Thyroid Gland

Aberrant thyroid tissue can also be found along the thyroglossal tract. This tract is commonly found in the base of the tongue above the hyoid bone. Because of the high iodine content in the thyroid tissue, it can readily be seen on CT (Fig. 4.6).[10] The thyroid tissue is characteristically seen as a round, well-demarcated ball of high density, close to the midline and either deep or more superficial, causing a bulge of the dorsal surface of the base of the tongue. Removal of a lingual thyroid is recommended because of an increased risk of thyroid malignancy.[11] The work-up should include a nuclear medicine study to demonstrate all thyroid tissues with normal function. This is needed because the lingual thyroid may be the only functioning thyroid in such a patient.

MACROGLOSSIA

Macroglossia, or generalized enlargement of the whole tongue, can be seen in a variety of conditions. A few congenital syndromes are associated with macroglossia, for example, mucopolysaccharidosis (e.g., Hurler's syndrome), glycogen storage disease (e.g., Pompe's disease), Beckwith-Wiedemann syndrome, and Robinow syndrome.[12] The normal sized tongue should not be mistaken for macroglossia in patients with syndromes associated with micrognathia or facial hypoplasia.

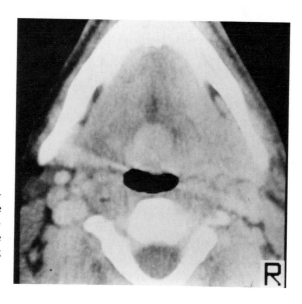

FIG. 4.6. Lingual thyroid. Axial scan through the mid-base of the tongue. A round iodine-containing ball of tissue can be seen in the tongue base causing slight bulging of the tongue surface.

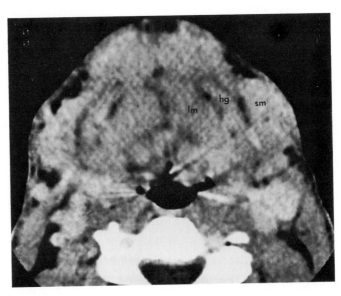

FIG. 4.7. Macroglossia. Semi-axial scan through the mid-base of tongue. The tongue shows generalized enlargement of the tongue musculature including the hyoglossus (hg) and the inferior longitudinal muscle (lm). The enlarged tongue is causing some encroachment on the airway as well as outward displacement of the submandibular glands (sm).

Macroglossia can also be seen in endocrine disturbances such as juvenile hypothyroidism (cretinism) and acromegaly. A metabolic disturbance such as amyloidosis (especially the primary form) may also affect the tongue and cause macroglossia.

Benign tumors such as lymphangiomas may also cause macroglossia when the involvement is extensive. The enlargement is then composed of lymphatic vessels and blood vessels that infiltrate diffusely into the tongue musculature.[13] They are most commonly found at an early age and can sometimes be associated with a cystic hygroma.[11]

Computed tomography is not needed to diagnose macroglossia, since that usually is evident by clinical exam. CT is, on the other hand, sometimes used in the clinical work-up of craniofacial anomalies. Observing an enlarged tongue during such an exam can help with the differential diagnosis. Macroglossia in an adult causes the submandibular glands to become both palpable and visible despite their normal size, because the enlarged tongue causes displacement of surrounding structures (Fig. 4.7).

LINGUAL ABSCESS

One case of a lingual abscess monitored by CT has recently been reported.[14] The history given was that of dysphagia, low-grade fever, and a painful swollen tongue. The CT scan revealed a low density midline lesion with a staining rim after contrast enhancement. With the location described, one has to remember that a thyroglossal duct cyst can also become infected and first manifest itself as a lingual mass under such circumstances.

CARCINOMA OF THE BASE OF THE TONGUE

Squamous cell carcinomas account for approximately 95 percent of the malignant lesions of the base of the tongue. Adenocarcinoma accounts for approximately 1–2 percent and lymphoma another 1 percent.[15] The rest consist of minor salivary gland malignancies, plasmacytomas, and other rare tumors.

Carcinomas arising from the base of the tongue are usually less well differentiated as a group than those arising from the oral tongue. Since the base of the tongue is difficult to assess clinically, these tumors also tend to go undetected longer than those of the oral portion. Therefore, 40 percent of base-of-tongue cancers have reached a size of more than 4 cm in diameter when they are detected;[16] in addition, 70 to 75 percent of these cancers have metastasized to lymph nodes by the time the diagnosis is made.[16,17]

Treatment of base-of-tongue cancers varies from center to center, but irradiation is the more commonly prescribed treatment since it produces less disability than surgery. If surgical removal of a base of tongue tumor is to be attempted, local excision or at the most hemiglossectomy is the procedure of choice. Total glossectomy is a disabling procedure with a high postoperative mortality rate because of complications leading up to terminal chest infections.[18] If hemiglossectomy is chosen as the mode of treatment, the surgeon has to assess, and make sure, that one hypoglossal nerve and one lingual artery can be preserved. The superior laryngeal nerve also has to be preserved to avoid postoperative aspiration problems.[18] The margins have to be at least 1 cm for a satisfactory removal of the tumor.

To evaluate the local extent of tumors of the base of the tongue, it was previously necessary to rely on physical examination by inspection and palpation. Sometimes general anesthesia had to be utilized together with multiple blind biopsies to map the local extension of the tumor. With CT we now have a tool to evaluate the base of the tongue. The tomograms can help guide the referring physician in evaluating these tumors.

Between the years 1980 and 1983 a total of 13 patients with base-of-tongue carcinomas were seen at our institution. All these patients had CT as a part of their pretreatment work-up. Well-known predisposing factors like alcoholism and heavy smoking were also present in the majority of our cases. The location and extension of the primary tumor is summarized in Table 4.1. Like carcinoma of the oral tongue, most base-of-tongue carcinomas are found along the lateral borders. Therefore, the muscles most commonly involved besides the intrinsic musculature are those of the hyoglossus–styloglossus complex. As the tumor continues to infiltrate, it will also involve the genioglossus muscle. It is well known that base-of-tongue carcinomas cross the midline early. This is probably true with regard to the more superficial mucosal portions of the tumor. Superficial spread across the midline could be demonstrated in one

TABLE 4.1 Local extension of the primary tumor in 13 patients with base of tongue carcinoma

Location	Number patients with involvement
Anterior belly of the digastric muscle	2
Mylohyoid muscle	4
Geniohyoid muscle	4
Genioglossus muscle	5
Hyoglossus muscle	10
Intrinsic musculature	11
Fibrous lingual septum	
Displaced	12
Infiltrated	1
Anterior tonsillar pillar	8
Posterior tonsillar pillar	4
Vallecula/pre-epiglottic space	3

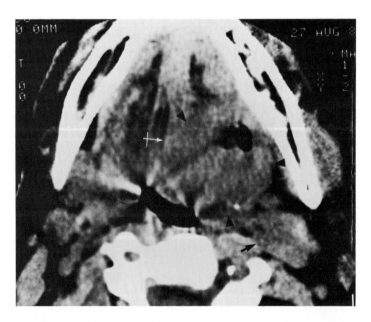

FIG. 4.8. Carcinoma of the base of the tongue. Axial scan through the mid-base of the tongue. A large tumor (▶) with an ulceration is invading the base of the tongue as well as the tonsillar fossa. The tumor can be seen coming up to the fibrous lingual septum (+—→), which is displaced. Metastatic lymph nodes (—→) have merged with the carotid sheath.

patient in our series. It seems that the deeper portion of the fibrous lingual septum forms a barrier to direct tumor extension. In the same series only one patient, where the tumor started in the midline, low in the tongue base, had involvement of the fibrous lingual septum. Instead, displacement of the fibrous lingual septum was seen in a majority of cases even if the tumor had reached considerable size (Fig. 4.8). When the tumors infiltrate, they do so by growing down into the loose areolar tissue of the tongue base. On CT this can be shown as tumor replacement of the relative low density ball of tissue made up of the intrinsic musculature, particularly the oblique and transverse muscles.[1] After infusion of contrast the tumor will enhance and therefore stand out even more. As the tumor infiltrates, the extrinsic muscles show enlargement as well as contrast enhancement (Fig. 4.9).

Computed tomography readily shows enlarged or abnormal lymph nodes.[19,20] Regional lymph nodes should therefore also be evaluated when studying the base of the tongue. Ten to twenty percent of patients with base-of-tongue carcinomas have clinically negative lymph nodes that show histological metastatic disease.[21] CT can correctly demonstrate metastatic lymph nodes if they have reached a size of more than 1 cm in diameter. One should remember that contralateral spread of metastatic disease occurs early. In 3 of our 13 patients clinically occult contralateral metastases were only detected by CT. This actually changed the nodal staging of these patients.

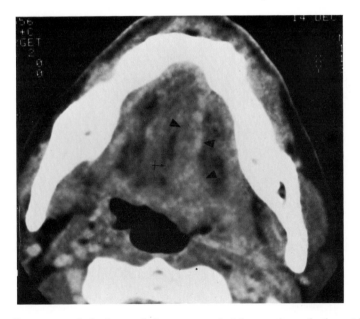

FIG. 4.9. Carcinoma of the base of the tongue. Axial scan through the mid-base of the tongue. An infiltrating tumor showing contrast enhancement (▶) is invading the genioglossus muscle, which is thickened. The fibrous lingual septum (+—→) is slightly displaced.

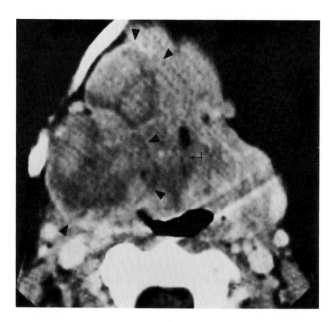

FIG. 4.10. Neurofibromatosis. Axial scan through the low base of the tongue. Two large rounded neurofibromas with nonhomogeneous contrast enhancement (▶) can be seen causing displacement of the fibrous lingual septum (←—+).

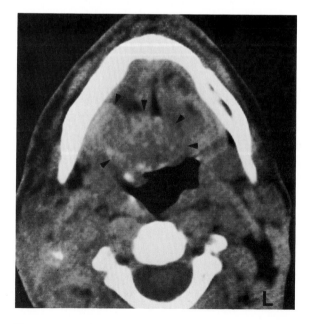

FIG. 4.11. Thyroid cancer metastatic to the base of the tongue. A large mass is invading the base of the tongue and crossing the midline (▶). Nodal metastases can also be seen obliterating the fascial planes of the right neck. Note the scattered calcifications throughout both masses.

Computed tomography has also come into use in the search for the 'unknown' head and neck primary in patients that present with metastatic neck nodes.[22] The base of the tongue, together with the nasopharynx and pyriform sinus, is one of the more common origins for such a tumor. Such a study should therefore include these three areas. Depending on the result a more directed biopsy can be performed instead of triple endoscopies and blind biopsies.

Biopsy of any head and neck lesion causes varying amounts of tissue edema with resulting mass effect and dissolution of the fascial planes. Therefore, CT should be performed before such biopsy.[2] This is also valid for the base of the tongue. If biopsies have been performed, there should be a delay of at least 7 to 10 days before CT is attempted. Otherwise the tumor size can be overestimated since the tumor cannot be separated from the coexisting tissue edema.

MISCELLANEOUS TUMORS

The base of the tongue harbors both mucous and accessory salivary glands. Tumors originating in these structures—both of the benign and the malignant variety—can therefore also be encountered. Tumors originating from other soft tissue components of the base of the tongue—for example, neurofibromas, rhabdomyosarcomas, and other sarcomatous tumors—may also occur (Fig. 4.10). Metastatic disease, although rare, can also spread to the base of the tongue (Fig. 4.11).

REFERENCES

1. Larsson SG, Mancuso A, Hanafee W: Computed tomography of the tongue and floor of the mouth. Radiology 143:493, 1982.
2. Schaefer SD, Merken M, Diehl J, et al.: Computed tomographic assessment of squamous cell carcinoma of oral and pharyngeal cavities. Arch Otolaryngol 108:688, 1982.
3. Muraki AS, Mancuso AA, Harnsberger HR, et al.: CT of the oropharynx, tongue base and floor of the mouth: normal anatomy and range of variations, and applications in staging carcinoma. Radiology 148:725, 1983.
4. Gardner E, Gray DJ, O'Rahilly R: Anatomy. A Regional Study of Human Structure. WB Saunders, Philadelphia, 1960.
5. Hollinshead WH: The head and neck. p. 414. In Anatomy for Surgeons. Vol. 1. Harper & Row, Hagerstown, Maryland, 1982.
6. Last RJ: Anatomy, Regional and Applied. 6th Ed. Churchill Livingstone, New York, 1978.
7. Gromet M, Homer MJ, Carter BL: Lymphoid hyperplasia at the base of the tongue. Spectrum of a benign entity. Radiology 144:825, 1982.
8. Ellis PDM, van Nostrand AWP: The applied anatomy of thyroglossal tract remnants. Laryngoscope 87:765, 1977.
9. Rabinov K, Van Orman P, Gray E: Radiologic findings in persistent thyroglossal tract fistulas. Radiology 130:135, 1979.
10. Machida K, Yoshikawa K: Aberrant thyroid gland demonstrated by computed tomography. Case report. J Comput Assist Tomogr 3:689, 1979.
11. Batsakis JG: Tumors of the Head and Neck. Clinical and Pathological Considerations. Williams & Wilkins, Baltimore, 1979.

12. Taybi H: Radiology of Syndromes and Metabolic Disorders. Year Book Medical Publishers, Chicago, 1983.

13. Giunta J, Suklar G, McCarty PL: Diffuse angiomatosis of the tongue. Arch Otolaryngol 93:83, 1971.

14. Eames FA, Peters JC: CT findings in lingual abscess. J Comput Assist Tomogr 7:344, 1983.

15. Frazell EL, Lucas JC: Cancer of the tongue. Report of the management of 1,554 patients. Cancer 15:1085, 1962.

16. Spiro RH, Strong EW: Surgical treatment of cancer of the tongue. Surg Clin North Am 54:759, 1974.

17. Leipzig B, Hokanson JA: Treatment of cervical lymph nodes in carcinoma of the tongue. Head Neck Surg 5:3, 1982.

18. Lam KH, Wong J, Lim STK, Ong GB: Carcinoma of the tongue: factors affecting the results of surgical treatment. Br J Surg 67:101, 1980.

19. Mancuso AA, Maceri D, Rice D, Hanafee W: CT of cervical lymph node cancer. AJR 136:381, 1981.

20. Silver AJ, Mawad ME, Hilal SK, et al.: Computed tomography of the cervical lymph nodes: use of intravenous contrast enhancement. AJNR 4:861, 1983.

21. Wang CC: Radiation Therapy for Head and Neck Neoplasms. Indications, Techniques and Results. John Wright–PSG Inc, Bristol, 1983.

22. Mancuso AA, Hanafee WN: Elusive head and neck carcinomas beneath intact mucosa. Laryngoscope 93:133, 1983.

5 Paranasal Sinuses and Pterygopalatine Fossa

PETER SOM

Over the past few years CT scanning has been instrumental in creating a new interest in the field of head and neck radiology. This reflects the greater imaging ability that the radiologist now has, as well as a recent awareness of the afflictions that affect this region of the body and of how influential the information attainable on imaging can be to the planning of treatment and the care of these patients.

Of the various types of pathology that can occur in this area probably the most familiar to radiologists and clinicians are the diseases affecting the paranasal sinuses and nasal cavity. Such familiarity is primarily due to the inflammatory conditions, especially the viral diseases (common cold); however, many of the malignant neoplasms are also well known. Although they represent less than 1 percent of all malignancies, their tendency to cause extensive local destruction without any significant symptomatology has given them a deservedly frightening reputation.

It is precisely the paucity of symptoms associated with many conditions affecting the nasal cavity and paranasal sinuses that makes the radiology of this area so important. Since the clinician can visualize only small portions of the nasal cavity, the radiologist plays a vital role in mapping out the extent of disease. This, in turn, provides essential information that will help to determine the operability of the patient and the surgical procedure to be used, or will allow an accurate follow-up of the response to radiation and chemotherapy.

To be able to detect early pathological changes the radiologist must have a familiarity with the normal anatomy. To this end, this chapter will suggest a protocol for the CT examination of the region and review the normal CT anatomy. An approach to analyzing inflammatory and malignant diseases will be presented, as will some criteria for when to suggest to the clinician that a CT scan be obtained. Lastly, a CT analysis of the postoperative patient will be given.

SCANNING PROTOCOL

One of the most important concepts in CT scanning is that all the margins of a pathological region must be visualized on the study. Usually this means the cranial and caudal edges, since the majority of patients are first scanned in the axial projection. To routinely include the vast majority of the pathological processes that can involve the nasal cavity and paranasal sinuses, a protocol consisting of contiguous 5-mm scans from the maxillary alveolus to the top of the frontal sinuses should be used. These can easily be set up by marking the scan plane and limits on a lateral scout image (Fig. 5.1).[1]

When these images are reviewed, with the patient still on the scanner, attention must be directed to determine if any margin of the pathology is still not entirely included in the study (the first and last scans of the series). If it is not, further contiguous scans in either or both directions must be taken.

The recommended scanning angle for performing these axial scans is parallel to the inferior-orbito-meatal (IOM) plane. These IOM scans cause minimal distortion of the paranasal sinus anatomy and in addition are the suggested views for the axial orbital studies and the best visualization of the optic nerve.[2,3]

Coronal Scans

Most cases require only axial scans; however, because of the thickness of each scan slice, the possibility exists that an averaging error will occur in the region of any bone oriented parallel to the CT scan plane. That is, small focal bone erosions or minimal soft tissue disease immediately above or below the bone may be indiscernable. Because of this, if it is suspected that disease has spread across the hard palate, the floor, or roof of the orbit, the nasal cavity, or the ethmoid or sphenoid sinuses (all of which are approximately parallel to the axial plane), a coronal scan must be obtained.[1]

This is a very important concept to remember, especially in tumor cases where the spread of an antral lesion into the orbit may mean an orbital exenteration and where tumor spread intracranially means either an extensive combined neurosurgical–ENT procedure or inoperability.

In many patients it is impossible to obtain 90° (to the IOM plane) coronal scans because of two factors. First, the patient may be unable to extend the neck sufficiently so that the combination of head tilt and gantry angle will not give a 90° coronal plane. Secondly, metallic dental fillings that lie directly below the paranasal sinuses will degrade the CT images taken through them. The usual compromise angle (60–80 percent) is a "modified coronal" scan.[4] The exact plane can best be judged by obtaining a supine or prone extended neck lateral scout image and then choosing a scan plane that runs from the most anterior metallic filling on its caudal margin to the most posterior sinus region to be investigated on its cranial margin (Fig. 5.2).

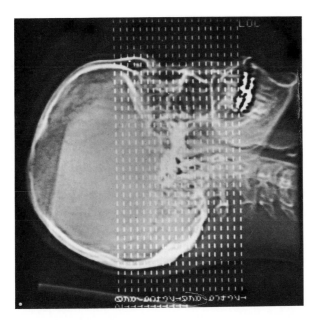

FIG. 5.1. Lateral scout film showing paranasal sinus protocol contiguous scans from maxillary alveolus to top of frontal sinuses.

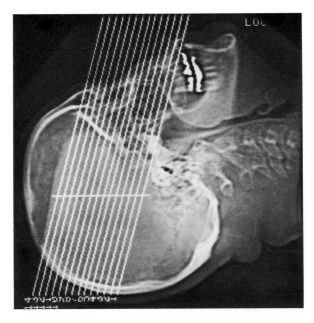

FIG. 5.2. Lateral supine extended head scout film showing recommended modified coronal study angle of the paranasal sinuses in this patient with numerous metallic dental fillings.

Contrast

Differentiating between a tumor mass and adjacent inflammatory or normal tissue is of the utmost importance in planning treatment. By utilizing any differential contrast enhancement characteristics, a distinction between adjacent, otherwise indistinguishable soft tissues may be possible.[1,5] Because of this, intravenous contrast material should ideally be used in all cases; the only exception being patients with histories of allergy to the contrast agents. Usually enhancement correlates with vascularity so that the greater the enhancement, the more vascular the lesion. A good way to easily assess abnormal enhancement is to compare the lesion with muscle tissue. If the muscle is "denser" than or as "dense" as the lesion, the pathological process should be considered to have no significant enhancement.

Window Settings

The last major point to remember is that in the paranasal sinuses and nasal cavity, the radiologist is equally concerned with both soft tissue and bone disease. If the CT scans are photographed only at wide window settings (1000 or greater), bone pathology will be best revealed and the air–soft tissue contours of any masses will be optimally seen. However, any differential contrast enhancement will be obscured (burned out). On the other hand, if the scans are photographed only at soft tissue windows (150–350), differential contrast enhancement will be easily seen, but focal bone erosions and the presence and true size and contour of soft tissue disease can be obscured (whited out). Because of this, all paranasal sinus CT scans should be reviewed at both "bone" and "soft tissue" window settings.

These are basic and important concepts and only by careful attention to them will errors in interpretation of paranasal sinus CT scans be minimized and the most diagnostic information be gained.

NORMAL ANATOMY

The normal mucosa in any of the paranasal sinuses is so thin that it is not imaged on CT. Instead, the air appears to abut directly on the bony sinus walls. Thus, any soft tissue that is seen lining the sinus walls (separating the air from the bone) is abnormal. It may be inflamed, infiltrated with tumor, or simply scarred and fibrosed.[1,5] As will be discussed below, further differentiation between these various entities is often possible by evaluating the surface configuration and the enhancing characteristics of the soft tissues.

Frontal Sinus

The frontal sinuses for all practical purposes are not present at birth. They develop progressively from anterior ethmoid cells so that in the average child the cephalad margin of the sinus is at the level of the superior orbital rim by the age of 8 years. Usually by age 10 years, the frontal sinuses are well up into the vertical plate of the frontal bone.[6] However, if the sinuses do not develop at this rate, or if they remain hypoplastic, there is no reason to invoke a pathological explanation. Asymmetrical development of the left and right frontal sinuses appears to be the rule and various degrees of hypoplasia are common. Even bilateral aplasia is considered to be a variant present in about 4 percent of people. Although bilateral aplasia has been associated with mucoviscidosis, the exact causal relationship is unclear and in general, sinus size appears to have no direct pathological implication.[1,7]

On CT scans, the sinuses must be viewed at high window settings. If not, differentiation between a hypoplastic sinus and an opacified, well-developed sinus will be impossible (Fig. 5.3). The latter may be a critical finding in acute frontal sinusitis, because the possibility exists for intracranial spread of the infection via the rich emissary veins that are present in the posterior frontal sinus wall.[8]

The integrity of the anterior and especially the posterior sinus walls is easily and best evaluated in the axial projection. The soft tissues of the forehead region should also be examined paying special attention to preservation of the subcutaneous fat planes.

The frontal sinuses can also pneumatize the horizontal or orbital plates of the frontal bones. This is not an unusual finding and once recognized should not create a diagnostic problem for the CT interpreter. Pneumatization is best

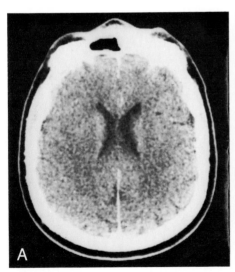
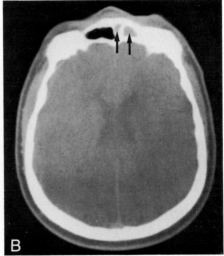

FIG. 5.3.   (A) Axial CT through the level of the frontal sinuses reveals a well aerated right frontal sinus and an apparent hypoplastic left frontal sinus. (B) Same CT scan as in (A) except viewed at wide window setting. The "hypoplastic" left frontal sinus is seen to actually be an opacified (infected) sinus (arrows).

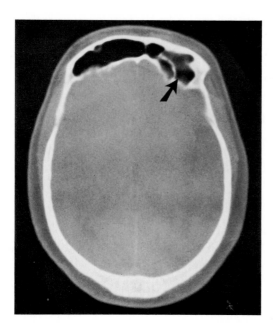

FIG. 5.4. Axial CT scan through the lower frontal sinuses reveals pneumatization of the orbital roof on the left side (arrow).

appreciated in the axial view, where the sinus contour can be easily traced into the orbital plate (Fig. 5.4). Often, because of averaging artifact, this horizontal plate recess appears to extend directly into the orbit. This misinterpretation can be avoided by taking coronal scans through the region.[1]

Supraorbital Ethmoid Sinuses

Anterior ethmoid cells can extend up independently to pneumatize the orbital plates of the frontal bone. This is best appreciated on coronal CT scans, where the sinus air cells can be seen arching upward into the medial orbital roof (Fig. 5.5). The distinction between frontal sinus and supraorbital ethmoid pneumatization of the orbital roof is of more than academic interest. This is because the surgical approach to this area differs greatly depending on which sinus is involved. This problem is usually related to inflammatory disease and in these cases both axial and coronal scans are necessary to resolve the problem with certainty.

Ethmoid Sinuses

These are the only sinuses fully developed at birth. The ethmoid complex usually has 15 to 18 cells on each side, with the posterior cells larger than the anterior ones. The overall ethmoid configuration is wedge-shaped, with the anterior portion narrower than the posterior.[9] This is easily seen in the

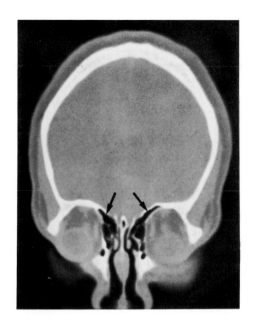

FIG. 5.5. Coronal CT scan reveals extension of the ethmoid sinuses (supraorbital cells) (arrows) up into the orbital roof.

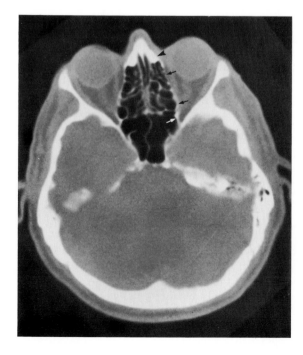

FIG. 5.6. Axial CT scan reveals the lacrimal bone (arrowhead), the lamina papyracea (black arrows), and the sphenoid sinus contribution (white arrow) to the medial orbital wall. The ethmoid complex is narrower anteriorly.

axial view. The lamina papyracea or ethmoid plate should be identified. This is the thin bone forming the lateral wall of the ethmoid, separating the ethmoid cells from the orbit. The medial wall of the orbit is formed by three bones. The lacrimal bone forms approximately the most anterior fifth and directly behind this the ethmoid lamina papyracea forms almost the entire remaining medial wall except for a few millimeters at the most posterior margin, which is formed by the sphenoid sinus (Fig. 5.6). This is an important few millimeters, however, because it means that anatomically the sphenoid sinus is related to the orbital apex and can thus be related to orbital apex pathology.[10]

The two ethmoid sinuses are separated by the nasal cavity. In the most cephalad portion, the nasal cavity narrows into two slit-like recesses, the olfactory recesses, which extend up to the roof of the nasal cavity, the cribriform plate. These recesses are separated by the midline nasal septum, which extends up to the nasal cavity roof (Fig. 5.7). Resting directly on the cribriform plate is the crista galli, which is an intracranial structure. The middle turbinates attach to either side of the nasal roof. Thus the crista galli, nasal septum, and middle turbinates all localize the thin (often difficult to image) cribriform plate.

On the upper ethmoid axial scans, the soft tissues of the midline base of the anterior cranial fossa can simulate a nasal cavity mass. Visualization of the crista galli, however, indicates the true intracranial location of the scan (Fig. 5.8). If there is any question of disease spread across the nasal cavity–ethmoid roof, a coronal scan should be obtained (Fig. 5.9).[1]

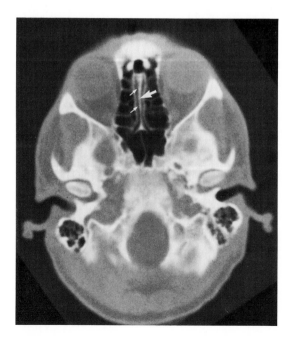

FIG. 5.7. Axial CT scan reveals the olfactory recesses (small white arrows on right recess) separated by the nasal septum (large arrow).

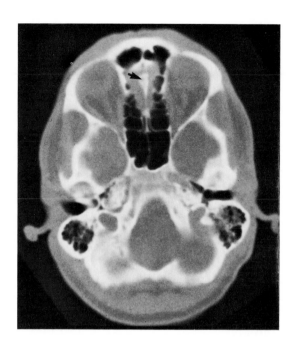

FIG. 5.8. Axial CT scan just above the level of the cribriform plate reveals the crista galli (arrow) and the surrounding soft tissues of the midline anterior cranial fossa.

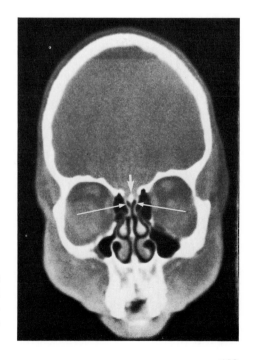

FIG. 5.9. Coronal CT scan reveals the crista galli (small arrow) resting on and the middle turbinates (long arrows) attaching to either side of the cribriform plate.

MAXILLARY SINUSES

These sinuses are statistically the most often involved by infection, trauma, and tumor. Although they are present at birth, they are very small. In the average child, the sinuses enlarge to pneumatize the maxilla laterally and reach to the level of the infraorbital canal by age 2 years, and extend laterally to these canals by age 4 to 5 years. The sinuses, or antra, pneumatize part of the body of the zygomatic bones by 9 years of age.[11] The relatively flat medial and anterior walls can be easily seen on axial scans (Fig. 5.10). The sigmoid, or "S" shaped, posterolateral wall should be carefully observed. Directly behind it is a thin layer of fat, which forms the anterior border of the infratemporal fossa. This is an important region, because disease spread from the sinus into this fossa (obliterating this fat plane) portends a graver prognosis. The most caudal portion of the maxillary sinus is the alveolar recess. In approximately 66 percent of people, this recess extends inferior to the plane of the hard palate.[11] The roots of the three molar teeth almost always project up into the sinus base. Slightly less often, the roots of the two premolar and the canine teeth also project into the sinus. It is because of this anatomic relationship that about 10 percent of antral disease is related to the teeth.[12] Similarly, many people are aware of sinusitis presenting clinically as pain in the upper teeth.

The roof of the antrum is the orbital floor. This surface is angled cephalad so that its highest point is in the posteromedial aspect of the orbit. Directly under this point the air in the upper recess of the underlying maxillary sinus can be seen as a round- to ovoid shaped lucency on axial CT scans. This

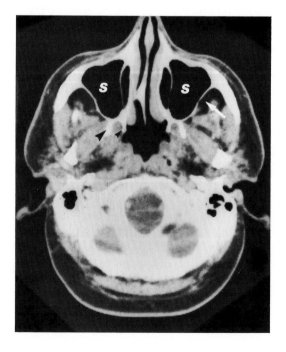

FIG. 5.10. Axial CT scan reveals normal maxillary sinuses (S) with air abutting directly upon the bone. The infratemporal fossa fat (arrow) is well visualized, as are the medial (small arrowhead) and lateral (large arrowhead) pterygoid plates.

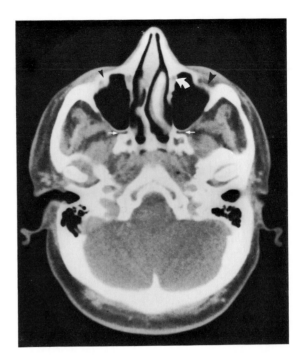

FIG. 5.11. Axial CT scan reveals the bone forming the lowest portion of the orbital floor (small arrowhead) and an apparent erosion of the anterior antral wall that actually is the most inferior periorbital soft tissue (large arrowhead). The pterygopalatine fossae are well visualized (small arrows). Curved arrow points to the nasolacrimal duct.

area should be clearly noted as representing the uppermost antrum and not an ethmoid cell or an area of destruction. The flattest, or most horizontal, portion of the orbital floor is the anterolateral margin and the bone forming this region can often be seen merging with the anterior antral wall on axial scans simulating bony pathology (Fig. 5.11).

If there is any question concerning erosion of the orbital floor, a coronal scan should be obtained. The infraorbital canal usually can be identified in the antral roof and anteriorly the nasolacrimal duct can be followed from its medial orbital margin down to the inferior meatus of the nasal cavity (Fig. 5.11).

Because the inferior orbital rim is concave upward, axial scans just above the lowest point of the rim can simulate the appearance of focal bone erosion of the anterior antral wall (Fig. 5.11). Viewing the normal antral bone on the immediately adjacent caudal scan should clarify this situation.

Directly behind the medial–posterior recess of the maxillary sinus are the pterygoid plates. These appear on axial scans as upside-down "V" shaped bones (Fig. 5.10). The medial plate forms the anterior border of the nasopharynx and the internal and external pterygoid muscles can be clearly identified extending from the pterygoid plates laterally to the inner surface of the mandibular ramus and condyle, respectively. Along the lower (caudal) one half to two thirds of the line of contact between the back of the maxilla and the front of the pterygoid plates, these bones appear fused together on the scans. However, in the upper (cephalad) one half to one third of this region, a clearly definable space between the pterygoids and the back of the maxilla is seen. This space is largest just under the base of the skull (the greater wing of the sphenoid bone) and is called the pterygopalatine fossa (Fig. 5.11). It has great clinical importance because it communicates with five different areas in the head: the mouth via the pterygopalatine canal, the nose via the sphenopalatine canal, the orbit via the inferior orbital fissure, the infratemporal fossa via the pterygomaxillary fissure (retromaxillary fissure), and intracranially via the pterygoid (vidian) canal and the foramen rotundum. All these canals are traversed by nerves and vessels, and once disease has invaded the pterygopalatine fossa, spread to any or all of the regions is probable.[13]

THE SPHENOID SINUS

This sinus is very small at birth and progressively develops to pneumatize the sphenoid bone. In almost all cases, the adult sinus extends posteriorly to lie under the anterior wall of the sella turcica. This is an important relationship to note if a transsphenoidal hypophysectomy is contemplated. In the rare case that the sinus does not extend back to the anterior sella wall, such surgery cannot be performed.[6,14,15]

About half the population has only a main sphenoid sinus cavity, which is usually asymmetrically divided by the intersinus septum.[16] This septum is in the midline anteriorly but can deviate far to one side or the other, creating two unequally sized sphenoid sinus cavities. This asymmetry, however, is never so great that a well-developed sinus will be seen on one side with no sinus present on the other side. When this appearance is encountered, usually the "aplastic sinus" is present but opacified and the only way to diagnose such a situation is to view the CT scan at bone window settings (Fig. 5.12).[1]

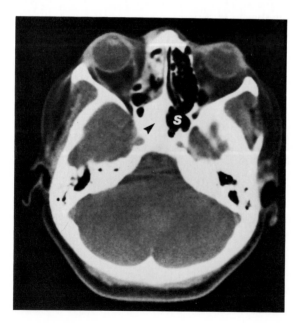

FIG. 5.12. Axial CT scan reveals an apparent solitary left sphenoid sinus cavity (S). Scan of the "aplastic" right sinus viewed at wide window settings (arrowhead) revealed the presence of an osteoma that completely filled a fully developed right sinus.

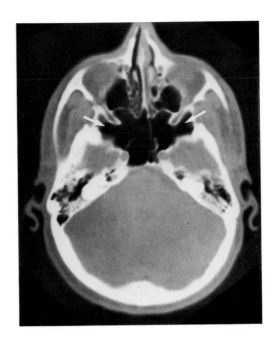

FIG. 5.13. Axial CT scan reveals sphenoid sinus lateral pneumatization of the floor of the middle cranial fossa (arrows) in the greater sphenoid wings.

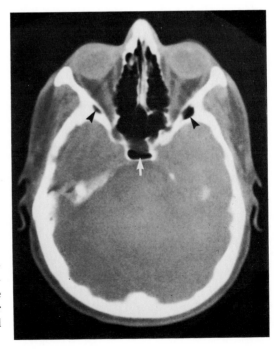

FIG. 5.14. Axial CT scan just caudal to that in Fig. 5.13 reveals sphenoid sinus pneumatization of the posterior orbital walls (greater sphenoid wing) (arrowheads) and the dorsum sellae (arrow).

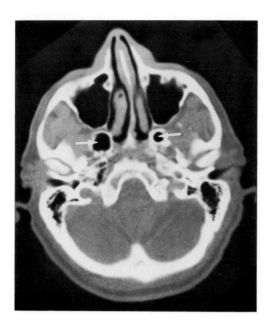

FIG. 5.15. Axial CT scan reveals pneumatization of the pterygoid plates (arrows).

In about half the population, lateral recesses develop from the main sphenoid sinuses. They can extend asymmetrically out into the floor of the middle cranial fossa and up into the posterior orbital wall (greater sphenoid wing) (Figs. 5.13, 5.14), up into the anterior clinoid process region (lesser sphenoid wing) or down into the pterygoid plates (Fig. 5.15). Familiarity with the CT appearance of these recesses will avoid mistakenly referring to them as areas of erosion.

INFECTION AND ALLERGY

Viral infections of the nasal cavity are probably the most common inflammatory diseases of this region. Although the turbinates may become edematous, the sinuses are rarely involved and these patients usually improve clinically before a CT scan is warranted.

Bacterial sinusitis most probably occurs on a sinus-by-sinus basis after either a transient or a more permanent obstruction of the sinus ostium has occurred. The mucosa becomes infiltrated and swollen and can be identified on CT as separating the sinus air from the bony sinus wall (Fig. 5.16). In more extreme cases, the mucosa can become heaped on itself, creating a polypoid appearance. In active infection, mucosal enhancement is seen.[1]

Mucosal thickening of similar CT appearance can be seen with fibrosis and scarring following either chronic infection or previous radiation therapy. This type of mucosal pathology usually does not enhance on contrast CT studies.

The sinus cavity may also fill with mucoid secretions that can either create an air–fluid level or total sinus opacification (Fig. 5.17). The density of these

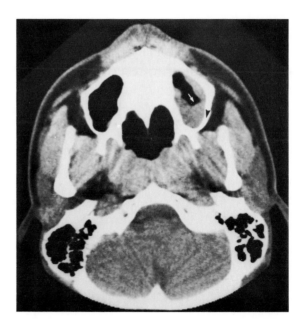

FIG. 5.16. Axial CT scan reveals thickened mucosa separating the sinus air (arrow) from the sinus wall (arrowhead).

secretions is lower than muscle but greater than fat (about 15–20 HU) and only very rarely is seen to enhance.

The sinus distribution of bacterial disease is usually asymmetrical. That is, one maxillary sinus alone or several unilateral sinuses may be involved with minimal disease affecting the opposite sinuses.[7] Occasionally, a pansinusitis

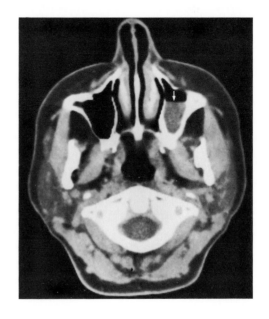

FIG. 5.17. Axial CT scan reveals an air–fluid level in the left maxillary sinus (arrow). Note the thickened left antral wall on the left side (compared with the normal right side). This suggests the presence of chronic infection.

can occur and in these cases of symmetrical sinus disease, distinguishing allergic sinusitis is impossible.

Allergic disease tends to involve the paranasal sinuses uniformly and symmetrically. There often is associated nasal polyposis, the presence of which may be a helpful sign to suggest the underlying allergic etiology (Fig. 5.18).[7] This has clinical importance only in that allergy can be a forgotten cause of sinusitis and treatment directed at this underlying cause can on occasion be initiated at the suggestion of the radiologist.

Air–fluid levels are rarely seen in allergic disease and the most common cause of such air–fluid levels is acute bacterial sinusitis.[1,7] Although these levels are apparent in less than half the patients with acute infections, there are so many of these patients that bacterial sinusitis represents the most common cause of such fluid levels. The second most common cause is antral lavage, the therapeutic washing of the antrum with a warm saline solution as a treatment for acute infection. It takes 3 to 4 days for this saline to drain out of the sinus. If a CT examination is performed prior to this time, the saline fluid level will be imaged, and differentiation from recurrent acute inflammatory secretions is impossible. The clinician should be asked to wait at least 4 days after antral washing before ordering a follow-up study.

Other causes of air–fluid levels include hemorrhage with or without a sinus wall fracture, barotrauma,[17] and blood dyscrasias such as Von Willebrand's disease.

The mucus retention cyst results from obstruction of a mucus-secreting gland in the sinus mucosa. These cysts are found in 10 percent of the population and cannot be distinguished from a sinus polyp on CT (Fig. 5.19).[18] They

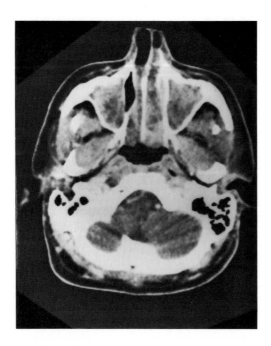

FIG. 5.18. Axial CT scan reveals that both maxillary sinuses are totally opacified. Polypoid swelling of the nasal turbinates is also present.

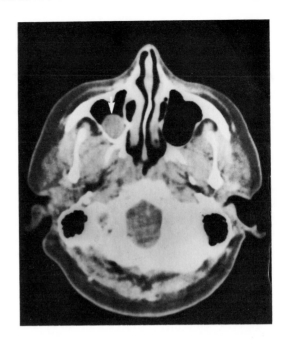

FIG. 5.19. Axial CT scan reveals a typical smooth, convex right maxillary retention cyst or polyp (arrow).

both have a smooth, convex margin and are homogeneous, soft tissue density lesions. Most are found in the maxillary sinuses, but they can be located in any of the paranasal sinuses. They usually are asymptomatic and come to clinical attention only as incidental CT findings or when there is an associated sinus infection. They can grow to completely fill the sinus; however, even in

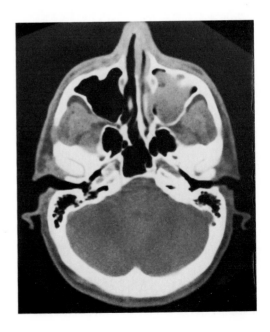

FIG. 5.20. Axial CT scan reveals a large left antral polypoid mass. Note the air separating the polyp margins from the sinus wall.

these cases small pockets of air are usually visible around the upper margins of the lesion that allow the diagnosis to be made on CT (Fig. 5.20). On rare occasions, these cysts or polyps can expand the sinus cavity. Usually, they are not associated with nasal polyps; however, one clear exception to this general rule is the antrochoanal polyp, which represents about 7 percent of all nasal polyps. These lesions arise in the antrum, bulge through the sinus ostium, and present as a nasal mass (Fig. 5.21).[1,19]

The mucocele is the most common expansile lesion to occur in any paranasal sinus and results from ostial obstruction and accumulation of mucoid, sterile secretions. The classical CT appearance is that of a mucoid-filled, nonenhancing, expanded sinus (Fig. 5.22).[1,20-24] Without sinus cavity enlargement, one can only suggest that a mucocele is present; however, differentiation from an obstructed, infected, fluid-filled sinus may at times be impossible.

About 65 percent of mucoceles occur in the frontal sinuses, 25 percent occur in the ethmoid sinuses, 10 percent occur in the maxillary sinuses, and only isolated cases occur in the sphenoid sinuses. If a mucocele becomes infected, it is referred to as a pyocele and CT usually shows a thin rim of enhancement around the margin of the mucocele with the central mucoid density remaining unchanged.[1]

The granulomatous diseases as a group tend to present first in the nasal cavity, from which they secondarily spread into the maxillary, ethmoid, and sphenoid sinuses. The frontal sinuses are involved far less frequently. The

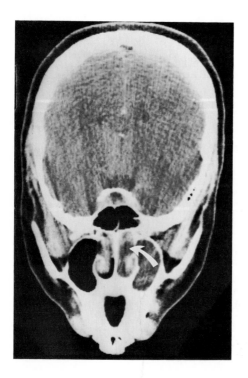

FIG. 5.21. Coronal CT scan reveals a left antrochoanal polyp (arrow). The mucoid density polyp fills the antrum and extends into the nasal cavity.

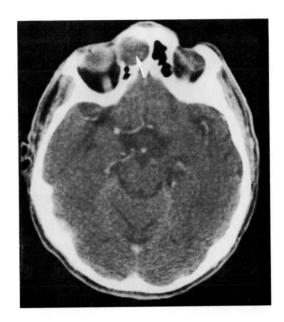

FIG. 5.22. Axial CT scan reveals an expansile right frontal sinus nonenhancing mass (arrow). This mucocele has caused typical inferolateral displacement of the globe.

soft tissue nasal changes can be small mucosal nodules or bulky soft tissue masses. They are usually bilateral, and focal areas of bone erosion can present in the nasal bones, nasal septum, and lateral nasal vault. In general, there is no specific pattern that correlates with a specific disease (Fig. 5.23). The changes of mucormycosis, tuberculosis, Wegener's granulomatosis, lethal midline granu-

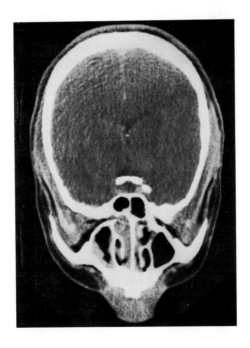

FIG. 5.23. Coronal CT scan reveals nonspecific nodular soft tissue changes in both nasal cavities and in the right antrum. The diagnosis is mucormycosis.

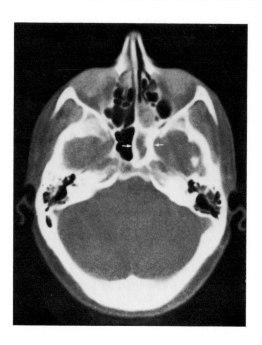

FIG. 5.24. Axial CT scan reveals soft tissue clouding of the left sphenoid sinus and posterior ethmoid sinuses. Sclerotic thickening of the walls of the sphenoid sinus (arrows) is evident, indicating the presence of chronic infection.

loma, and sarcoid are indistinguishable from each other and from the more exotic inflammatory granulomatous diseases that affect the head and neck.[25] Included in the CT differential diagnosis must always be lymphoma, which can present exactly the same CT findings. Focal destruction of the anterior nasal septum with little surrounding soft tissue disease should also raise the possible diagnosis of cocaine abuse.

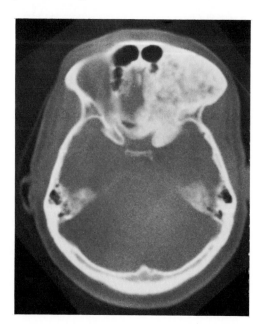

FIG. 5.25. Axial CT scan reveals massive bony expansion of the left orbital roof extending into the left sphenoid sinus and anterior clinoid process. Small lower density areas are seen scattered throughout the increased bone mass. The diagnosis is fibrous dysplasia.

In the presence of chronic inflammatory disease, the adjacent bone becomes thickened and fairly uniformly sclerotic in appearance. This CT finding is most often seen in the walls of the maxillary sinus but can occur anywhere (Figs. 5.17 and 5.24).[26] The differential diagnosis of this bone appearance includes radiation osteitis, metastatic prostate, and Paget's disease.

Fibrous dysplasia and ossifying fibroma primarily widen bone by expanding the diploic space.[27] The inner and outer tables are not eroded. On CT, the diploic space can have either large well-defined bony and fibrous areas, increased bone density with small, well-defined, fibrous cystic areas, or appear as a "ground glass" density in which the fibrous areas are numerous and very small (Fig. 5.25).[1] In almost all cases, these entities can be differentiated from the more uniform, less expanded bone appearance of Paget's disease, metastatic prostate carcinoma, and osteitis.[28]

MALIGNANCY

Malignancies of the paranasal sinuses include a wide variety of both primary and metastatic lesions. Although the radiologist in most cases cannot provide the surgeon with a precise histological diagnosis, analysis of the type of bone destruction, the location of the tumor, the enhancement characteristics, and the clinical setting can allow a preferred list of differential diagnoses to be made. Often this list coincides with the clinician's impression and the biopsy histology. However, on occasion the CT pattern of disease suggests that a different tumor is present. This is especially important when histologically the lesion is anaplastic in appearance. In these cases, the surgeon should take a second biopsy for electron microscopy and histochemical testing in order to establish a definitive diagnosis.[29]

Besides helping to establish a diagnosis, the radiologist plays a very important role in the mapping and staging of the tumor.[30] Precise localization of tumor margins is the primary information utilized to determine patient operability. Accurate mapping is also necessary to set correct radiation therapy fields and to follow tumor response to both radiation and chemotherapies.

The easiest and best method for assessing tumor growth or regression is to compare old and new scans. If surgery has been performed, a postoperative CT scan should be obtained 6 to 8 weeks after the operation. This will establish a new base line normal for this patient. The 6 to 8 week time interval allows any postoperative hemorrhage and edema to subside so that they will not be confused with tumor.[31]

The type of bone destruction that is present is helpful in suggesting a diagnosis. If the bone is aggressively destroyed, either squamous cell carcinoma, an aggressive sarcoma (i.e., angiosarcoma), or metastases from lung, breast, or the distal genitourinary tract is the likely tumor. If the bone is partially remodeled, that is, if CT shows that the involved tumor cavity is expanded, with major portions of the bony walls pushed outward, a different set of lesions is usually responsible. These include the minor salivary gland tumors, the lymphomas, most sarcomas, and rare lesions such as esthesioneuroblastomas and ameloblastomas. Most of these tumors enhance minimally or only to a moderate degree.[31,32] If the cavity is expanded and the tumor is very vascular (intensely enhancing), lesions such as extramedullary plasmacytoma, melanosarcoma, meningioma, and metastatic hypernephroma are most often responsible. If disorganized calcifications or bone formations are seen, tumors such as osteogenic sarcomas, chondrosarcomas, mesenchymomas, and in the maxillary sinus odontogenic tumors should be included in the differential diagnosis.[1,26,33-35]

A good rule to keep in mind when correlating the CT scan findings with the clinical aspects of the case is that pain is associated almost solely with infection. Large areas of tumor bone destruction and soft tissue disease can be present without any complaint of pain. In these cases, the patient usually presents with symptoms related to the mass and position of the tumor (e.g., nasal obstruction, change in voice quality, diplopia). Diagnostically, however, infection often coexists with tumor and differentiating between them may at times be impossible both clinically and on CT.

A more precise differential diagnosis can be made by correlating the CT findings with clinical information. A brief review of some of the more clinically important tumors will illustrate these points.

Squamous cell carcinoma is the most common tumor to involve the nasal cavity and paranasal sinuses. It represents nearly 80 percent of all malignancies in that area. Most squamous cell carcinomas (80 percent) occur in the maxillary sinuses and present with aggressive bone destruction. Although occasionally some bone remodeling can be seen, this tumor is the classical aggressive bone-destroying lesion (Fig. 5.26). It usually enhances slightly and is seen in patients over 40 years of age.[1,4,5,24,28,36,37]

Inverting papilloma is a polypoid unilateral nasal tumor that expands the

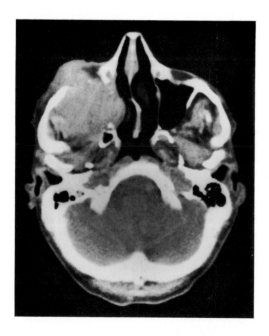

FIG. 5.26. Axial CT scan reveals an extensive squamous cell carcinoma of the right maxillary sinus that has infiltrated the cheek and infratemporal fossa. The sinus walls are destroyed and not displaced.

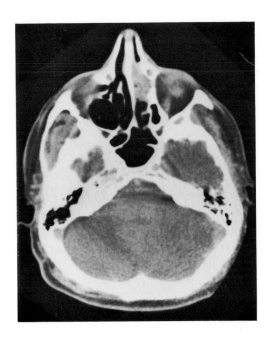

FIG. 5.27. Axial CT scan reveals a left nasal cavity slightly expansile nondestructive mass. Inverting papilloma.

nasal vault and can bulge into the ipsilateral antrum and ethmoid sinuses. It is almost always contained by an intact, albeit remodeled, nasal septum. The lesion is usually minimally to moderately enhanced (Fig. 5.27).[38-40] There is a 10 to 13 percent association with squamous cell carcinoma either in the lesion, arising adjacent to the papilloma, or developing after the papilloma is surgically removed.[28] Because of this, patients with inverting papilloma should be followed routinely with CT scans.

Esthesioneuroblastomas occur mainly in people 20 to 40 years of age, a younger patient population than for squamous cell carcinoma. They are unilateral, expansile, moderately enhancing nasal cavity tumors that extend into the maxillary and ethmoid sinuses in a similar pattern to that seen in patients with inverted papilloma. However, between 10 and 15 percent of these tumors erode through the cribriform plate. The radiologist must pay special attention to this area because the surgical treatment of the tumor depends on whether or not any intracranial extension has occurred.[41,42]

The minor salivary gland tumors arise primarily in the nasal cavity and the main tumor spread involves the antrum and the ethmoid and sphenoid sinuses. They usually enhance only moderately and remodel bone (Fig. 5.28). This group includes adenocystic carcinoma (cylindroma), malignant mixed tumor, and probably should include the adenocarcinomas. This last group occurs mainly in the ethmoid sinuses and its incidence is high in patients who have been working with hardwoods (furniture industry) for many years.[1,28,43]

Embryonal rhabdomyosarcoma occurs primarily in young patients, under 20 years of age. This lesion usually remodels bone to some degree and enhances moderately. It can be confused histologically with anaplastic carcinoma, mela-

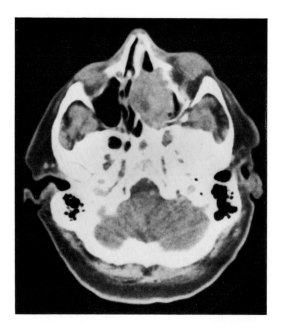

FIG. 5.28. Axial CT scan reveals a nonenhancing expansile nasal cavity mass. The nasal septum is intact but bowed to the right. Cylindroma.

nosarcoma, histiocystic lymphoma, esthesioneuroblastoma, and extramedullary plasmacytoma. Electron microscopy and histochemical testing are the only accurate ways to differentiate between these lesions. Most of the paranasal sinus rhabdomyosarcomas involve the ethmoid and maxillary sinuses.[28,44]

The majority of extramedullary plasmacytomas, melanomas, and lymphomas that involve the paranasal sinuses originate in the nasal cavity and extend into the maxillary and ethmoid sinuses. Bone remodeling is present. The plasmacytomas and melanomas are vascular lesions that are markedly enhanced on CT studies (Fig. 5.29). The lymphomas are not vascular and exhibit moderate enhancement.[1,45]

These malignancies that predominantly cause bone remodeling may often look like benign lesions on CT; however, one cannot always equate the pattern of bone involvement (aggressive destruction versus bone remodeling) with the biological nature of the tumor. The adenoidcystic carcinomas, adenocarcinomas, and melanomas all have worse prognoses than the more aggressive-appearing squamous cell carcinomas.

In the maxillary sinus, an expansile lesion can also be of odontogenic origin. If a displaced tooth is identified along the margin of the lesion, a dentigerous cyst is present. Of all the odontogenic malignancies, the one most likely to invade the antrum is the ameloblastoma. These usually expansile tumors have minimal enhancement and always involve the alveolar recess of the sinus. In fact, if a tumor involves only the upper portion of the maxillary sinus, it cannot be of primary odontogenic origin.[46,47]

Metastases to the paranasal sinuses are rare. Excluding direct extension of basal cell carcinomas, squamous cell carcinomas, and melanomas of the skin,

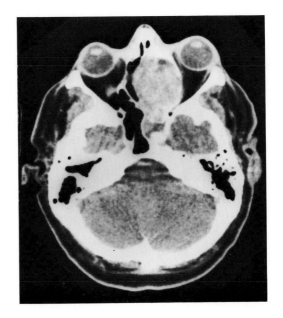

FIG. 5.29. Axial CT scan reveals an enhancing expansile nasoethmoid mass. The lamina papyracea is bowed to the left and the nasal septum is bowed to the right. The sphenoid sinus is filled with nonenhancing secretions, suggesting that it is obstructed by the mass rather than invaded. Plasmacytoma.

most metastases are from primary tumors of the breast, lung, and genitourinary tract.[28] These lesions are aggressive bone-destroying metastases that are usually impossible to differentiate on CT from primary paranasal sinus squamous cell carcinoma. When metastatic hypernephroma involves the central skull base (as it often does), it may be indistinguishable from a sphenoid sinus or nasopharyngeal carcinoma. However, when the maxillary sinus or nasal cavity is involved, the lesion is both expansile and vascular (marked enhancement). Whenever such a CT appearance is seen, the possibility of metastatic hypernephroma or melanoma must be thought of and the appropriate clinical and diagnostic work-up considered. Extramedullary plasmacytomas of the antrum also have a similar CT appearance; however, they are primary and not metastatic lesions. Other vascular tumors such as angiosarcomas are aggressive bone-destroying lesions and the angiofibromas are nasopharyngeal tumors that encroach secondarily on the maxilla.[48] Angiofibromas invariably extend from their nasopharyngeal origin anteriorly into the nasal cavity and insinuate themselves into the pterygopalatine fossa. This results in widening of this fossa, with anterior bowing of the posterior antral wall (Fig. 5.30). Although other lesions can occasionally widen this fossa,[49] the combination of a nasopharyngeal enhancing mass and a widened pterygopalatine fossa is virtually diagnostic for angiofibroma.

Another sign suggestive of metastases is the presence of two or more noncontiguous areas of bone erosion in a patient who clinically does not have osteomyelitis. When primary neoplasms involve bone, they virtually always erode bone without skip areas. The appearance on serial CT scans is one of a progressively enlarging area of bone destruction, not of two or more separate areas of erosion.[1]

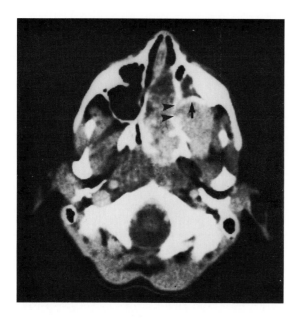

FIG. 5.30. Axial CT scan reveals an enhancing left nasopharyngeal mass that has widened the left pterygopalatine fossa (arrowheads), bowed the antral wall anteriorly (arrow), and extended laterally into the infratemporal fossa. Angiofibroma.

The evaluation of the postoperative patient has been made remarkably more accurate by the use of CT. Prior to CT scanning, the surgical removal of the bony sinus margins eliminated the main landmarks necessary for evaluating the sinuses. The postoperative soft tissue changes were extremely difficult to see and detection of early recurrent disease was virtually impossible. The early

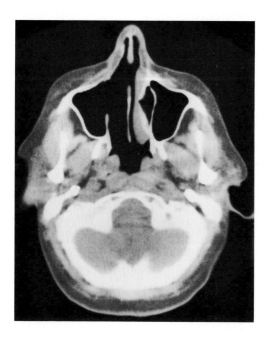

FIG. 5.31. Axial CT scan after partial right medial maxillectomy. The right inferior turbinate was also removed. Note the normal smooth mucosal margins leading into the cavity and the normal appearance of the remaining antrum.

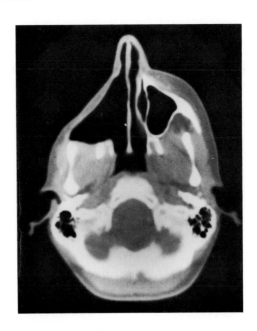

FIG. 5.32.   Axial CT scan after right total maxillectomy. The postoperative cavity is smooth.

changes of tumor recurrence are at least brought within the realm of radiographic diagnosis by using the CT scanner. This is especially so if a baseline postoperative CT scan is obtained as a reference study (see above).

The maxillary sinuses are the sinuses most often operated on and are the easiest of the paranasal sinuses to evaluate on CT. In part this is because of their large size and the fact that air normally fills the postoperative cavity.

The ethmoid sinuses are narrower than the antra and postoperative scarring commonly causes total or partial sinus opacification. This makes the detection of early tumor recurrence very difficult. The frontal and sphenoid sinuses are rarely involved by malignancy and even more rarely are these patients considered suitable candidates for surgery.

The normal postoperative maxillary sinus has a smooth mucosal surface. In the case of a partial maxillectomy this mucosa may be the remaining original sinus lining (Fig. 5.31). In the case of a total maxillectomy, a split-thickness skin graft is applied to the inner surface of the cheek to form the new mucosal lining (Fig. 5.32). On CT, any mucosal nodularity must be considered suspect of tumor recurrence, especially if such nodularity was not seen on a baseline scan (Figs. 5.33 and 5.34). The surgeon can be directed to these suspicious areas for a specific biopsy, rather than obtaining blind biopsies that might miss a small lesion. CT has been shown to detect these small lesions with a greater sensitivity than clinical examination.[31] The aim of studying these patients is to provide the clinician with the earliest possible notification of tumor recurrence so that more of these patients can be saved.

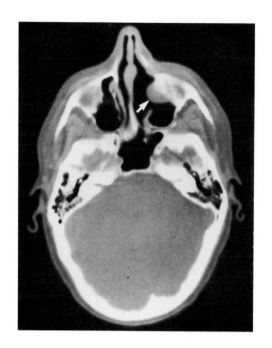

FIG. 5.33. Axial CT scan after left partial maxillectomy. A smooth convex mass is seen on the lateral wall (arrow). Retention cyst in nonresected antral mucosa.

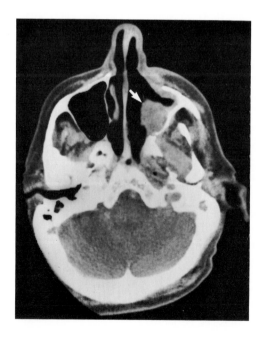

FIG. 5.34. Axial CT scan after left partial maxillectomy. An irregular nodule, which represents a recurrence of tumor, is present in the left antrum.

REFERENCES

1. Som PM: The paranasal sinuses. pp. 1–142. In Bergeron RT, Osborn AG, Som PM (eds.): CV Mosby, St. Louis, 1984.

2. Unsold R, Degroot J, Newton TH: Images of the optic nerve: anatomic CT correlation. AJR 135:767–773, 1980.

3. Unsold R, Newton TH, Hoyt WF: CT examination technique of the optic nerve. Technical note. J Comput Assist Tomogr 4:560–563, 1980.

4. Carter BL: Computed tomography. Part III. pp. 212–240. In Valvassori GE, Potter GD, Hanafee WN, et al.: Radiology of the Ear, Nose and Throat WB Saunders, Philadelphia, 1982.

5. Mancuso AA, Hanafee WN: Computed tomography of the Head and Neck. pp. 203–243. In Mancuso AA and Hanafee WN (eds): Paranasal Sinuses—Normal Anatomy, Methodology and Pathology. Williams and Wilkins, Baltimore, 1982.

6. Caffey J: Pediatric X-ray Diagnosis Ed. 7, Vol. 1. pp. 111–118. Year Book Medical Publishers, Chicago 1980.

7. Dodd GD, Jung BS: Radiology of the Nose, Paranasal Sinuses and Nasopharynx. Williams & Wilkins, Baltimore, 1977.

8. Remmler D, Boles R: Intracranial complications of frontal sinusitis. Laryngoscope 90:1814–1824, 1980.

9. Gray's anatomy, Ed. 36, Williams PL, Warwick R (eds): WB Saunders, Philadelphia, 1980.

10. Fujii K, Chambers SM, Rhoton AL Jr: Neurovascular relationships of the sphenoid sinus: a microsurgical study. J Neurosurg 50:31–39, 1979.

11. Alberti PW: Applied surgical anatomy of the maxillary sinus. Otolaryngol Clin North Am 9(1):3–20, 1976.

12. Potter GD: Sectional Anatomy and Tomography of the Head. Grune and Stratton, New York, 1971.

13. Van Alyea OE: Nasal Sinuses: Anatomic and Clinical Consideration. Baltimore, 1942. Williams and Wilkins,

14. Fujioka M, Young LW: The sphenoid sinuses: radiographic patterns of normal development and abnormal findings in infants and children. Radiology 129:133–136, 1978.

15. Radiology of the Skull and Brain, The Skull. Newton TH, Potts DG (eds): CV Mosby, St. Louis, 1971.

16. Etter LE: Atlas of Roentgen Anatomy of the Skull. Charles C Thomas, Springfield, ILL, 1955.

17. Fagan P, McKenzie B, Edmonds C: Sinus barotrauma in divers. Ann Otolaryngol Rhinol Laryngol 85:61–64, 1976.

18. Fascenelli FW: Maxillary sinus abnormalities: radiographic evidence in an asymptomatic population. Arch Otolaryngol 90:190–193, 1969.

19. Smith CJ, Echevarria R, McLelland CA: Pseudosarcomatous changes in antrochoanal polyps. Arch Otolaryngol 99:228–230, 1974.

20. Som PM, Shugar JMA: Antral mucoceles: a new look. J Comput Assist Tomogr 4:484–488, 1980.

21. Som PM, Shugar JMA: The CT classification of ethmoid mucoceles. J Comput Assist Tomogr 4:199–203, 1980.

22. Gore RM, Weinberg PE, Kim KS, Rainsey RG: Sphenoid sinus mucoceles presenting as intracranial masses on computed tomography. Surg Neurol 13:375–379, 1980.

23. Osborn AG, Johnson L, Roberts TS: Sphenoidal mucoceles with intracranial extension. J Comput Assist Tomogr 3:335–338, 1979.

24. Hesselink JR, New PFJ, Davis KR, et al.: Computed tomography of the paranasal sinuses and face—Part II—Pathological Anatomy. J Comput Assist Tomogr 2:568–576, 1978.

25. Harrison TR: Harrison's principles of internal medicine, ed. 9, McGraw-Hill, New York, 1980.

26. Bilaniuk LT, Zimmerman RA: Computed tomography in evaluation of the paranasal sinuses. RCNA 20:51–66, 1982.

27. Fu Y-S, Perzin KH: Non-epithelial tumors of the nasal cavity, paranasal sinuses, and nasopharynx: a clinicopathologic study. Cancer 33:1289–1305, 1974.

28. Batsakis JG: Tumors of the Head and Neck: Clinical and Pathological Considerations, ed. 2. Williams and Wilkins, Baltimore, 1979.

29. Som PM, Shugar JMA: When to question the diagnosis of anaplastic carcinoma. Mt Sinai J Med 40:230–235, 1981.

30. Jeans WD, Gilani S, Bullimore J: The effect of CT scanning on staging of tumors of the paranasal sinuses. Clin Radiol 33:173–179, 1982.

31. Som PM, Shugar JMA, Biller HF: The early detection of antral malignancy in the post-maxillectomy patient. Radiology 143:509–512, 1982.

32. Som PM, Shugar JMA: The significance of bone expansion associated with the diagnosis of malignant tumors of the paranasal sinuses. Radiology 136:97–100, 1980.

33. McCoy JM, McConnel FMS: Chondrosarcoma of the nasal septum. Arch Otolaryngol 107:125–127, 1981.

34. Waga S, Tochio H, Yamagiwa M, Nishioka H: Chondrosarcoma of the ethmoid sinus extending to the anterior fossa. Surg Neurol 16:324–328, 1981.

35. Singh J, Gluckman JL, Kaufman RA, Wakely PE: Osteosarcoma of the nasal bone in a child. Head Neck Surg 4:246–250, 1982.

36. Conley J: Concepts in Head and Neck Surgery. George Thieme. Verlag, Stuttgart, 1970.

37. Larsson LG, Martensson G: Maxillary antral cancers. JAMA 219:342–345, 1972.

38. Kelly JH, Joseph M, Carroll E, et al.: Inverted papilloma of the nasal septum. Arch Otolaryngol 106:767–771, 1980.

39. Momose KJ, Weber AL, Goodman M, et al.: Radiological aspects of inverted papilloma. Radiology 134:73–79, 1980.

40. Wilson WR, Carroll ED, Bentkover SH, Schuknecht HF: Inverted papilloma. Arch Otolaryngol 106:54–61, 1980.

41. Burke DP, Gabriel TO, Knake JE, et al.: Radiology of olfactory neuroblastoma. Radiology 137:367–372, 1980.

42. Pagani JJ, Thompson J, Mancuso A, Hanafee W: Lateral wall of the olfactory fossa in determining intracranial extension of sinus carcinomas. AJR 133:497–501, 1979.

43. Ramsden D, Sheridan BF, Newton NC, DeWilde FW: Adenoid cystic carcinoma of the head and neck: a report of 30 cases. Aust NZ J Surg 43:102–108, 1973.

44. Ogura JH, Schenck NL: Unusual nasal tumor problems in diagnosis and treatment. Otol Clin North Am 6:813–837, 1973.

45. Fierstein JF, Thawley SE: Lymphoma of the head and neck. Laryngoscope 88:582–593, 1978.

46. Dayal VS, Jones J, Noyek AM: Management of odontogenic maxillary sinus disease. Otolaryngol Clin North Am 9:212–222, 1976.

47. Stafne EC, Gibilisco JA: Oral roentgenographic diagnosis. Ed 4. WB Saunders, Philadelphia, 1975.

48. Sessions RB, Bryan RN, Naclerio RM, Alfrod BR: Radiographic staging of juvenile angiofibroma. Head Neck Surg 3:279–283, 1981.

49. Som PM, Shugar JMA, Cohen BA, Biller HF: The non-specificity of the antral bowing sign in maxillary sinus pathology. J Comput Assist Tomogr 5:350–352, 1981.

6 The Orbit and Globe

ALFRED L. WEBER
ROBERT OOT

Eye and orbital lesions comprise a multitude of diverse pathological entities that eluded precise diagnosis in the pre-CT era. The usefulness of plain films and conventional tomographic examinations is limited in many eye and orbital diseases.[1]

In a series of 220 patients, reported by Dallow and Weber, an accurate diagnosis was provided in 19 percent (equivocal 6 percent) of cases by plain films and in 28 percent (equivocal) by conventional tomography. This applied particularly to the inflammatory lesions. In most reported series, they constituted about 50 percent of cases where exophthalmos was the predominant finding.[1] In some cases, invasive procedures (orbital venography and arteriography) were utilized to map out lesions prior to exploratory surgery. Today, orbital venography is specifically used to outline a venous malformation. Arteriography is used to delineate the vascular anatomy in vascular tumors, aneurysms, and arteriovenous (AV) malformations and shunts. The introduction of CT in 1971[2-5] and the subsequent development of third and fourth generation scanners (with high resolution capability) have significantly changed the diagnostic approach to evaluating eye and orbital lesions. Abnormalities in the eye and orbit are readily detected, because their specific anatomy consists of a spectrum of different densities (fat, muscles, vessels, nerves, vitreous, lens, uveoscleral coat, and bone). High-resolution CT, with thin sections (1–2 mm) is capable of depicting the various eye lesions.[6] It is especially useful for detecting lesions in eyes that defy accurate fundoscopic examination.

This synopsis is intended to present a survey of the CT findings for the most common eye and orbital lesions.

TECHNIQUE

Computed tomography has revolutionized the radiology of the orbit and has become the standard by which other diagnostic imaging modalities must be measured. The role of nuclear magnetic resonance (NMR) in evaluation of

131

the orbit has yet to be defined. However, early experience with NMR scanners indicates that this technique may provide high quality images that will be capable of supplying physiological as well as anatomic information about the orbit.[7]

CT evaluation of the orbit should begin with axial images. With the patient supine, the head should be placed in a slightly hyperextended position and a lateral view digital radiograph should be obtained. Although images obtained in the plane parallel to the Reid's baseline provide satisfactory images, the optic canal and axis of the orbit subtend an angle of approximately $-30°$ with the Reid's baseline and images along this plane display the optic nerve to best advantage.[8] This plane is approximated by a line drawn from the anterior clinoid (or tuberculum sellae if the clinoid cannot be identified) to a point just cranial to the inferior orbital rim. Prior to initiation of each scan for assessment of the optic nerve, the patient should be instructed to look upward, a position that tends to straighten out most of the optic nerve. A slice thickness of approximately 5 mm is adequate for evaluating the orbit in most cases and a total of approximately 10 to 12 images will include the entire orbit. In certain cases, thinner sections of approximately 1.5 to 2 mm may be required, but such exquisite detail is not routinely necessary.

Although axial images detect and adequately demonstrate most orbital pathology, coronal images may provide additional information. Coronal images may be necessary to display subtle abnormalities involving (1) the orbital apex (because of the close proximity of its structures) and (2) the superiorly and inferiorly placed muscles (because of their close relationship with the bony orbital margins).[9] Coronal imaging may also best demonstrate pathological processes that involve both the orbit and the adjacent structures, such as the nasal cavities and the ethmoid or maxillary sinuses. It may also more accurately define the overall extent of lesions and their relationship to the optic nerve.

The current software programs included with most scanners allow axially obtained data to be reformatted into coronal or sagittal planes,[10] although some loss of anatomic definition and spatial resolution invariably occurs in the computer generated images. In cases where coronal imaging is impossible, such as in a severely traumatized patient, the axial raw data can be reformatted into coronal and/or sagittal reconstructions.

Images are usually obtained during the intravenous infusion of iodinated contrast material. Infusion is initiated prior to positioning the patient. Bolus injections of contrast material are not routinely administered but may be of value in evaluating highly vascular lesions.

The IV contrast medium does not significantly increase the visibility of normal intraorbital structures but does improve visualization of the optic chiasm and parasellar region. Its use is crucial in cases where a combined intraorbital–intracranial lesion is suspected. Each case, however, must be evaluated individually. In some cases, contrast enhancement is unlikely to be of value, such as in the evaluation of intraorbital foreign objects or of Graves' disease.

Radiation Dosimetry[11]

Later generation CT scanners not only provide higher quality images but also can accomplish this with a lower radiation dose. With a highly collimated beam, scatter is minimal. The dose delivered to the given slice should not increase by more than a factor of two, regardless of the number of contiguous sections that are imaged. The critical organ is the ocular lens and a series of 25 1.5 mm contiguous axial CT sections through the orbit (600 mA, 9.6-sec scans) gives the lens a dose of $\times$ 3.6 rads.[10] However, the addition of coronal images would obviously increase the total lens dose.

ANATOMY OF THE ORBIT[12-14]

Because of the large amount of fat surrounding the various components of the orbit, small structures can routinely be visualized. The ability to visualize individual structures depends on the resolution of the CT scanner, the section plane, and the thickness (Figs. 6.1, 6.2).

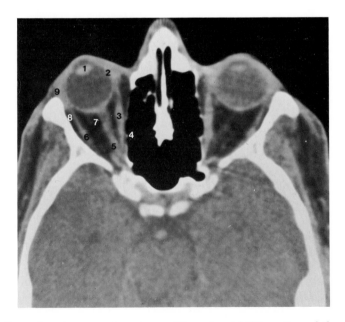

FIG. 6.1. Scan showing normal anatomy. Normal axial CT section of the mid-orbits: (1) lens, (2) sclera, (3) medial rectus muscle, (4) lamina papyracea, (5) optic nerve, (6) lateral rectus muscle, (7) intraconal space, (8) extraconal space, and (9) lacrimal gland.

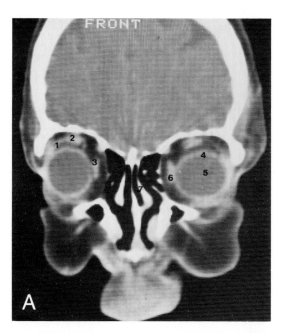

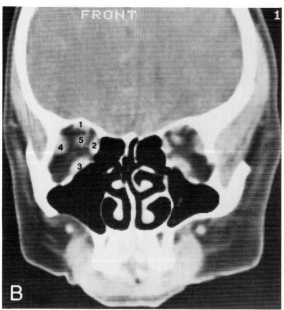

FIG. 6.2. Scans showing normal anatomy. (A) Normal coronal CT section through the anterior orbit and globe: (1) intramuscular fascia, (2) superior rectus muscle, (3) medial rectus muscle, (4) uveoscleral coat, (5) vitreous, (6) medial wall of the orbit, and (7) ethmoid sinus. (B) Normal coronal section through the posterior portion of the orbit: (1) superior rectus muscle, (2) medial rectus muscle, (3) inferior rectus muscle, (4) lateral rectus muscle, and (5) optic nerve.

Bony Orbit

The overall configuration of the bony orbit is that of a quadrangular pyramid, with its base facing forward. Above, the orbit is intimately related to the floor of the anterior cranial fossa and the frontal sinus; below, to the maxillary sinus; medially, to the ethmoid sinus; posterolaterally, to the temporal fossa; and posteromedially, to the middle cranial fossa. The optic canal is located at the apex of the pyramid and communicates with the middle cranial fossa. The plane of the optic canal subtends an angle of approximately 30° with the plane of Reid's baseline.

Extraocular Muscles

There are six extrinsic ocular muscles: two obliques and four recti. The four rectus muscles arise from a common origin, the annulus of Zinn, a tendinous ring that encircles the optic foramen and the medial aspect of the superior orbital fissure. Each muscle extends forward as a separate bundle, ultimately inserting on the globe. The muscles are joined by an intermuscular fascial membrane, dividing the orbit into intraconal and extraconal components. The medial rectus (the largest muscle) and the lateral rectus muscles are well demonstrated on the axial images. The superior and inferior recti run in close relation to the bony orbital roof and floor, respectively. Although the superior and inferior recti are demonstrated on axial images, subtle abnormalities involving these muscles may be best demonstrated on coronal images.

The superior oblique muscle is the longest and thinnest of the extraocular muscles. It originates in relation to the orbital apex, superomedial to the optic foramen. It passes anterior to the trochlea, at which point its tendon turns sharply medially and inserts into the globe below the superior rectus. The inferior oblique is the only extrinsic muscle that does not originate from the orbital apex but arises from the anteromedial aspect of the orbit, near the orifice of the nasolacrimal duct, and inserts on the posterolateral aspect of the globe. Although the obliques can occasionally be defined on axial images, they are most convincingly displayed in the coronal plane.

An additional muscle, the levator palpebrae superioris, can usually be seen, passing forward immediately above the superior rectus to insert into the upper eyelid.

Orbital Fascia

An understanding of the anatomy of several components of the orbital fascia is relevant to the interpretation of orbital CT. The orbital septum, a membranous sheet attached to the edge of the orbit and continuous with the periosteum, is an important barrier in the spread of preseptal eyelid inflammation to the posterior compartment, the orbit proper.

The Tenon's capsule is a thin, fibrous membrane that envelops the globe from the corneal margin to the optic nerve and is separated from the sclera by a potential space, the episcleral space. This capsule is related to the aponeuroses and ligaments of the extraocular muscles, conjunctiva, and globe, facilitating the extension of tenonitis to the orbital tissue.

Optic Nerve

Anatomically, the optic nerve is a part of the brain proper and serves as a fiber tract joining the retina and the lateral geniculate body of the thalamus. It is not surrounded by Schwann cells like other peripheral nerves but is enveloped by meninges. Its total length is 4 to 5 cm and consists of four parts, including an intracranial and an intraocular part. Its long axis is at an angle of 30° with respect to the Reid's baseline. Scans obtained along this plane will maximally display the nerve. The optic nerve's appearance is also a function of gaze and is best "straightened out" in extreme upward gaze.[8]

Orbital Vessels

Orbital vessels can be routinely seen on high-resolution CT studies.[15] If resolution of the orbital vascular structures is clinically important, it is imperative that thin (1.5–2 mm) sections be obtained.

The ophthalmic artery originates from the internal carotid artery and runs inferolateral to the optic nerve as it traverses the optic canal. Soon after entering the orbit proper, it usually crosses over the nerve, between the nerve and the superior rectus muscle. It courses anteriorly, lying between the medial rectus and the superior oblique and gives off a number of variable branches, some of which may be visualized by CT.

Orbital venous drainage occurs mostly via the superior ophthalmic vein and this structure is routinely visualized as it courses obliquely through the superior aspect of the orbit.[15] The inferior ophthalmic vein is less routinely identified.

Lacrimal Gland

The lacrimal gland is about the size of an almond and is divided into two lobes, a larger orbital lobe and a smaller palpebral lobe. It is routinely visualized on the medial surface of the zygomatic process of the frontal bone and extends down almost to the lateral angle of the globe.[12]

INTRACRANIAL LESIONS EXTENDING INTO THE ORBIT

Meningioma

Meningioma is the most common intracranial tumor to involve the orbit. It accounts for approximately 5 percent of orbital mass lesions.[16] Although orbital symptomatology is most frequently the first clinical sign of these lesions,[17] the orbital neoplasm usually represents the propagation of an intracranial tumor.[17,18]

The most common intracranial sites of origin are the lesser wing of the sphenoid and the parasellar region. Meningiomas, for the most part, invade the orbit via foraminal and fissural openings or cause exophthalmos secondary to hyperostotic encroachment on the orbit (Fig. 6.3).[18] An occasional, more aggressive meningioma can destroy bone, especially in relation to the sphenoid wing, and enter the orbit directly.[18,19] Meningiomas arising from a subfrontal location, or from other uncommon sites such as the nasal fossa, the pterygopalatine space, or the paranasal sinuses can also involve the orbit on occasion.[20,21]

Of the primary orbital meningiomas, the most common site of origin is the retrobulbar portion of the optic nerve. These tumors can also arise from (1) the ectopic arachnoid cells, located within the orbit but unattached to the optic nerve or orbital wall, (2) the periorbita of the orbital walls, or (3) the optic canal.[18] As with other central nervous system meningiomas, the tumor shows a female preponderance and most commonly occurs in middle age. There is, however, an association between optic nerve sheath meningiomas and neurofibromatosis. In this class of patients, the tumor tends to present at a younger age[16] and can occasionally present bilaterally.[22]

The CT appearance of meningiomas parallels their histopathology. These lesions usually appear as homogeneous areas of high density with sharply defined borders on non-contrast-enhanced scans.[19,23] They frequently contain calcification, often psammomatous in nature,[24,25] and macroscopic areas of calcification may be seen in approximately 20 percent of cases.[23] Because meningiomas are vascular lesions, often demonstrating a protracted capillary blush on arteriography, virtually all meningiomas that are not markedly calcified demonstrate contrast enhancement.[19] Meningiomas arising near the bone have a tendency to excite osteoblastic reaction and these changes can readily be demonstrated on CT (Fig. 6.3). However, meningiomas can be locally aggressive and cause bony inversion. When bony destruction changes are seen in relation to a presumed meningioma, one can suspect that the meningioma is atypical and may behave in a more aggressive fashion.[23,25]

Orbital meningiomas, arising in relation to the sphenoid wing, tend to show hyperostotic and/or bony erosive changes, with a contiguous soft tissue mass usually present in relation to the anterior portion of the middle cranial fossa.[23] Those meningiomas arising from the parasellar region similarly demonstrate

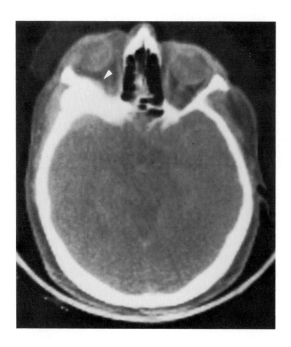

FIG. 6.3. Meningioma of the right sphenoid bone. Axial CT section through both orbits of 58-year-old woman with pain, swelling, and left proptosis reveals marked hyperostosis of the posterior wall of the right orbit. Note small hemispherically shaped soft tissue mass arising from the hyperostotic bone (arrowhead). Note proptosis of the right globe.

a parasellar soft tissue mass, in addition to the orbital component, and frequent bony changes.

On CT an optic nerve sheath meningioma usually manifests as an enlargement of a portion or all of the optic nerve (Fig. 6.4A). On plain scan, the tissue may appear at a slightly higher density than the optic nerve.[26] These differences may be accentuated by contrast infusion (Fig. 6.4B). A "railroad track" appearance may result, with the more densely enhancing tumor surrounding the more lucent optic nerve.[27] The optic canal may be expanded, and the presence of hyperostosis around the optic canal is virtually diagnostic of meningioma. Primary orbital meningiomas, arising from ectopic arachnoid cells within the orbit but unattached to the optic nerve, may present as focal masses and may cause adjacent hyperostosis or changes in adjacent sinuses, such as pneumosinus dilatans.[18]

Calcification occurs occasionally in optic nerve meningiomas. Differentiation of an optic nerve meningioma from an optic nerve glioma can be difficult. Optic nerve gliomas tend to cause a more fusiform enlargement of the optic nerve, as opposed to the more tubular appearance of an optic nerve meningioma (Fig. 6.5A). Although optic nerve gliomas can be confined to the orbit, they most frequently demonstrate spread along the optic pathway and commonly involve the optic chiasm and optic radiations (Fig. 6.5B). They tend to be of lower density and show less contrast enhancement than optic nerve meningiomas, essentially never demonstrating the "railroad track" sign.[28,29]

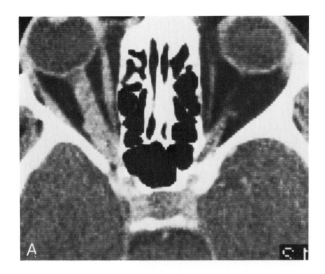

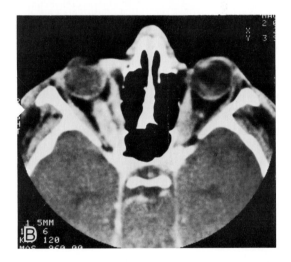

FIG. 6.4. Optic nerve sheath meningioma in 26-year-old man with progressive loss of vision in the right eye. (A) Axial precontrast CT section reveals diffuse thickening of the right optic nerve from the apex to the globe. (B) Postcontrast CT reveals diffuse enhancement of the right optic nerve. Note low density center secondary to optic nerve ("railroad track" sign).

Aneurysms

Aneurysms of the ophthalmic artery are uncommon and usually occur at the origin of the internal carotid artery.[30] Aneurysms arising at this site, as well as intracavernous carotid artery aneurysms,[17] can present with orbital and/or visual symptoms. Expansion of the aneurysm can cause compression of cranial nerves with paresis of the sixth, third, and/or fifth nerves, in that order of frequency. Other symptoms may include progressive visual failure, quadrantic or hemianoptic field defects, and exophthalmos.[30,31]

Small aneurysms may be difficult to resolve by CT. The appearance of large aneurysms varies, depending on the presence or absence of thrombosis.[32,33]

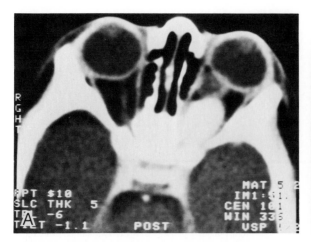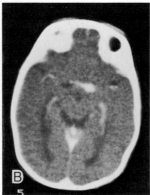

FIG. 6.5. Optic nerve glioma with intracranial extension in 4-year-old boy with proptosis and decreased vision on the left. (A) Axial CT section through the midorbit reveals a spindle-shaped mass involving the entire left optic nerve. The tumor is enhanced in the mid and posterior third. (B) Axial scan through the suprasellar cistern reveals tumor in the left chiasm.

Most commonly, larger aneurysms are partially thrombosed. They may demonstrate areas of calcification and following contrast infusion the unthrombosed portion of the aneurysm will demonstrate homogeneous enhancement. Completely thrombosed aneurysms usually present on nonenhanced scans as sharply demarcated areas of slightly increased density. The aneurysm wall may enhance following contrast enhancement. Nonthrombosed aneurysms tend to demonstrate slightly increased density on plain scans and demonstrate homogeneous contrast enhancement (Fig. 6.6).

Intraorbital ophthalmic artery aneurysms are very rare and are usually related to trauma.[30] They should appear as well-defined contrast-enhancing mass lesions.

Neurofibromatosis

Neurofibromatosis is inherited as an autosomal dominant trait with a penetrance exceeding 80 percent. The clinical manifestations include cafe au lait spots, subcutaneous neurofibroma, and other malformations, as well as neoplasms of neuroectodermal origin.[34] This disease affects the orbital–facial region in a number of ways, including formation of orbital neoplasms, plexiform neurofibroma, orbital osseous dysplasia, and congenital glaucoma (buphthalmos).[35,36]

Orbital tumors have been discussed separately; however, in a recent review of 24 neurofibromatosis patients, who presented with exophthalmos and/or facial disfigurement, 10 patients harbored orbital tumors including optic gliomas

FIG. 6.6. Bilateral intracavernous carotid artery aneurysms in 83-year-old woman with 5-month history of diplopia; right facial pain; and first, second, and sixth nerve palsy on the right. (A) Axial postcontrast CT section through the sella reveals sharply defined homogeneous enhancing lesions in the cavernous sinus bilaterally, slightly larger on the right. (B) AP digital angiogram shows these lesions to be bilateral intracavernous carotid artery aneurysms.

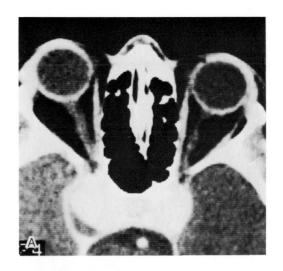

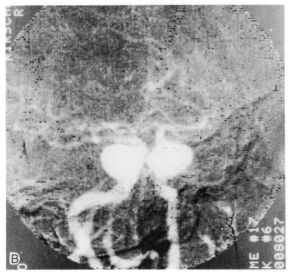

(3 cases), neurofibromas (2 cases), neurofibrosarcoma (2 cases), perioptic meningiomas (2 cases) and rhabdomyosarcoma (1 case).[35]

The plexiform neurofibroma is a poorly circumscribed tumor that involves segments and branches of nerves. The temporalis muscles and eyelids are commonly involved in tumors that present with orbital–facial findings (Fig. 6.7). The tumor can extend into and involve any part of the eye and orbit, with the most common locations being the choroid, ciliary body, conjunctiva, iris, and limbus.[37] In a recent series, a high percentage of these plexiform neurofibromas extended into and enlarged the cavernous sinus area, suggesting involvement of cranial nerves III, IV, V, or VI.[36]

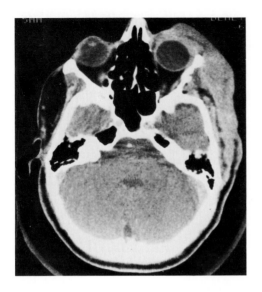

FIG. 6.7. Plexiform neurofibroma of the left temporal fossa with extension into the anterior orbit in 33-year-old man with neurofibromatosis and masses in the left facial area and neck. Axial CT sections through the orbit and adjacent intracranial cavity reveal a homogeneous, slightly undulated mass in the left temporal fossa with extension into the lid of the left eye.

In cases of orbital osseous dysplasia, the greater sphenoid wing is severely hypoplastic and the lesser wing is hypoplastic with a more medial and vertical position. Also invariably present is associated deformity of the sella and ethmoids. This bony defect allows the temporal lobe to herniate into the orbit, which is frequently enlarged, and these patients may present with pulsating exophthalmos.[35]

In buphthalmos, the intraocular pressure is elevated because of obstructed outflow of the aqueous humor. On CT the globe demonstrates overall enlargement in all dimensions.[35]

SECONDARY AND METASTATIC TUMORS OF THE EYE AND ORBIT

Metastatic disease to the eye and orbit has been reported by Henderson[38] to occur in 9 percent of orbital tumors. Tumor metastases to the orbit occur much less frequently than metastases to the globe. In a series reported by Ferry and Font in 1974,[39] the eye was involved with metastatic carcinoma in 88 percent of 227 cases, and involvement of the optic nerve was the rarest. The vast majority of orbital and ocular metastases in adults arise from the breast and lung. The most common sources of orbital metastases in children are neuroblastoma, Ewing's sarcoma, and Wilms' tumors.[40] These tumors seem to metastasize exclusively to the orbit, rather than to the globe.[41] However, sarcomas rarely metastasize to the eye. The posterior segment of the globe, especially the choroid, is a very common site for metastases. Patients with ocular metastases present with blurred vision because of retinal detachment. Exophthalmos is the most common symptom of metastases to the retrobulbar soft tissues and is associated with pain, a decrease in vision, periorbital edema, ophthalmo-

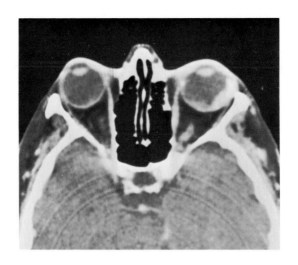

FIG. 6.8. Carcinoma of the breast with metastasis to the eye in 73-year-old woman with widespread metastatic disease from carcinoma of the breast. Axial CT scan through both globes reveals polypoid masses arising from the left uveoscleral coat with projection into the adjacent vitreous.

plegia, and diplopia. The metastases became symptomatic before the primary tumor in more than half of the cases.[39] Metastatic lesions may present on CT as a localized or diffuse thickening of the uveoscleral coat. Another mode of presentation on CT is a polypoid mass, single or multiple, that projects into the vitreous with or without extrascleral extension (Fig. 6.8).[41]

There are no specific findings to differentiate metastatic tumor from other growths in the eye, including melanoma. Following infusion of contrast material, there may be slight contrast enhancement of metastatic lesions. Most metastatic lesions of the orbit are homogeneous and appear as discrete masses, occasionally with irregular margins.[42] An infiltrating mass within the orbit, with enophthalmos, is characteristic of scirrhous carcinoma of the breast.[43] Bony metastases occur most frequently in the sphenoid bone; they often are found in both the orbit and the adjacent intracranial cavity and occasionally in the temporal fossa (Fig. 6.9).

The secondary tumors that most frequently invade the orbits originate from the paranasal sinuses.[44,45] The majority of malignant tumors of the paranasal sinuses are carcinomas, which most often arise from the antrum and ethmoid sinuses. Among a series of 200 malignant paranasal sinus tumors, orbital invasion occurred in 40 percent,[45] because malignant tumors of the paranasal sinuses destroy bone and invade the extraconal space of the orbit. Because of the late diagnosis of many of these lesions, the tumor may progress into the intraconal space and, in advanced cases, involve the entire orbit. This is reflected clinically by proptosis, decreased vision, and extraocular muscle motility abnormalities. These tumors rarely invade the coat of the eye. CT does not allow differentiation of the various histological tumor types. The degree of enhancement following infusion of the contrast medium is variable.[45] Marked enhancements may be encountered in vascular tumors, such as hemangiopericytoma. In advanced cases, simultaneous intracranial involvement may be demonstrated

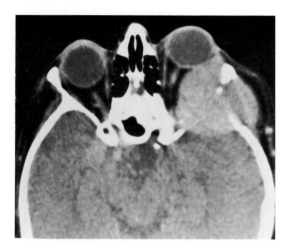

FIG. 6.9. Oat cell carcinoma metastatic to orbit and intracranial cavity in 64-year-old woman with metastatic oat cell carcinoma who complained of proptosis of the left eye and ptosis. Axial CT section through the orbits reveals a marked degree of proptosis caused by a homogeneous, sharply defined mass within the left orbit, adjacent middle cranial fossa, and temporal fossa. Note diffuse, ill-defined bone destruction involving the left sphenoid bone.

and in these cases enhancement can differentiate the tumor from the surrounding brain.[43]

Other lesions that may secondarily involve the orbits are malignant tumors from the nasopharynx, which most often invade the orbit via the inferior orbital fissure. In advanced cases, they may extend into the orbit, via the middle cranial fossa and parasellar area.[46] Benign lesions such as angiofibroma, by virtue of their slow growth and expansion, extend into the orbit through the inferior orbital fissure.[47]

Tumors of the superficial facial structures, predominantly basal cell carcinomas, can extend into the orbit secondarily.

INTRAORBITAL LESIONS

Lacrimal Gland Masses

The lacrimal gland is located in the lacrimal fossa, in the superior lateral aspect of the orbit adjacent to the tendons of the superior and lateral rectus muscles. It is almond shaped, extraconal in position, and extends deep into the orbital septum. The lacrimal gland consists of two portions: (1) a large orbital or superior portion and (2) a small palpebral or inferior portion, which, however, is continuous behind. The histology of the lacrimal glands is similar to that of the salivary glands and, therefore, involved by similar disease processes.[14]

Epithelial tumors represent 50 percent of the tumors involving the lacrimal gland; half of these are pleomorphic adenomas, the other half malignant lesions. The malignant tumors include adenoid cystic carcinoma, malignant mixed tumor, epidermoid carcinoma, adenocarcinoma, squamous cell carcinoma, and undifferentiated (anaplastic) carcinoma. The remaining 50 percent of lacrimal gland lesions are of the lymphoid inflammatory type and represent a spectrum from the benign dacryoadenitis to malignant lymphoma. Tumors of the lacrimal gland and adjacent soft tissues may present with fullness of the eyelid, ptosis, or unilateral exophthalmos.[38]

Benign mixed tumors are the most common tumors of the lacrimal gland.[48] They may be small in size with a smooth surface, but larger tumors may show bosselation. Recurrent mixed tumors often have a nodular surface.

On CT pleomorphic adenomas may be homogeneous and enhance moderately following infusion of contrast material.[48] Lesions with cystic components often appear heterogeneous and may not enhance. As a result of slow growth, the lacrimal gland fossa and adjacent bone may be excavated (Fig. 6.10A). On rare occasions, a slight sclerotic reaction may be noted. The tumor margins are usually smooth and well defined, and the globe is displaced medially and inferiorly (Fig. 6.10). If the tumor extends posteriorly along the extraconal space, medial displacement of the medial rectus muscle or optic nerve may occur. Extension along the lateral rectus muscle may simulate a primary lesion

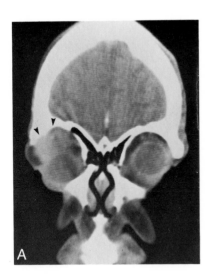
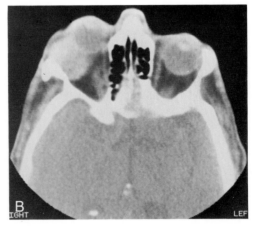

FIG. 6.10. Pleomorphic adenoma of the right lacrimal gland with indentation of the bony roof of the orbit in 74-year-old man with slowly progressive right exophthalmos. (A) Homogeneous mass in the upper lateral portion of the orbit causes marked inferior and medial displacement of the right globe. Note bilobed indentation of the roof of the orbit secondary to pressure from the adjacent tumor (arrowheads). (B) Axial CT section through the orbit demonstrates the homogeneous, sharply defined lacrimal gland tumor causing proptosis of the right globe.

in the muscle. A variable amount of proptosis is caused by large lacrimal gland lesions.[49]

Among the lacrimal gland tumors, adenoid cystic carcinoma represents the most common malignant tumor.[48] These tumors are infiltrative and are not surrounded by a capsule. Because of nerve involvement, pain is a common symptom. Frequently, the tumor extends into the bone and causes irregular destruction of the adjacent bony margins. The tumor may extend to the sclera and flatten the globe, which accounts for visual changes. In advanced cases the tumor invades the base of brain, including the pituitary gland. Metastases are not common and cervical and/or preauricular lymph nodes may be involved, although infrequently.

In addition to the adenoid cystic variety, miscellaneous malignant tumors are encountered.[48] Usually, these various malignant lesions cannot be differentiated by CT (Fig. 6.11). They all may cause bone destruction and extend widely through the orbit and adjacent structures, including the intracranial cavity.

CT can demonstrate the exact location and extension of these malignant lesions (Fig. 6.11). They show various attenuation values and may reveal contrast enhancement.[49] They invade adjacent orbital soft tissues and in advanced cases may extend into the temporal fossa and intracranial cavity. Their margins may be poorly defined and bone destruction can be identified, using the bone window technique.

The lacrimal gland can be involved by a diverse group of inflammatory lesions that have a variable appearance on the CT scan. Most of these lesions have a well-defined margin and a homogeneous appearance. The pathological spectrum extends from acute dacryoadenitis, showing smooth enlargement of

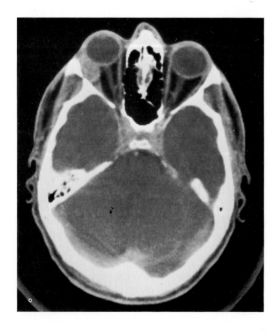

FIG. 6.11. Adenoid cystic carcinoma of the right lacrimal gland in 33-year-old man with right orbital fullness, proptosis, and pain. Axial CT section through the midorbits shows a homogeneous mass in the region of the right lacrimal gland with extension along the lateral rectus muscle. The tumor envelops the globe medially and causes proptosis.

one or both lacrimal glands, to lymphoid hyperplasia, Sjögren's syndrome, pseudotumor, or malignant lymphoma.

Epidermoid–Dermoid Cysts

Dermoid and epidermoid cysts are relatively common orbital lesions. They occur predominantly in the anterior portion of the orbit, especially in the superotemporal area. These cysts manifest an intermittent growth behavior. They are distributed through the pediatric and adult age group with the preponderance of patients under 20 years of age.[47]

The designation of these cysts as dermoids or epidermoids is largely based on the histological studies. There are no characteristic CT features that differentiate the two types. Epidermoids, in time, cause local pressure, erosion with a sharply defined rim, and, occasionally, a sclerotic reaction. Because of the high fat content, the majority of these lesions manifest as well-circumscribed cystic space-occupying lesions with a low absorption center (Fig. 6.12).[50] High density material may collect in the cystic cavity and produce a layering effect with a cystic area anteriorly and an isodense area posteriorly.[51] If the debris in the cyst cavity predominates, an isodense, sharply marginated mass may be found.[52] Medial displacement of the rectus muscles occurs when the cyst extends posteriorly. Bony abnormalities can be well delineated on CT by changing the window level and width.

Rhabdomyosarcoma

Embryonal rhabdomyosarcoma is the most common primary malignant orbital tumor of childhood. The tumor arises from the embryonic mesenchyma within the orbital soft tissues, rather than from the extraocular muscles.[53] Seventy-five percent of cases present before the age of 10 and only very rarely does the tumor present after the age of 25.[48] The tumor most often presents with exophthalmos. A palpable mass may be felt through the lids or conjunctiva, but the tumor is most often retrobulbar in location.[54,55] CT scanning is currently the best means of evaluating the tumor's extent. The tumor is usually of average density on plain scan and shows mild to moderate contrast enhancement.

At the time of presentation the tumor usually involves both the intraconal and extraconal spaces. The lesion is usually distinct from the globe and causes proptosis. Bony destructive changes may be present.[53]

Orbital Lymphoid Tumors

Lymphoid tumors are classified into benign pseudolymphomas (reactive lymphoid hyperplasia) and malignant lymphomas. Pathologically they are characterized by monomorphous sheets of lymphocytes lacking fibrotic stroma.[56,57]

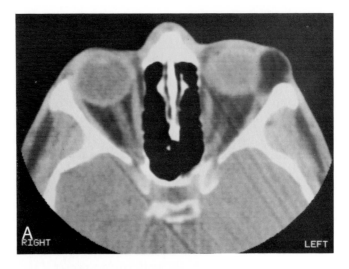

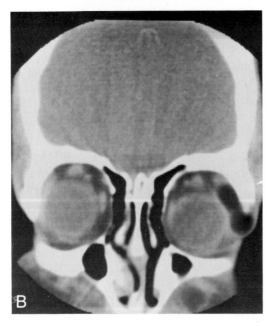

FIG. 6.12. Epidermoid cyst in the upper lateral portion of the left orbit in 28-year-old man with a mass in the upper lateral lid of the left orbit, which was noted since age 4 years. (A) Axial CT section through the mid-portion of the left orbit discloses a sharply defined low density mass in the anterior lateral portion of the orbit. (B) Coronal section reveals the same mass in the upper lateral portion of the orbit, causing no indentation of the globe, which is slightly displaced medially and inferiorly.

The incidence of lymphoid tumors ranges from 30 to 79 years of age, with a peak incidence in the sixth and seventh decades. The symptoms, in decreasing order of frequency, include proptosis, periocular swelling, diplopia, tearing, diminished visual acuity, and pain.[58] The onset of symptoms is slowly progressive, with a mean duration of 7.5 months. The proptosis measures about 5 mm and in the majority of patients ranges from 2 to 6 mm. Lymphoid tumors may be located in any part of the orbit but are situated most frequently in the upper portion of the orbit (Fig. 6.13). If the tumor is located anteriorly

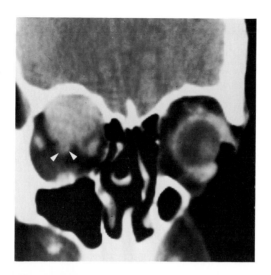

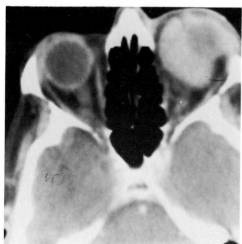

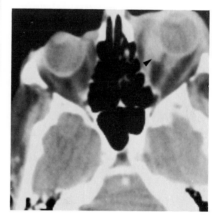

FIG. 6.13. Well-differentiated lymphocytic lymphoma of the left orbit in 88-year-old man with noted left ptosis and progressive exophthalmos over a period of 4 years. (A) Coronal CT section of the orbit demonstrates a homogeneous, sharply defined mass in the upper half of the right orbit. Note inferior displacement of the optic nerve (small arrowheads). (B) Axial CT sections through the upper orbits show an oval-shaped homogeneous mass adjacent to the posterior and medial aspect of the globe. (C) Axial scan through the mid-orbits reveals that the mass is partially intraconal (small arrowhead). The mass envelops the lateral portion of the globe and is partially extraconal anteriorly. Note proptosis of the globe.

(lacrimal gland, conjunctival tissue, lids), a mass may be palpated. CT demonstrates the location and extension of lymphoid neoplasms. Density characteristics, pre- and postcontrast, reveal no specific findings to suggest a histological diagnosis. Lymphoid lesions do not cause indentation of the globe (Fig. 6.13C). They frequently envelop the globe and extend posteriorly along muscles and fascial planes with an extra- and an intraconal component (Fig. 6.13). They are, in a small number of cases, confined to the intraconal space. If lymphoid tumors are limited in location to a muscle or lacrimal gland, difficulties may arise in the differential diagnosis. Bone erosion or excavation is rarely found in orbital lymphoma. The margin of the tumor is usually well defined but may be slightly knobby in some cases. Differentiation from other benign and malignant tumors cannot be determined by CT.

Vascular Neoplasms

Vascular lesions, the most common of which are cavernous hemangiomas and lymphangiomas, represent 10 to 15 percent of all orbital neoplasms.[59]

Hemangiomas

Cavernous hemangiomas are among the most common orbital tumors in adults. The neoplasm is encapsulated and is usually intraconal in location.[60,61] These tumors grow slowly and usually become manifest in the second to fourth decade, with exophthalmos the most common presenting symptom. On CT studies the tumors tend to demonstrate high absorption values on plain scan and show moderate contrast enhancement. Calcifications may occasionally occur.[61] The tumors tend to be oval or round in shape and have smooth, well-defined margins.[60] The vast majority of lesions are intraconal in location and two-thirds are localized lateral to the optic nerve. Bony expansion of the orbit was seen in 17 of 18 cases, indicative of the slow growing, benign nature of the tumor.[61]

Lymphangiomas

Lymphangiomas consist of a delicate network of vascular channels that resemble lymphatics. These spaces are usually filled with clear fluid, although blood can sometimes be found as well. The tumors are not well encapsulated and are usually infiltrative in nature.[61] They progress slowly and most commonly present in children and young adults. Lymphangiomas are usually highly absorptive on plain CT scan but tend to be heterogeneous in appearance. They usually demonstrate little or no contrast enhancement. The margins of the lesions are irregular and poorly defined. The tumor is most commonly extraconal in location, but both components of the retrobulbar space may be involved. Lymphangiomas are equally likely to occur anterior or posterior to the globe, and the majority are medial to the optic nerve. Since these tumors are slow growing, expansion of the bony orbit can occur.[61]

Hemangiopericytoma

Hemangiopericytoma is a distinct tumor entity arising from pericytes. The majority of lesions are slow growing. However, variation in growth rates ranging from 3 weeks to 30 years have been encountered.[62] Many of the tumors are well circumscribed, dark red-to-purple blue lesions with thin capsules or pseudocapsules. They have a rich vascular supply and a tendency to bleed during surgery. Focal areas of hemorrhage and cyst formation are encountered. The tumor has no preferred location in the orbit. Clinical features are dependent on the location of the tumor. Progressive, painless exophthalmos, with occasional lid edema, is the most frequent clinical presentation. Complete surgical excision is mandatory to prevent recurrence. Distant metastases occur in a certain number of cases. On the basis of histology, it is difficult to predict whether the tumor will be benign or malignant in behavior. Hemangiopericytomas appear well defined on CT. They have high absorption areas on plain CT scan and show a variable degree of enhancement.[63] The increased enhancement effect, reflecting the vascular nature of the lesion, is best demonstrated on CT by a bolus injection followed by intravenous infusion.

Arteriovenous Malformation and Carotid Cavernous Fistulas

Isolated arteriovenous (AV) malformations of the orbit are rare. Lesions in this area are usually associated with intracranial AV malformations.[64,65] The Wyburn-Mason syndrome consists of an AV malformation that extends from the region of the midbrain anteriorly, down the visual pathways to involve both the orbit and retina. AV malformations localized to the orbit may be secondary to trauma.[2]

Clinically, pulsatile exophthalmos is frequently seen and an associated bruit may be audible to the patient. Chronic mass effect and pulsations may lead to optic atrophy and gliosis.

On CT orbital AV malformations appear as irregular tortuous structures that demonstrate marked contrast, and the ophthalmic artery may appear prominent. Within the orbit AV malformations can be located in both the intraconal and extraconal compartments and an intracranial component of the malformation may often be demonstrated.[52,65,66]

Carotid–Cavernous Sinus Fistula

Carotid–cavernous fistulas (CCFs) are abnormal communications between the carotid artery and the cavernous sinus (Fig. 6.14A). The spontaneous ones are secondary to a dural arteriovenous malformation or the rupture of an intracavernous carotid aneurysm.[67]

Clinically CCFs usually present with pulsatile exophthalmos and orbital congestion. The optic nerve can be stretched, leading to visual loss or blindness, and increased pressure within the cavernous sinus can lead to cranial nerve palsies.

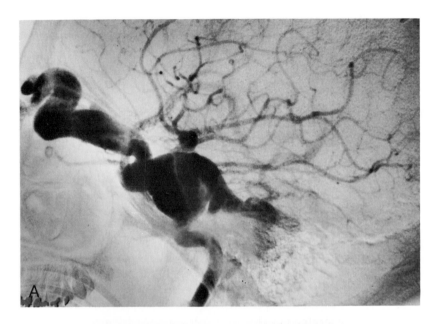

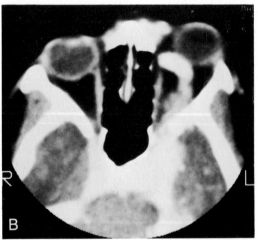

FIG. 6.14. Left carotid cavernous sinus fistula in 19-year-old woman with posttraumatic pulsatile exophthalmos. (A) Subtraction, lateral angiographic study reveals a markedly dilated cavernous sinus and superior ophthalmic vein caused by the carotid cavernous sinus fistula. Also note some reflux into the petrosal veins posteriorly. (B) Moderately enlarged superior ophthalmic vein extending via the superior orbital fissure into an enlarged left carotid cavernous sinus. Note proptosis of the left globe.

On CT, proptosis and an enlarged superior ophthalmic vein are the most common findings (Fig. 6.14B). In addition, irregular tortuous vessels that demonstrate marked contrast enhancement are demonstrated in both the intra- and extraconal compartments. Along with these findings, prominence of the ipsilateral cavernous sinus may be evident (Fig. 6.14B). The extraocular muscles may also enlarge, presumably secondary to venous hypertension and vascular engorgement.[68]

ORBITAL INFECTION AND ITS CEREBRAL COMPLICATIONS

Bacterial inflammatory disease of the orbit is most often due to sinus infection,[69-71] skin infection, insect bite, impetigo, or the presence of a foreign body.[72] A distinction should be made between preseptal and postseptal infections of the orbit. The orbital septum, a periosteal reflection from the anterior bony margin of the orbit, inserts on the tarsal plates of the eyelids and acts as a barrier to the spread of infection into the orbit.[70,73] The infection may spread into various compartments of the orbit via venous intercommunications (thrombophlebitis), foramina, or congenital osseous dehiscences. The crossover of infection from the sinuses, particularly the ethmoid sinus, is facilitated by the lack of valves in the veins between the orbit and sinus cavities. Infection of the orbit can be located in the subperiosteal space (between the bony orbital wall and its periosteal lining) or the extraconal and intraconal spaces. CT provides information concerning the location and extent of orbital infection. Preseptal cellulitis is reflected by considerable swelling of the eyelids and conjunctiva (Fig. 6.15). If the infectious process extends into the subperiosteal space, the periosteal lining is displaced medially and may slightly enhance following

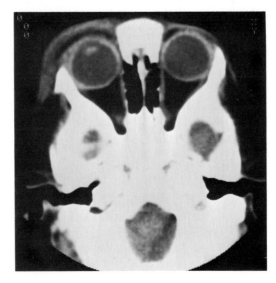

FIG. 6.15. Preseptal right orbital cellulitis. 8½-month-old baby girl with 8-hr history of right periorbital swelling. Horizontal CT scan demonstrates marked periorbital swelling of the lid and conjunctiva of the right eye. Note normal ethmoid sinuses.

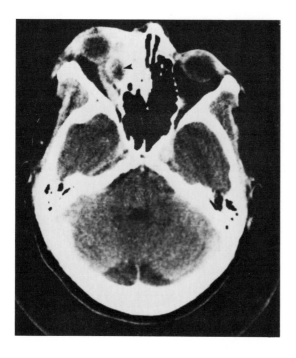

FIG. 6.16. Orbital subperiosteal abscess with orbital cellulitis secondary to right ethmoid sinusitis in 33-year-old woman with history of a LeFort II fracture on the right. She developed swelling and pain of right orbit together with redness of right cheek. Axial CT sections through the mid-portion of the orbits outlines a subperiosteal inflammatory mass enveloping the proptotic right globe. Some lateral displacement of the optic nerve is present. Note oval-shaped, low density area adjacent to the medial wall of the right orbit in the mid third secondary to an abscess (arrowhead).

contrast infusion. A hemispherical shaped inflammatory mass is usually seen projecting into the medial aspect of the orbital cavity (Fig. 6.16). A low density area with an enhancing rim suggests an abscess in the subperiosteal space. The adjacent medial rectus muscle is often edematous and enlarged. Associated uveoscleral thickening may occur from the adjacent inflammatory process. Gas may also be found within the abscess cavities, either in the subperiosteal space or in the orbital and periorbital soft tissue structures. Inflammation within the intraconal space obliterates the sharp outline of the optic nerve and muscle and causes increased density of the fatty tissue. If the inflammatory mass increases in size, considerable proptosis and displacement of the globe will occur. When the infection remains unchecked, palsies of the third, fourth and sixth cranial nerves may ensue. Intracranial extension is indicated by meningimus, retro-orbital pain with severe proptosis, and signs of septic cavernous sinus thrombosis.

Graves' Disease

In adults Graves' disease is the most common cause for unilateral or bilateral exophthalmos. It accounts for approximately 16 percent of patients presenting with unilateral proptosis and for a great majority of cases with bilateral proptosis. The disease is most commonly encountered in middle-aged females, with a female-to-male incidence of 4:1. It also occurs in children and accounts for 14 percent of all causes of exophthalmos in patients younger than 15 years of age.[74] Endocrine ophthalmopathy may occur before, during, or after the phase of systemic hyperthyroidism. Pathologically, one finds an abundance of mucopolysaccharides (hyaluronic acid), collagen, and glycoproteins. The osmotic pressure in the orbit is increased by the capacity of hyaluronic acid to bind water. In the initial stages of Graves' disease, the fat content may increase considerably and lead to prolapse of fat anteriorly, with anterior displacement of the orbital septum. In the late stages, however, fibrous tissue is laid down to replace the orbital fat and muscles. Muscle enlargement in the posterior portion of the orbit leads to compression of the optic nerve with resultant loss of vision.

Extraocular muscle thickening is reported to be bilaterally symmetrical in 70 percent of cases. It is asymmetrical, either unilateral or bilaterally, in 30 percent.[75] Unilateral disease occurs in about 6 percent of cases. The inferior and medial rectus muscles are the most frequently involved and are the most severely affected. The CT reveals muscle enlargement with a fusiform configuration in the axial projection, which should be supplemented with a coronal projection (Fig. 6.17). Minimal muscle enlargement is difficult to determine on CT. In addition, orbital fat is increased, with forward bulging of the orbital septum. In the late stages of Graves' ophthalmopathy, the optic nerve may be enlarged. Slight bony displacement of the medial wall of the orbit or even bony erosion, presumably as the result of direct pressure from large extraocular muscles, has been reported.[76]

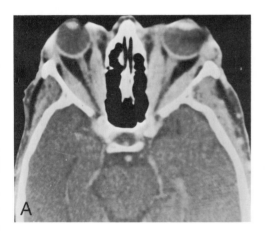
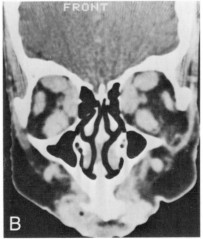

FIG. 6.17.   Grave's disease in 80-year-old woman with bilateral proptosis. (A) Axial CT sections through both orbits reveals marked enlargement of the medial and lateral rectus muscles and bilateral proptosis. (B) Coronal scan through the mid-orbits demonstrates marked enlargement of all rectus muscles in both orbits but predominantly in the superior, medial, and lower rectus muscles.

Orbital Pseudotumor

Pseudotumor constitutes an idiopathic inflammatory process without identifiable cause. The disease process may be localized or diffuse and can involve any site, tissue, or group of tissues of the orbit. The disease may also involve the globe, in conjunction with orbital involvement. Histological examination reveals a polymorphous inflammatory cell infiltrate with a significant reactive fibrovascular component. In cases where lymphocytes predominate, a diagnosis of reactive lymphocytic hyperplasia is made. In this latter category, the possibility of lymphoma must be considered and close follow-up is indicated.[77]

Males and females appear to be equally afflicted and there is no racial predilection. The disease is most common in middle age, but can affect children as well as patients in the sixth and seventh decades of life. The disease process tends to be unilateral. If the lesion involves both sides, systemic disease or endocrine exophthalmos should be considered. The disease develops most often in a matter of months, usually less than 6, but has a rapid onset in acute cases. Proptosis and pain are the main features. Swollen lids, pain, vascular engorgement (predominantly at the insertions of the rectus muscles), limitation of extraocular muscle movement, papilledema, and optic neuropathy are other clinical findings. Patients also display constitutional symptoms such as malaise and distress. Pseudotumor may have a remitting course or respond to steroid

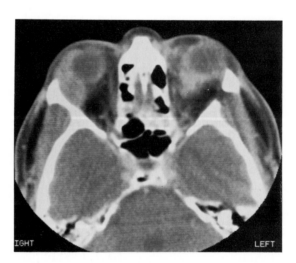

FIG. 6.18.   Bilateral pseudotumor of the orbits in 20-year-old man with recurrent swelling in the region of the left lacrimal gland 3 years prior to admission and swelling of the right eye on the present admission. Axial CT section demonstrates marked enlargement of the right lacrimal gland. Some ill-defined increase in density in the remaining soft tissue structures of the right orbit, together with slight thickening of the uveoscleral coat, is also present. Note ill-defined increase in density in the left orbit, predominantly in the retroocular space medial to the optic nerve. Also note thickening of the uveoscleral coat.

treatment. In some cases, multiple recurrences or a progressive course with loss of vision and progressive proptosis are observed, despite treatment. A lesion may be limited to one muscle or may involve the entire orbit, including the lacrimal gland. In cases with myositis, the inferior rectus muscle is most frequently involved, either alone or with other muscles. Visual loss is a serious complication in pseudotumor.

The various types of pseudotumor can be accurately localized by CT.[78] Nugent et al.[79] have classified pseudotumors into five anatomic patterns: (1) anterior, (2) posterior, (3) diffuse, (4) lacrimal, and (5) myositic. The anatomic distribution correlated well with the clinical features of acute pseudotumor. The authors noted that lacrimal and myositic pseudotumors resolved more rapidly with steroid therapy than did the remaining groups.

Anterior pseudotumor is localized in the retrobulbar space adjacent to the posterior pole of the globe, whereas the posterior variety is situated in the apex of the orbit. Both the anterior and posterior types of pseudotumor obliterate segments of the optic nerve. The diffuse form of pseudotumor involves the entire orbit, causing effacement of muscles and the optic nerve (Fig. 6.18). The myositic form of pseudotumor is often limited to one or more muscles, which are enlarged and often irregular in outline (Fig. 6.19). Enlargement of

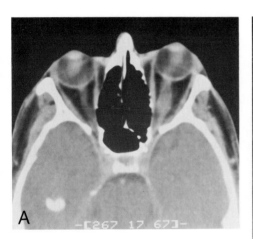
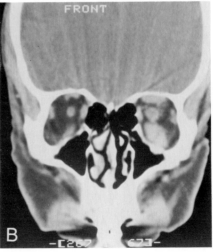

FIG. 6.19. Pseudotumor of the left orbit involving the muscles and optic nerve in 60-year-old man with left proptosis, pain, and conjunctival injection. (A) Axial CT scan through the mid-portion of both orbits shows diffuse, moderate thickening of the left optic nerve together with left proptosis. (B) Axial CT section through the mid-portion of both orbits reveals diffuse enlargement of the superior and inferior rectus muscles along with enlargement of the optic nerve. Compare with normal right side.

the optic nerve may also occur (Fig. 6.19). Pseudotumor may be limited to the lacrimal gland and cause diffuse enlargement.

Enlarged extraocular muscles are encountered in a variety of pathological conditions.[80] Enlarged muscles are found in Graves' disease, carotid–cavernous sinus fistula, AV malformation, and primary or metastatic tumors. In vascular abnormalities, the superior ophthalmic vein is enlarged in conjunction with an increase in muscle size. Muscle enlargement in Graves' disease is usually smooth and often asymmetrical.

OPTIC NERVE LESIONS

A large number of conditions can involve the optic nerve and most frequently manifest themselves as enlargement of the optic nerve, either focally or diffusely (Table 6.1).[81]

Optic Nerve Gliomas

Optic nerve gliomas account for approximately 3 percent of all orbital tumors and outnumber optic nerve meningiomas by 3 or 4 to 1. The peak incidence of this tumor is in the 2- to 6-year age group, with 75 percent of cases presenting in the first decade and 90 percent in the first two decades of life. There is an increased incidence of this tumor in patients with neurofibromatosis. In this age group the incidence in males and in females is essentially equal and the most common initial symptoms are decreased visual acuity and exophthalmos, which is usually mild.[82] Optic gliomas of adulthood behave in a more aggressive invasive fashion and are more common in males.[83]

Anatomically, the optic nerve is not comparable with other peripheral nerves but is, in fact, more similar to fiber tracts of the brain. It differs from other central nervous system fiber tracts in that it has its own surrounding meningeal sheath and is divided into bundles by extensions of pial tissue. Optic nerve gliomas are essentially brain tumors and are most frequently grade I astrocytomas; however, pathologically most optic gliomas of adulthood are glioblastoma multiforme.[83]

Optic nerve gliomas may occur anywhere along the optic pathway. In a recent series of gliomas of the anterior optic pathway, the intraorbital optic nerves were involved either unilaterally or bilaterally in approximately two-thirds of cases and the optic chiasm was involved in 95 percent of cases.[28] Thus it appears that although a glioma can involve just the intraorbital optic nerve, associated involvement of the chiasm is much more common.[28]

By CT intraorbital optic nerve gliomas appear as either a fusiform or sausage-shaped enlargement of the optic nerve (Fig. 6.5A). The margins of the lesion tend to be smooth and the lesions are usually isodense with the optic nerve, which is not separable from the tumor. If the tumor is large and occupies much of the intraconal space, differentiation from other intraconal lesions such as a cavernous hemangioma can be difficult, although in this instance, contrast enhancement may be of help, making it possible to separate the enhancing hemangioma from the normal but displaced optic nerve.[45,81,89]

Calcification may rarely occur.[55] Optic nerve gliomas do often demonstrate contrast enhancement, but the degree of enhancement usually varies from imperceptible to moderate and is generally less intense than the enhancement seen with meningiomas.[52,54,81] The "railroad track" sign seen with meningiomas has not been reported in gliomas.

Optic Neuritis/Papilledema

Optic neuritis is an acute inflammation of the optic nerve. Although it may be associated with other inflammatory diseases, it is most frequently associated with multiple sclerosis. Patients with optic neuritis commonly go on to develop clinically definite multiple sclerosis although there is a dispute over the frequency of this evolution, with figures ranging from 13 to 85 percent having been reported in the literature. A recent review seems to support the point of view that optic neuritis is a form of multiple sclerosis, with approximately 50 percent of patients going on to develop multiple sclerosis.[85]

By CT the optic nerve may appear enlarged and demonstrate increased tortuosity in optic neuritis.[81,86,87] Contrast enhancement of the optic nerve can occasionally be seen, presumably secondary to increased vascular permeability.[81] The above changes may be reversible as the neuritis subsides. The optic nerve may, however, appear normal in optic neuritis; one investigation has reported seeing definite optic nerve abnormalities in 20 percent of patients with the clinical diagnosis of optic neuritis.[81] In another large series, the optic nerve appeared normal in 12 of 19 cases of optic neuritis.[88]

The subarachnoid space continues into the orbit as part of the optic nerve sheath and enhancement of the optic nerve may be seen during metrizamide CT cisternography.[89] Frequent enlargement of the optic nerves in cases of intracranial hypertension has been shown,[88] and it is postulated that this reflects transmission of the elevated pressure into the orbital optic nerve sheath, causing enlargement of this space.[81,88]

EYE LESIONS

Retinoblastoma

Retinoblastomas occur in about 1/17,000 to 1/34,000 of live births.[90] They usually present in the first 2 years of life, although cases have been recorded in adults.[91] Most cases result from spontaneous mutation; the familial incidence is approximately 10 percent.

The clinical signs and symptoms consist of a white pupillary reflex (leukocoria), strabismus, painful red eye with or without glaucoma, nystagmus, hyphema, uveitis, heterochromia iridis, mydriasis, and orbital cellulitis. Exophthalmos is less common and is encountered when the tumor extends into the orbit. About 34 percent of patients have independent foci within the eye. In 30 percent of patients, bilateral lesions are found. Pathological examination can differentiate between endophytic and exophytic growth, with spread by implantation to the choroidal, retinal, and posterior corneal surfaces. The endophytic type is the most common and growth extends into the vitreous. Optic nerve invasion has been reported in 12.7 percent of cases[92] and orbital extension in 8 percent.[77]

CT reveals densities with high absorption values, which are usually well defined in small to moderate sized lesions (Fig. 6.20).[93,94] The high densities with high absorption values are secondary to calcium deposits, which may be focal or involve the entire tumor.[95] Calcific deposits are rarely encountered in extraglobal retinoblastomas.[94] Large tumors present as irregular masses that may occupy a large area of the vitreous. Noncalcified areas of tumor may be of low density and enhance following contrast infusion. Retinoblastomas that are confined to the globe have been reported to occur in 80 to 90 percent of cases in which pathologic specimens were obtained.[96] Extraglobal extensions are readily detected by CT. Thickening of the optic nerve is a reflection of the tumor spread along the nerve, which may advance into the intracranial cavity via the subarachnoid pathway.

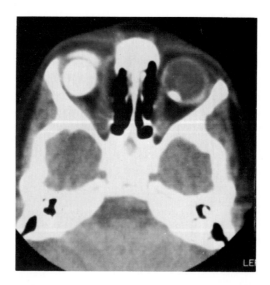

FIG. 6.20. Bilateral retinoblastomas. 11-month-old girl had enucleation of the right eye for a large retinoblastoma. Patient also had a tumor in the left eye (well circumscribed) inferonasally and greater than 10 disc diameters. The patient received radiation for tumor in left eye. Axial CT section through the orbits reveals a prosthesis on the right. On the left, there is an oval-shaped, high density area in the retina slightly medial to the optic nerve disc.

CT following radiation therapy shows reduction of the tumor mass, with consolidation of the calcific deposits. Secondary retinal detachment may diminish or resolve.[95]

Extrusion of the previously satisfactory prosthesis following enucleation may suggest an orbital recurrence of retinoblastoma and indicate the need for follow-up examinations.

Malignant Melanoma

Malignant melanomas occur in all adult age groups, but most frequently in the sixth and seventh decades of life.[97] They are almost always single and unilocular and are located in the choroid. Malignant melanomas may invade the local structures and cause blood-borne metastases.

Cure rates are adversely affected by large tumor size and infiltration to the angle, sclera, ciliary body, optic nerve, and extraglobal tissues.[98]

A high resolution CT with 1- to 2-mm sections provides valuable information regarding tumor size, location, and extension, predominantly outside the globe and into the optic nerve (Fig. 6.21).[41] In early lesions, the only finding may be slight thickening of the uveoscleral layers. Absorption values of the tumor and enhancement patterns, following infusion of contrast material, are nonspecific and do not allow differentiation from other tumors such as metastatic deposits.

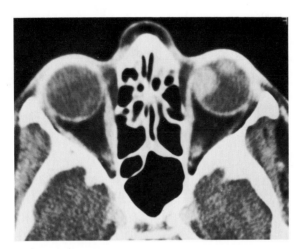

FIG. 6.21. Melanoma of the left globe in 43-year-old woman. A mass was noted within the right globe nasally on ophthalmological examination. Axial CT section reveals a polypoid, sharply defined homogeneous mass arising from the medial aspect of the choroid between 8 o'clock and 11 o'clock. There is no extrascleral extension.

Optic Nerve Drusen

Optic nerve drusen are hyaline bodies found on the optic disc or deep within the substance. They increase in size by accretion, often calcify, and result in a laminated structure.[99] They have been described in association with tuberous sclerosis, angioid streaks, pseudoxanthoma elasticum, pigmentary degeneration of the retina, optic atrophy, and renal dysfunction.

Optic nerve drusen have a waxy, white, glistening, irregular appearance when they are located in the superficial portion of the disc. If the papilla is raised and has a blurred margin, the condition may be confused with papilledema.[100] The condition is often familial, occurring in siblings and parents. Other than causing confusion with papilledema, the process is seldom of any importance. Occasionally, visual field defects, arcuate in nature, are caused by nerve fiber damage. CT in the axial and coronal planes reveals well-defined punctate lesions of high density in one or both of the optic nerve heads (Fig. 6.22).[101] Buried drusen, not ophthalmoscopically evident, have been shown by CT. It is not certain at what age disc elevation develops or at what stage calcification can be detected by CT.

Choroidal Osteoma

Choroidal osteomas are composed of mature bone with a hypocellular marrow.[102,103] They occur predominantly in females but have been reported in males. They arise in the juxtapapillary choroid and manifest as orange to orange-white, sharply defined elevations of the retina.

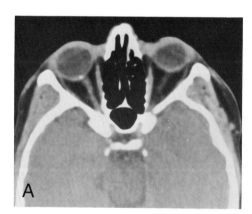
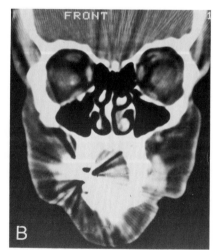

FIG. 6.22. Optic nerve disc druse in 43-year-old woman with slowly progressive visual loss in right eye accompanied by optic atrophy. (A) Axial CT section reveals a sharply marginated, punctate calcific density at the right optic nerve disc. (B) Coronal CT scan localizes this density to the inferior lateral portion of the optic nerve disc.

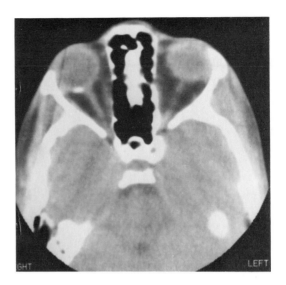

FIG. 6.23. Choroid osteoma of the right globe lateral to the optic nerve disc. The patient was found to have a subretinal neovascular membrane in right eye, lateral to the globe and overlying the choroid osteoma. Axial CT section reveals an oval-shaped bony density lateral to the optic nerve disc within the choroid.

The patients are usually asymptomatic in childhood, but may present with central or paracentral scotoma in later life.

CT demonstrates a sharply marginated, high density area, round to oval in shape, and located in the posterior globe (Fig. 6.23). The lesion may be single or multiple and may be present in either one globe or bilaterally.

Phthisis Bulbi

Phthisis bulbi represents the end stage of diffuse ocular disease caused by a variety of conditions.[104] The most common etiologies are longstanding inflammatory disease, glaucoma, foreign bodies, trauma, severe global damage and rupture, or as a complication following surgery.[96]

The globe is markedly atrophied and the ocular structures are shrunken and disorganized. In the course of time, calcium is deposited within the cataractous lens, sclera, uvea, and gliotic retina.

CT shows a shrunken irregular globe, with multiple globular or linear calcific densities (Fig. 6.24).

Staphyloma

A staphyloma is characterized by localized or general ectasia of the scleral tissue, with uveal tissue present within the tissue bulge. The staphyloma can be localized in various parts of the globe.

CT demonstrates the ectasia of the globe and the location and size of the staphyloma (Fig. 6.25).

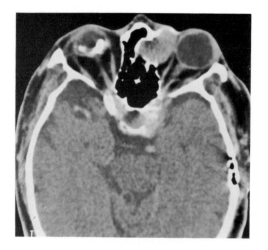

FIG. 6.24. Phthisis bulbi of the right globe. 55-year-old man was blinded in the right eye by a traumatic accident sustained at age 14. Axial CT section reveals a shrunken globe with posterior calcification. Incidental note is made of a mucocele in the anterior left ethmoid sinus.

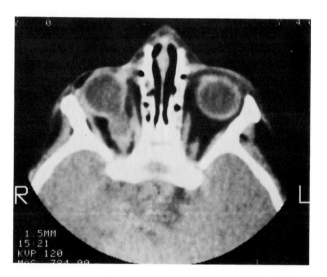

FIG. 6.25. Staphyloma in the posterior globe in 2-year-old boy with right microphthalmos and staphyloma in the posterior globe; no vision is present in right eye. Axial CT sections of both orbits reveal microphthalmos on the right with localized ectasia of the uveolsceral coat into the optic nerve.

SUMMARY AND CONCLUSION

CT of the eye and orbit is the most important imaging modality utilized today in orbital diagnosis. The advent of high resolution scanners has made the CT assessment of several eye diseases, other than retinoblastoma and melanoma, possible. With further technical improvements, more disease entities will be added to this list. It is mandatory to add coronal sections to the baseline axial sections for (1) evaluating diseases adjacent to the roof and floor of the orbit, (2) defining the relationship of masses to the optic nerve, (3) determining the superoinferior dimension of lesions, particularly tumors, (4) better defining the muscle enlargement secondary to Graves' disease and pseudotumor, and (5) delineating optic nerve enlargement and separating the nerve fibers from the thickened optic nerve sheath in meningioma.

Administration of an intravenous contrast medium (42 g iodine) adds a further dimension to the diagnosis of orbital lesions, predominantly tumors. Marked enhancement ensues in vascular tumors (hemangioma, hemangiopericytoma), aneurysms, AV malformations, and shunts (carotid cavernous sinus fistulas).

Low density lesions (epidermoid, lipoma) are fairly characteristic and allow a specific diagnosis. Exophthalmos caused by inflammatory disease (Graves' disease, pseudotumor, complications of sinus disease) can often be accurately assessed, in conjunction with the clinical findings. Calcifications and bone densities found in etiologically unrelated conditions are well defined by CT (meningioma, retinoblastoma, choroid osteoma, drusen, phthisis oculi). The sensitivity of CT is much greater for detecting calcific densities, as is exemplified in the diagnosis of retinoblastoma. CT has played an important role in evaluating pathological conditions that extend into the orbit secondarily from the paranasal sinuses (infection, benign and malignant tumors) and the intracranial cavity (meningioma, neurogenic tumors, pituitary lesions, and a miscellaneous group of rarer lesions). It becomes clear from this discussion that the ultimate diagnosis is the synthesis of all parameters: clinical evaluation, size, shape and location of lesions, density characteristics, and enhancement patterns.

REFERENCES

1. Dallow RL, Weber AL: Combined ultrasonography, computerized tomography and radiology in evaluation of orbital disease. pp. 15–23. Proceedings Third International Symposium in Orbital Disorders, Amsterdam, 1977.
2. Dilenge D: Angiography in angiomas of the orbit. Radiology 113:355–361, 1974.
3. Newton TH, Hoyt WF: Dural arteriovenous shunts in the region of the cavernous sinuses. Neuroradiology 1:71–81, 1971.
4. Weisberg CA: Computed tomographic findings in carotid–cavernous sinus fistula. Comput Tomogr 5:31–36, 1981.
5. Lloyd GA, Wright JE, Morgan G: Venous malformations in the orbit. Br J Ophthalmol 55:505–516, 1971.
6. Mafee MF, Goldberg MF, Valvassori GE, Capek V: Computed tomography in the evaluation of patients with persistent hyperplastic primary vitreous (PHPV). Radiology 145:713–717, 1982.
7. Hawkes RC, Holland GN, Moore WS, et al.: NMR imaging in the evaluation of orbital tumors. AJNR 4:254–256, 1983.
8. Hammerschlag SR, O'Reilly GV, Naheedy MH: Computed tomography of the optic canals. AJNR 2:593–594, 1981.
9. Tadmor R, New PF: Computed tomography of the orbit with special emphasis on coronal sections. Part 1. Normal anatomy. J Comput Assist Tomogr 2:24–34, 1978.

10. Forbes GS, Earnest F, Waller RR: Computed tomography of orbital tumors including late-generation scanning techniques. Radiology 142:387–394, 1982.

11. Beck TJ, Rosenbaum AE, Miller NR: Orbital computed tomography: technical aspects. Int Ophthal Clin 22:7–43, 1982.

12. Unsöld R: Computed tomographic anatomy of the orbit. Int Ophthalmol Clin 22:45–80, 1982.

13. Grove AS (ed): Computed tomography in ophthalmology. Int Ophthalmol Clin 22:1–240, 1982.

14. Warwick R: Eugene Wolff's Anatomy of the Eye and Orbit. 7th Ed. WB Saunders, Philadelphia, 1976.

15. Weinstein MA, Modic MT, Risius B, et al.: Visualization of the arteries, veins and nerves of the orbit by sector computed tomography. Radiology 138:83–87, 1981.

16. Henderson JW, Farrow GM: Primary orbital hemangiopericytoma. Arch Ophthalmol 96:666, 1978.

17. Vladyka, Vladykova J, Ciganek L: Diagnosis and therapeutic possibilities in orbital meningiomas. OFTAC 39:123–127, 1983.

18. Lloyd GAS: Primary orbital meningioma. A review of 41 patients investigated radiologically. Clinical Radiology 33:181–187, 1982.

19. New PFS, Aronon S, Hesselink JR: National Cancer Institute Study. Evaluation of computed tomography in the dx of intracranial neoplasms. IV. Meningioma. Radiology 136:665–675, 1980.

20. Godel V, Yoram S, Shanon E, et al.: Maxillary meningioma appearing as exophthalmos. Arch Otolaryngol 107:626–628, 1971.

21. Nakagawa H, Lusins JO: Biplane computed tomography of intracranial meningioma with intracranial extension. J Comput Assist Tomogr 4:478–483, 1980.

22. Hart WM, Burde RM, Klingele TG, et al.: Bilateral optic nerve sheath meningioma. Arch Ophthalmol 98:149–151, 1980.

23. Claveria LE, Sutton D, Tress BM: The radiological diagnosis of meningiomas. The impact of EMI scanning. Br J Radiol 50:15–22, 1977.

24. Robbins SL.: Pathologic basis of disease. WB Saunders, Philadelphia, 1974.

25. Kernohan JW, Sayre GP: Tumors of the central nervous system. Section X. Fasc 35, Atlas of Tumor Pathology. Armed Forces Institute of Pathology, Washington, DC, 1952.

26. Taveras JM, Wood EH: Diagnostic Neuroradiology. Williams & Wilkins, Baltimore, 1976.

27. Daniels DL, Williams AL, Sylverstein A, et al.: CT recognition of optic nerve sheath meningioma and abnormal sheath visualization. AJNR 3:181–183, 1982.

28. Savoiardo M, Harwood-Nash DC, Tadmor R, et al.: Gliomas of the intracranial anterior optic pathways in children. Radiology 138:601–610, 1981.

29. Byrd SE, Harwood-Nash DC, Faz CR, et al.: Computed tomography of intraorbital optic nerve gliomas in children. Radiology 129:73–78, 1978.

30. Nabwi P, Tan WS, Spigus DG.: Carotid ophthalmic artery aneurysm: a report of two cases. Radiolog 23:137–138, 1983.

31. Weber AL, Davis KR, Ojemann RG, et al.: Internal carotid artery aneurysm. Ann Otol Rhinol Laryngol 91:543–545.

32. Schubiger O, Valavanis A, Hazek J: Computed tomography in cerebral aneurysms with special emphasis on giant intracranial aneurysms. J Comput Assist Tomogr 4:24–32, 1980.

33. Pinto RS, Kricheff II, Butler AR, et al.: Correlation of computed tomographic angiographs and neuropathological changes in giant cerebral aneurysms. Radiology 132:85–92, 1979.

34. Wander JV, Das Gupta TK: Neurofibromatosis. Curr Probl Surg 14:1–81, 1977.

35. Zimmerman RA, Bilaniuk LT, Metzger RA, et al.: Computed tomography of orbital facial neurofibromatosis. Radiology 146:113–116, 1983.

36. Jacoby CG, GO RT, Beren RA: Cranial CT of neurofibromatosis. AJR 135:553–557, 1980.

37. Kobrin JL, Block FC, Weingiest TA. Ocular and orbital manifestations of neurofibromatosis. Surv Ophthalmol 24:45–51, 1979.

38. Henderson JW: Orbital Tumors. 2nd Ed. pp 136–143. Brian C. Decker, New York, 1980.

39. Ferry AP, Font RL: Carcinoma metastatic to the eye and orbit. I. A clinicopathological study of 227 cases. Arch Ophthalmol 92:276–286, 1974.

40. Albert DM, Rubenstein RA, Scheis HG: Tumor metastases to the eye. 1. Incidence in 213 adult patients with generalized malignancy. Am J Ophthalmol 63:723, 1967.

41. Bernardino ME, Danziger J, Young SE, Wallace S: Computed tomography in ocular neoplastic disease. AJR 131:111, 1978.

42. Hesselink JR, Davis KR, Weber AL, et al.: Radiological evaluation of orbital metastases with emphasis on computed tomography. Radiology 137:363–366, 1980.

43. Hesselink JR, Weber AL: Pathways of orbital extension of extraorbital neoplasms. J Comput Assist Tomogr 6:593–597, 1982.

44. Bilaniuk LT, Zimmerman RA: Computer assisted tomography: sinus lesions with orbital involvement. Head Neck Surg 2:291–301, 1980.

45. Weber AL, Stanton AC: Malignant tumors of the paranasal sinuses. Radiological, clinical and histopathological evaluation of 200 cases. Head Neck Surg 6:761–776, 1984.

46. Weber AL, Provenzano DE. Nasopharyngeal masses. Radiolog 2:1–32, 1982.

47. Bryan RN, Sessions RB, Horowitz BL: Radiographic management of juvenile angiofibromas. AJNR 2:157, 1981.

48. Foote FW Jr, Frazell EL: Tumors of the Major Salivary Glands. An Atlas of Tumor Pathology. Sect 4. Fascicle 11. Armed Forces Institute of Pathology, Washington, D.C., 1954.

49. Hesselink JR, Davis KR, Dallow RL, et al.: Computed tomography of masses in the lacrimal gland region. Radiology 131:143–147, 1979.

50. Blei L, Chambers JT, Liotta LA, et al.: Orbital dermoid diagnosed by computed tomographic scanning. Am J Ophthalmol 85:58–61, 1978.

51. Hammerschlag SB, Hesselink JR, Weber AL: Computed tomography of the Eye and Orbit. Appleton-Century Crofts, Norwalk, Connecticut, 1983.

52. Hilal SK, Trokel SL. Computerized tomography of the orbit using thin sections. Seminars in Roentgenology 12:137–147, 1977.

53. Danziger J, Handel S, Jing B, et al.: Computerized tomography in rhabdomyosarcoma of the head and neck. Cancer 49:463–467, 1979.

54. Smith VH: Tumors of the head: orbital tumors. Brit J Hosp Med 28:22–25, 1982.

55. Price HI, Danziger A: The computerized tomographic findings in paedriatric orbital tumors. Clin Radiol 30:435–440, 1979.

56. Jakobiec FA, McLean F, Font R: Clinicopathologic characteristics of orbital lymphoid hyperplasia. Ophthalmology 86:948, 1979.

57. Jakobiec FA: in discussion; Henderson JW, Fallow GM: Primary malignant mixed tumors of the lacrimal glands. Ophthalmology 87:473, 1980.

58. Yeo JH, Jakobiec FA, Abbott GF, Trokel SL: Combined clinical and computed tomographic diagnosis of orbital lymphoid tumors. Am J Ophthalmol 94:235–245, 1980.

59. Henderson JW: Orbital Tumors. WB Saunders, Philadelphia, 1973.

60. Forbes GS, Sheedy PF, Waller RR: Orbital tumors evaluated by computed tomography. Radiology 136:107–111, 1980.

61. Davis KR, Hesselink JR, Dallow RL, et al.: CT and ultrasound in the diagnosis of cavernous hemangiomas and lymphangiomas of the orbit. CT 4:98–104, 1980.

62. Searl SS, Chew N: Hemangiopericytoma. Int Ophthalmol Clin 22:141–162, 1982. In: Tumors of the Eyelid and Orbit: A Chinese-American Collaborative Study.

63. Cromwell LD, Kerber L, Margolis MT: Selective carotid angiography in the diagnosis of orbital hemangiopericytoma: report of two cases. AJR 129:730–733, 1977.

64. Salvoni U, Menichelli F, Pasquini U: Computer assisted tomography in 90 cases of exophthalmos. J Comput Assist Tomogr 1:81, 1977.

65. Wende S, Aulich A, Nover A, et al.: Computed tomography of orbital lesions. A cooperative study of 210 cases. Neuroradiology 13:123–134, 1977.

66. Kennerdell JS, Ghoshhajra K: Computed tomographic scanning of orbital tumors. Int Ophthalmol Clin 22:95–131, 1982.

67. Peeters PL, Kruger R: Dural and direct cavernous sinus fistulas. AJR 132:599, 1979.

68. Merrick R, Lathchaw RE, Gold LH: Computerized tomography of the orbit in carotid cavernous sinus fistulae. Comput Tomogr 4:127–132, 1980.

69. Gans H, Sekula J, Wlodyka J: Treatment of acute orbital complications. Arch Otolaryngol 100:329–332, 1974.

70. Gellady AM, Shulman ST, Ayoub EM: Periorbital and orbital cellulitis in children. Pediatrics 61:272–277, 1978.

71. Hawkins DB, Clark RW: Orbital involvement in acute sinusitis. Clin Pediatr 16:464–471, 1977.

72. Haynes RE, Cramblatt HG: Acute ethmoiditis. Am J Dis Child 114:261–267, 1967.

73. Kaplan RJ: Neurological complications of infections of the head and neck. Otolaryngol Clin North Am 9:729–749, 1976.

74. Youssefi B: Orbital tumors in children. A clinical study of 62 cases. J Pediatr Ophthalmol 6:177–185, 1969.

75. Enzmann DR, Donaldson SS, Kriss JP: Appearance of Grave's disease in orbital computed tomography. J Comput Assist Tomogr 3:815–819, 1979.

76. Healy JF, Metcalf JH, Brahme FJ: Thyroid opathalmopathy: bony erosion on CT and increased vascularity on angiography. AJNR 2:472–474, 1981.

77. Jones IS, Jakobiec FA (ed): Diseases of the Orbit. Harper and Row, Hagerstown, Maryland, 1979.

78. Trokel SL, Hilal SK: Computed tomographic scanning of orbital inflammation. Int Ophthalmol Clin 22(4):81–98, 1982.

79. Nugent RA, Rootman J, Robertson WD, et al.: Acute orbital pseudotumor: classification and CT features. AJR 137:957–962, 1981.

80. Trokel SL, Hilal SK: Recognition and differential diagnosis of enlarged extraocular muscles in computed tomography. Am J Ophthalmol 87:503–512, 1979.

81. Peyster RG, Hoover ED, Hershey BC, et al.: High resolution CT of lesions of the optic nerve. AJR 140:869–874, 1983.

82. Chuterian AM, Schwartz JF, Evans RA, et al.: Optic gliomas in children. Neurology 14:83–95, 1964.

83. Hoyt WF, Meshel LG, Lessell S, et al.: Malignant optic gliomas of adulthood. Brain 96:121–132, 1973.

84. Swenson SA, Forbes GS, Younge BR, et al.: Radiologic evaluation of tumors of the optic nerve. AJNR 3:319–326, 1982.

85. Ebers GC, Cousin HK, Feasby TE, Paty DW: Optic neuritis in familial MS. Neurology 31:1138–1142, 1981.

86. Howard CW, Osher RH, Tomsak RL: Computed tomographic features in optic neuritis. Am J Ophthalmol 89:699–702, 1980.

87. Howard CW, Osher RH, Tomsak RL: Computed tomographic features in optic neuritis. Am J Ophthalmol 89:699–702, 1980.

87. Cabanis EA, Salvolini U, Rodallec A, et al.: Computed tomography of the optic nerve: Part I. Normal results. J Comput Assist Tomogr 2 (2):141–149, 1978.

88. Cabanis EA, Salvolini U, Rodallec A, Menichelli F, et al.: Computed tomography of the optic nerve: Part II. Size and shape modifications in papilledema. J Comput Assist Tomogr 2:150–155, 1978.

89. Fox AJ, DeBrun G, Vinveia F et al: Intrathecal metrizamide of the optic nerve sheath. J Comput Assist Tomogr 3:653–659, 1979.

90. Kitchen FD: Genetics in retinoblastoma. pp. 125–132. In Reese AB (ed): Tumors of the Eye. Harper and Row, New York, 1976.

91. Mokely TA, Jr. Retinoblastoma and other neuroectodermal tumors of the retina. pp. 90–124. In Reese AB (ed): Tumors of the Eye. Harper and Row, New York, 1976.

92. Rootman J, Hofbauer J, Ellsworth RM, Kitchen D: A clinicopathological study of optic nerve invasion by retinoblastoma. Read before the Canadian Ophthalmological Society, June 1975.

93. Goldberg L, Danziger A: Computed tomographic scanning in the management of retino-blastoma. Am J Ophthalmol 87:380–382, 1977.

94. Danziger A, Price HI: CT findings in retinoblastoma. AJR 133:695, 1979.

95. Harris GJ, Williams AL, Reeser FH, Abrams GW: Intraocular evaluation by computed tomography. Int Ophthalmol Clin 22:197–217, 1982.

96. Zeiter HJ. Calcification and ossification in ocular tissue. Am J Ophthalmol 53:265, 1962.

97. delRegata JA, Apjeit HJ. Cancer of the Eye. pp. 160–181. In Cancer: Diagnosis, Treatment and Prognosis, 5th Ed. CV Mosby, St. Louis, 1977.

98. Spencer WH: Optic nerve extension of intraocular neoplasms. Am J Ophthalmol 80:465, 1975.

99. Boyce SW, Platia EV, Green WH: Drusen of the optic nerve head. Ann Ophthalmol 10:695–704, 1978.

100. Hoyt WF, Pont ME: Pseudo-papilledema: anomalous elevation of the optic disc. Pitfalls in diagnosis and management. JAMA 181:191–196, 1962.

101. Turner RM, Gutman T, Hilal SK: CT of Drusen bodies and other calcific lesions of the optic nerve: case report and differential diagnosis. AJNR 4:175–178, 1983.

102. Laibovitz RA: An unusual case of intraocular calcifications. Choroidal osteoma. Ann Ophthalmol 11:1077, 1979.

103. Gass JD, Guerry RK, Jacy RL, Harris G: Choroidal Osteoma. Arch Ophthalmol 96:428, 1978.

104. Duke-Elder WS (ed): Calcareous degeneration and ossification. Ch. 9. In Systems of Ophthalmology. Vol. 7. pp. 180–182. CV Mosby, St Louis, 1962.

7 The Temporal Bone

GALDINO E. VALVASSORI
MAHMOOD F. MAFEE

INTRODUCTION

Computed tomography is rapidly replacing multidirectional tomography as the radiographic study for assessing the temporal bone. Several factors are responsible for this new approach. First of all, the CT sections are easier to interpret because of the high contrast of the images and better recognition of soft tissue structures and pathology. In addition, through changes in the window width and window level CT makes it possible to assess various parameters of the image including adjacent intracranial and extracranial structures and pathology. Finally, CT is rapidly becoming the only tomographic equipment available in most institutions.

Three prerequisites are necessary for the study of the temporal bone: high definition, thin sections, and multiple projections.

High definition: in the latest generation of CT scanners the pixel has been reduced to 0.25 mm by special software reconstruction techniques.

Thin sections: by narrowing the collimation of the x-ray beam and the aperture of each detector, the slice thickness has been reduced to 1.5 mm. Serial sections at 1-mm increments can be obtained by 0.5-mm overlapping of the sections.

Multiple projections: the CT study of the temporal bone should always include at least two projections. The use of a single projection may lead to serious mistakes, since structures that are parallel to the plane of section are only partially or not at all visualized. For instance, the floor of the external auditory canal and the tegmen cannot be evaluated in the axial sections. The basic projection is of course the axial since it is the easiest to obtain (Fig. 7.1). Direct coronal sections in either the prone or the supine position can be obtained in most patients by extending the patient's head and tilting the gantry (Fig. 7.2.).

171

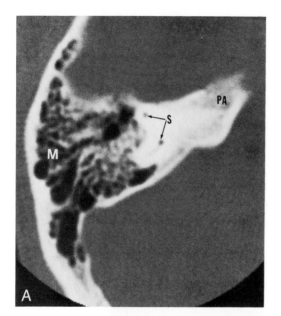

FIG. 7.1. Six representative axial sections of a normal right temporal bone from top to bottom. A, attic; C, cochlea; CA, cochlear aqueduct; CC, carotid canal; Ccr, common crus; CL, clivus; E, external auditory canal; F, facial nerve canal; H, horizontal semicircular canal; I, incus; IAC, internal auditory canal; J, jugular fossa; LA, lateral attic wall; LS, lateral sinus; M, mastoid; MA, mastoid antrum; ML, malleus; O, ossicles; OW, oval window; P, posterior semicircular canal; PA, petrous apex; RW, round window; S, superior semicircular canal; ST, sinus tympani; V, vestibule.

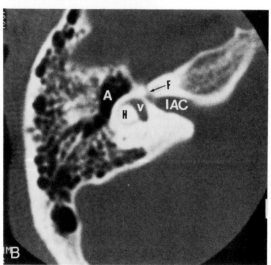

Direct lateral and oblique projections are extremely hard on the patient or are impossible. Whenever it is necessary, images in these projections are obtained by computer reformatting. However, reformatted images are always suboptimal because of intrinsic distortion and volume averaging and are further deteriorated by motion that may occur not only during scanning but also during the longer interscan time. For the last reason, whenever the need for reconstructed images is foreseen, we use the rapid sequential technique with automatic table incrementation. A series of 20–25 overlapping 1.5-mm pretargeted

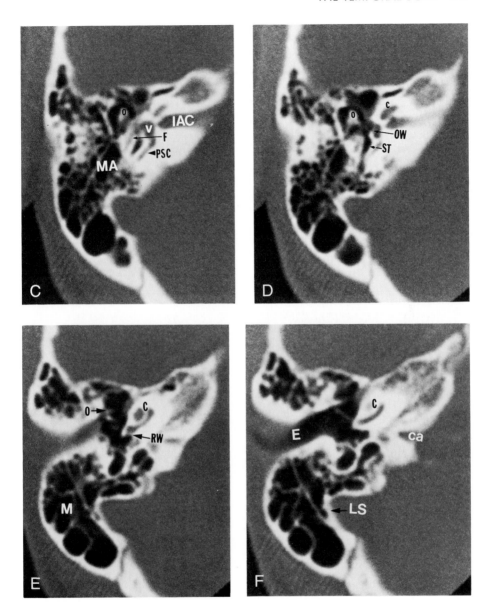

FIG. 7.1 (*Cont.*).

axial sections at 1-mm increments is obtained extending from the undersurface of the external auditory canal and petrous pyramid to the tegmen. The obtained block of data is then transmitted by telecommunication to the multiplanar diagnostic imaging center (MPDI) in California, where the original data are processed into sagittal or other plane images. The entire series of reformatted images is then transmitted back to us through the same network (Fig. 7.3).

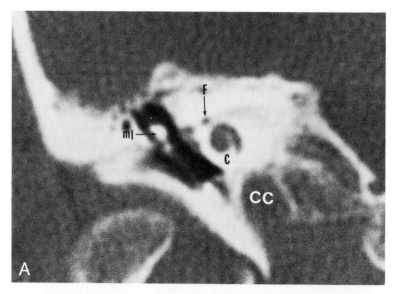

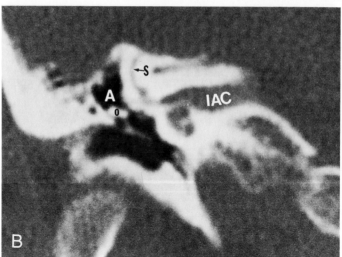

FIG. 7.2. Six representative coronal sections of a normal right temporal bone from front to back. (Refer to Fig. 7.1. for abbreviations.)

Table 7.1 can be used as a guide as the projection or projections necessary for the study of the various structures of the temporal bone.

Densitometric Analysis

This technique has been used in the attempt to differentiate different media (serous fluid, blood, soft tissues) obscuring the normally aerated spaces of the mastoid and middle ear. In addition we have tried to analyze various soft

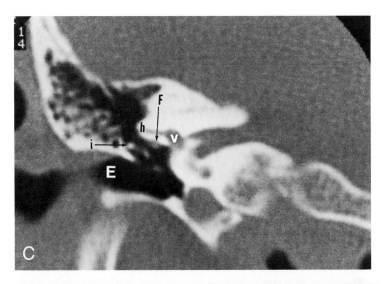

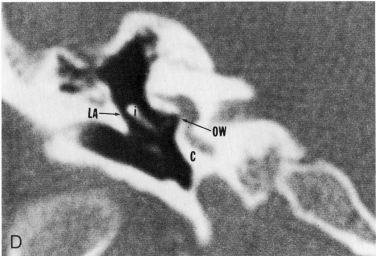

FIG. 7.2 (*Cont.*).

tissue pathologies occurring in the middle ear, such as granulation tissue, cholesteatoma, and tumors. In our experience densitometric analysis has been disap-
pointing in ears where the bony confines are intact and therefore the spaces
are not enlarged. In these cases, because of the anfractuosity of the walls of
the middle ear and mastoid and the presence of structures of different density
such as ossicles, tendons, and ligaments, the densitometric reading obtained
even with the smallest cursor is very often affected by partial volume averaging.
However, densitometric data become more precise whenever the middle ear
walls are smoothed out by disease, spaces are enlarged, and enclosed structures
are destroyed. Densitometric analysis is particularly important in the postsurgical ear where large cavities have been created.

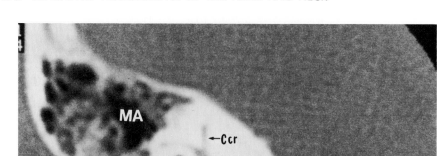

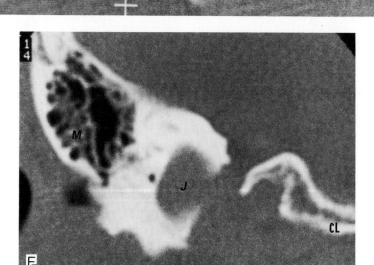

FIG. 7.2 (*Cont.*).

The following list summarizes densities of some common tissues found in the middle ear and mastoid.

Cholesteatoma: low density (25–45 HU) surrounded by a denser capsule.
Granulation tissue: higher density than cholesteatoma (45–65 HU).
Tympanosclerosis: very high density (80–120 HU) because of calcific deposits.
Tumor: the density varies with the type of neoplasm but usually ranges
   between 30 and 60 HU.

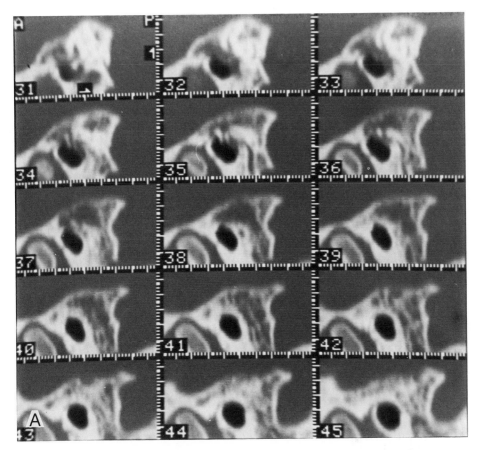

FIG. 7.3. (A), (B). Reformatted images in the sagittal plane. Image 19 is the medial section and image 45 is the most lateral. These sections are from a patient with fracture of the anterior wall of the external auditory canal (images 36, 37, 38) and separation of the ossicular chain at the incudomalleolar joint (images 35, 36).

Enhancement Study

A second series of scans performed in one or more projections following bolus and drip infusion of contrast material is mandatory whenever a vascular anomaly of the temporal bone or an otogenic brain abscess is suspected and in all tumors except for the osteoma. In these cases CT will demonstrate not only the involvement of the temporal bone but also the presence and extent of the intra- or extracranial component of the lesion.

The CT studies shown in this chapter were performed on a GE CT/T8800 unit using 1.5-mm collimation with 0.25-mm pixels and extended gray scales to 4,000 HU (+3000 − 1000).

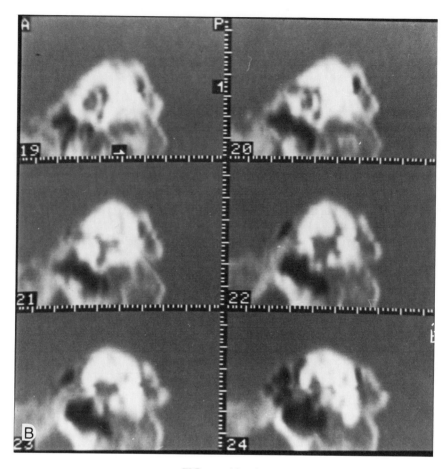

FIG. 7.3 (*Cont.*).

CONGENITAL ANOMALIES OF THE TEMPORAL BONE

A proper radiographic assessment is essential in all patients with congenital anomalies of the temporal bone. Otoscopy is of little value in atresia and aplasia of the external auditory canal and audiometry is unreliable in young children. The radiographic study should demonstrate the status of the anatomic structures of the ear, the development and course of the facial nerve canal, the position of the sigmoid sinus and jugular bulb, and the course of the carotid canal.[1] Such information is of value for the otologist in determining the proper treatment for conductive and sensorineural hearing losses.

The CT examination should always consist of axial and coronal sections. Sagittal reconstructed images should be added whenever the vestibular aqueduct and mastoid segment of the facial canal are under investigation.

TABLE 7.1 Projections used to study structures of temporal bone

Structure	Projection
Mastoid pneumatization	Axial
Tegmen and dura level	Coronal
Position of the lateral sinus	Axial
External auditory canal	Axial and coronal
Middle ear	Axial and coronal
Eustachian tube	Axial
Ossicular chain including oval window	Axial and coronal
Inner ear structures (except vestibular aqueduct)	Axial and coronal
Vestibular aqueduct	Axial and sagittal reconstruction
Internal auditory canal	Axial and coronal
Facial nerve canal, petrous and tympanic segments	Axial and coronal
Facial nerve canal, mastoid segment	Coronal and sagittal reconstruction
Jugular fossa	Axial and coronal
Carotid canal	Axial and coronal
Petrous apex	Axial

Anomalies of the Sound Conducting System

A good CT study provides the surgeon with the following basic information he needs in deciding if corrective surgery is feasible and in determining which type of surgery is indicated.

1. The degree and type of abnormality of the tympanic bone. These abnormalities range from relatively minor deformity to complete agenesis of the external auditory canal (Figs. 7.4, 7.5).
2. The degree and position of the pneumatization of the mastoid air cells and mastoid antrum.
3. The development and aeration of the middle ear cavity.
4. The status of the ossicular chain, the size and shape of the ossicles and the presence of fusion or fixation (Figs. 7.4, 7.5).
5. The patency of the labyrinthine windows.
6. The relationship of the meninges to the mastoid and the superior petrous ridge. The middle cranial fossa often forms a deep groove lateral to the labyrinth, which results in a low lying dura over the mastoid and epitympanum.

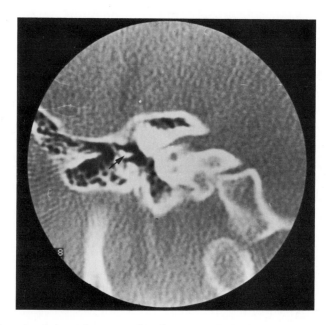

FIG. 7.4. Atresia of the right external auditory canal, direct coronal section. Agenesis of the right external auditory canal is present, with a thick atretic plate closing the tympanic cavity. Notice the malformation of the ossicles (arrow), which appear fused.

Anomalies of the Inner Ear

With the recent advances in cochlear implants for profound sensorineural deafness, assessment of the inner ear structures has become essential. Of course, only defects in the otic capsule are visible radiographically. Abnormal development of the membraneous labyrinth is not detectable by the present radiographic techniques.

Anomalies of the otic capsule may involve either a single structure or the entire capsule and may range from a minor hypoplasia to complete agenesis of the inner ear structures (Michel anomaly). A common deformity of the labyrinthine capsule is the Mondini type, which is characterized by an abnormal development of the cochlea associated with dilatation of the vestibular aqueduct and vestibule. The semicircular canals are often malformed and usually hypoplastic (Fig. 7.6).

Anomalies of the Facial Nerve

Anomalies of the facial nerve canal involve the size and the course of the canal. Complete or partial agenesis of the facial nerve canal with total paralysis may be present. Occasionally the facial nerve canal may be unusually narrow and hypoplastic. In these cases intermittent episodes of facial paresis may occur.

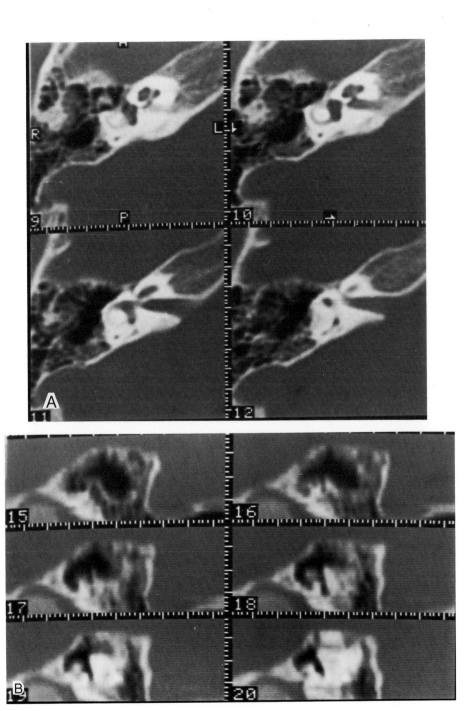

FIG. 7.5. Atresia of the right external auditory canal, (A) axial sections and (B) reformatted sagittal images. There is agenesis of the external auditory canal but normal development of the mastoid pneumatization and middle ear cleft. Notice the malformation of the ossicles (A9, B19 and 20) which appear fused and fixed to the atretic plate.

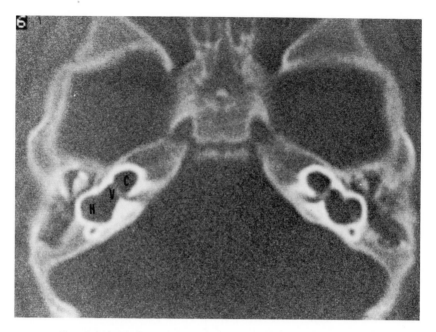

FIG. 7.6. Bilateral Mondini anomaly, axial section. The cochleas are empty because the bony partitions between the cochlear coils are not developed. There is lack of canalization of the horizontal semicircular canals, which form large pouches lateral to the dilated vestibules. C, cochlea; V, vestibule; H, horizontal semicircular canal.

The horizontal segment of the facial canal is at times displaced inferiorly to cover the oval window. Anomalies in the course of the mastoid segment are common in congenital atresia of the external auditory canal. The facial canal is usually rotated laterally. The rotation varies from a minor obliquity to a true horizontal course.

Vascular Anomalies

Whenever a vascular anomaly is suspected on the basis of the clinical findings or of the preinfusion CT examination, a repeat study following bolus and drip injection of contrast material is mandatory. Dynamic CT scanning of a single preselected plane or sequential CT with table incrementation is extremely useful in these cases. This technique has been previously described.[2-4] The most important vascular anomalies are

1. Anterior position of the vertical segment of the sigmoid sinus
2. High jugular bulb projecting into the hypo- or mesotympanum
3. Ectopic course of the internal carotid artery within the middle ear cavity

TEMPORAL BONE TRAUMA

Radiographic studies of the temporal bone following head trauma are indicated when cerebrospinal fluid otorrhea or rhinorrhea, hearing loss, or facial nerve paralysis is present.

The CT study should always include axial and, if possible, direct coronal sections. Lateral reconstructed images may be required in selected cases with longitudinal fractures or facial nerve paralysis. In acute trauma with unconsciousness or neurological findings, the CT study should be extended to the entire head and brain to rule out the possibility of intracranial hemorrhage. In addition, a series of scans obtained after intrathecal injection of metrizamide is often useful to demonstrate the site of the leak in a patient with cerebrospinal fluid otorrhea or rhinorrhea.

Temporal bone fractures are divided into longitudinal and transverse lesions depending on the direction of the fracture line. Longitudinal fractures occur more frequently than transverse fractures (5:1 ratio). However, this classification is somewhat arbitrary, since most fractures follow a serpiginous tract in the temporal bone.[1]

The typical longitudinal fracture involves the temporal squama and extends into the mastoid. The fracture usually reaches the external auditory canal and passes medially into the epitympanum where it produces a disruption of the ossicular chain (Fig. 7.7). From the epitympanum the fracture extends into the petrosal and follows an intra- or extralabyrinthine course. An intralabyrinthine course of the fracture is rare, since the labyrinthine bone is quite resistent to trauma. Extralabyrinthine extension occurs either anterior or posterior to the labyrinth, although anterior extension is more common.

A transverse fracture of the temporal bone typically crosses the petrous pyramid at a right angle to the longitudinal axis of the pyramid. The fracture usually follows the line of least resistence and runs from the dome of the jugular fossa through the labyrinth to the superior petrous ridge.

The fracture line disappears at certain levels only to reappear a few millimeters distant. This apparent gap is not caused by interruption of the fracture but rather by the fact that the plane of the fracture line changes course and becomes invisible in some of the sections.

Longitudinal fractures are best demonstrated in the axial sections and transverse fractures in the coronal images.

Traumatic disruption of the ossicular chain is most common in patients with longitudinal fractures but may occur even in the absence of an actual fracture. Dislocation of the malleus is rare because of its firm attachment to the tympanic membrane and the strong anterior malleolar ligament. The incus is most commonly dislocated, since its attachments to the malleus and stapes are easily torn. Fractures and dislocation of the footplate of the stapes are not directly recognizable but may be identified by the presence of air within the vestibule.[6]

Facial paralysis occurs immediately or after a period of a few hours or days following trauma. Immediate onset of facial paralysis is the result of bisection

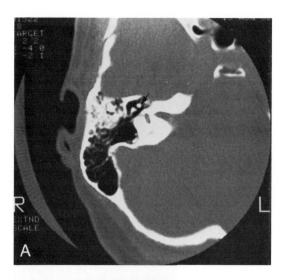

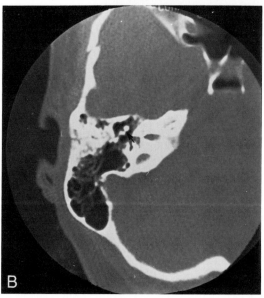

FIG. 7.7. Longitudinal fracture of the right temporal bone. Notice the fracture of the temporal squama and of the mastoid cortex. The fracture passes through the mastoid air cells, which appear cloudy because of hemorrhage, into the attic where it causes a separation of the ossicular chain at the incudomalleolar joint (arrow).

of the facial nerve by the fracture (Fig. 7.8). Delayed facial paralysis is due to fracture of the facial canal and posttraumatic edema of the nerve. Facial paralysis occurs in approximately 25 percent of longitudinal fractures and is of the delayed and often transient type in 50 percent of those cases. Facial paralysis is observed in 50 percent of the transverse fractures and is almost always of the immediate and permanent type. In some cases the site of involvement of the facial canal cannot be visualized in the CT sections. However, by evaluation of the course of the fracture line, the site of the lesion can be determined.

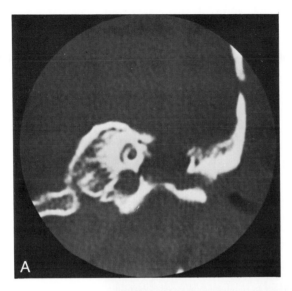

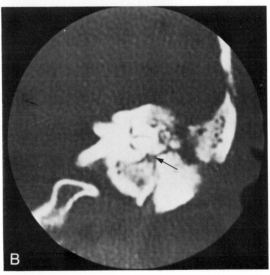

FIG. 7.8. Comminuted fracture of the left temporal bone with facial paralysis and meningoencephalocele, direct coronal sections. Multiple fractures of the temporal squama and mastoid are present. Notice the large defect in the tegmen (A) with a soft tissue mass protruding into the middle ear cavity. The fracture transects the mastoid segment of the facial canal (B, arrow).

INFLAMMATORY DISEASES AND CHOLESTEATOMAS OF THE MIDDLE EAR AND MASTOID

Acute Otomastoiditis

Acute otitis media is a clinical diagnosis and radiological examination is indicated whenever coalescent mastoiditis is clinically suspected (Fig. 7.9). If coalescence of cell walls occurs (usually not before the end of the 2nd week), the

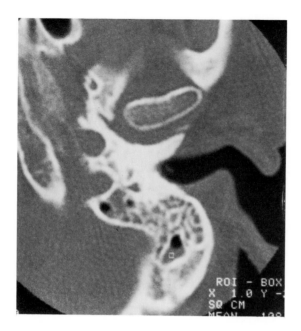

FIG. 7.9. Left acute otomastoiditis, axial section. The mastoid air cells are cloudy and several small air fluid levels are noticed within them.

bony septa are destroyed and an empyema develops (Fig. 7.10A). The coalescent infection may perforate the thin mastoid cortex and produce a variety of subperiosteal abscesses. If the sinus plate or tegmen are dehiscent or destroyed, intracranial complications such as sigmoid sinus thrombosis, perisinus abcess, epidural (Fig. 7.10B) and cerebellar (Fig. 7.11) abscesses may develop.

Chronic Otomastoiditis

Two groups of chronic ear disease (inflammation) can be distinguished: tubotympanic disease and attico-antral disease.

The tubotympanic type is a chronic tubotympanic mucositis. These infections are usually confined to the mucous membrane of the nasopharynx, the eustachian tube, and the tympanum. The mucosa of the meso- and hypotympanum is thick, exuberant, and edematous. Polyps may be present. These polyps may be associated with the necrosis of the ossicles, particularly the long process of the incus and its lenticular process.

In chronic attico-antral disease, the process is confined to the attic and mastoid air cells and is due to occlusion of the attic floor by a chronic pathological process.[5] Inflammatory changes of the middle ear cavity and mastoid antrum, with effusion or granulation tissue, can be readily visualized by CT (Fig 7.12).[6,7] Long-standing or repeated infections may produce concentric healing with tympanosclerotic plaques or new bone formation (Fig. 7.13).[6]

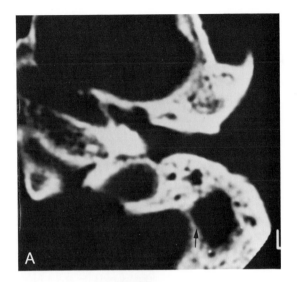

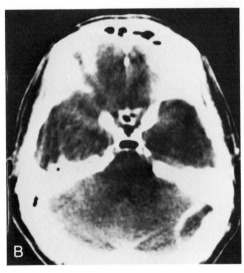

FIG. 7.10. Coalescent mastoiditis with epidural abscess, axial sections. A large area of coalescence is present in the posteroinferior portion of the mastoid with thinning and erosion of the adjacent sinus plate (A, arrow). Following the infusion of contrast material, a thick rim of enhancement is demonstrated around the posterior fossa epidural abscess (B).

Cholesteatomas of the Middle Ear and Mastoid

Congenital primary cholesteatoma is a rare form of middle ear cholesteatoma that is not related to infection in the ear. It originates from embryonic cell remnants in the tympanic cavity and is seen otoscopically as a white mass behind an intact tympanic membrane. CT is the radiographic method of choice to assess the location and extent of the disease. Cholesteatoma is seen as a soft tissue mass in an otherwise well-aerated tympanic cavity (Fig. 7.14).

In acquired cholesteatoma, high resolution CT used with the combination

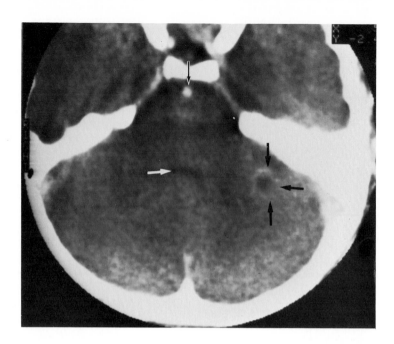

FIG. 7.11. Otogenic cerebellar abcess. Axial section of a 12-year-old boy with left acute mastoiditis who developed ataxia and cerebellar signs. Note the low density image with peripheral enhancement in the left side of the cerebellum.

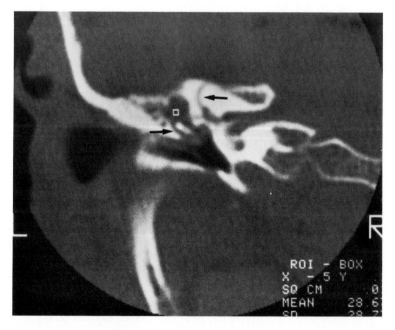

FIG. 7.12. Right chronic attico-antral disease, coronal section. There is nonhomogeneous clouding of the attic and posterosuperior quadrant of the tympanic cavity. The anterior and inferior portions of the mesotympanum are aerated. The scutum (arrow) is intact.

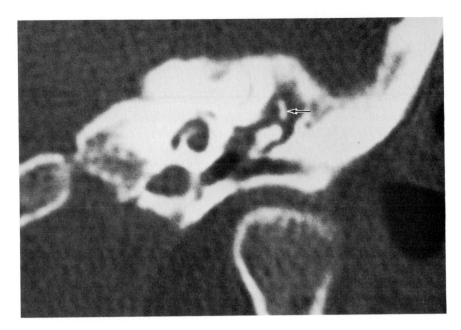

FIG. 7.13. Left chronic otitis media, coronal section. The attic and upper portion of the tympanic cavity are cloudy. A large tympanosclerotic plaque (arrow) is visible in the attic above the ossicles.

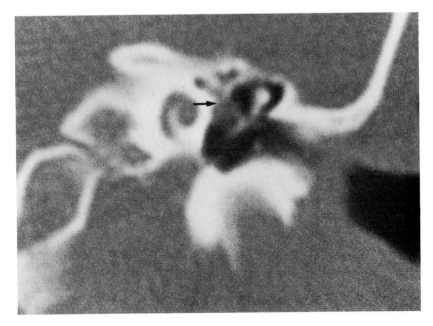

FIG. 7.14. Congenital cholesteatoma of the left middle ear, coronal section. A well-defined soft tissue mass (arrow) is visualized in the anterior portion of the tympanic cavity medial to the malleus handle.

of narrow slice thickness and extended bone CT scale provides valuable information regarding the size and extent of the lesion. Cholesteatomas may be mainly localized to the attic and antrum or may extend into the mesotympanum or even anteriorly into the eustachian tube. One of the advantages of CT is the possibility of tissue identification. The CT attenuation values of uninfected cholesteatomas are typically low (45 HU or less).

When a cholesteatoma is infected or buried within the granulation tissue and partially destroyed trabeculae, the CT attenuation values of the soft tissue mass may be quite high. In this situation other criteria, such as expansion of the attic, aditus, and antrum and extensive erosion of the lateral attic wall (Fig. 7.15), medial (labyrinthine) attic wall, and posterior superior external auditory canal wall are useful in arriving at the correct diagnosis.[2,6,8]

In cholesteatoma, multidirectional tomography and computed tomography of the temporal bone provide the following information, which are of assistance to the surgeon in determining the type of surgery and preventing complications:

1. Exact size and extent of the cholesteatomatous sac.
2. Erosion of the lateral attic wall, mastoid, tegmen, sigmoid sinus plate, ossicles, and of the posterosuperior canal wall with sagging.
3. Involvement of the facial nerve canal and presence of labyrinthine fistula (Fig. 7.16).

In our series CT proved to be the diagnostic method of choice for residual or recurrent postoperative mastoid and middle ear disease.[9]

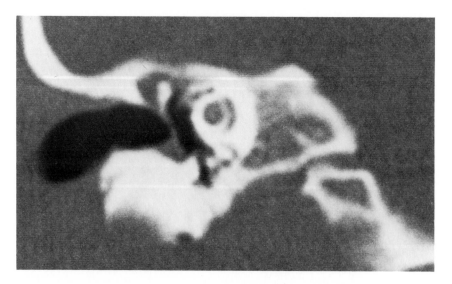

FIG. 7.15. Right acquired cholesteatoma, coronal section. The inferior portion of the lateral wall of the attic is eroded and a soft tissue mass extends into the attic lateral to the ossicles. The tympanic membrane is thickened but not retracted.

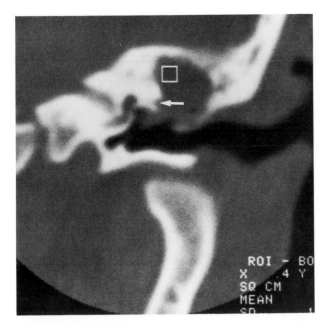

FIG. 7.16.   Left acquired cholesteatoma, coronal section. A large low density, soft tissue mass fills and expands the mastoid antrum and attic. Notice the erosion and fistula (arrow) of the horizontal semicircular canal.

CT is also an indispensable radiological imaging method for evaluating the pre- and postsurgical complications of otomastoiditis and cholesteatomas. Any mass protruding into the mastoid cavity from the tegmen must be considered as a possible meningoencephalocele until proved otherwise (Fig. 7.8A). CT is particularly useful in confirming a brain herniation and diagnosing abscess formation and cerebritis.

Epidermoid cysts or primary cholesteatomas of the petrous bone arise from epidermal cell rests laid down in the temporal bone during the early formation of this sense organ.[10] Intradural cerebellopontine angle and intraosseous petrous bone epidermoids or congenital cholesteatomas may cause minimal symptoms and usually have spread beyond the original site by the time they are found. Congenital cholesteatomas of the petrous bone are often responsible for slowly developing facial paralysis, sensorineural hearing loss, and vestibular disturbances.

The findings on multidirectional tomography and computed tomography are striking and usually specific. The petrous apex, undersurface of the petrous bone, adjacent occipital bone, and middle cranial fossa are often extensively involved. Typically, attenuation values on CT are low and do not increase following intravenous injection of contrast material except for moderate capsular enhancement (Fig. 7.17).[2,11]

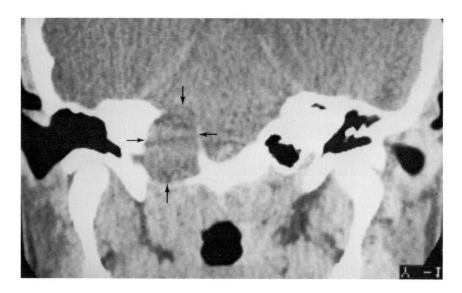

FIG. 7.17. Epidermoid cyst of the right petrous apex, coronal section. A large low-density lesion surrounded by a thin enhanced rim (arrows) has destroyed the right petrous apex and eroded the adjacent aspect of the clivus. Notice the defect of an old mastoidectomy in the right ear.

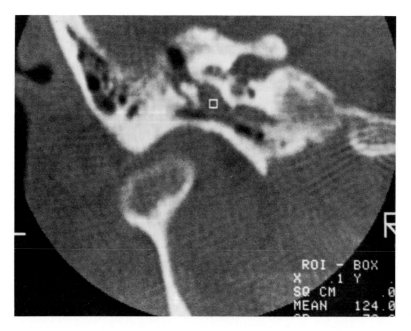

FIG. 7.18. Right glomus tympanicum, coronal section. The examination performed following the bolus injection of contrast material demonstrates a high density, soft tissue mass filling the tympanic cavity. There is no erosion of the hypotympanic floor.

GLOMUS COMPLEX TUMORS (CHEMODECTOMAS)

Chemodectomas, or paragangliomas, arise from paraganglionic glomus tissues (chemoreceptors). The four common sites are the carotid artery bifurcation (carotid body tumor), inferior ganglion (ganglion nodosum) of the vagus nerve (glomus vagale or vagal body tumor), jugular fossa (glomus jugulare), and middle ear (glomus tympanicum).

Glomus jugulare tumors are the most common. They arise from glomera of the chemoreceptor system located in the jugular foramen and jugular bulb region. The glomus tympanicum tumor arises over the promontory from glomus tissues situated in the adventitia of vessels along the tympanic branch (Jacobson nerve) of the glossopharyngeal nerve and auricular branch (Arnold nerve) of the vagus nerve (Fig. 7.18). They are benign tumors histologically, but they may be locally invasive and cause significant morbidity and even mortality.

Improved microsurgical techniques in association with preoperative embolization permit complete resection of these vascular tumors in many cases with minimal blood loss.[12,13]

Radiographic techniques are valuable not only to ascertain the correct diagnosis but also to determine the extent of the bone destruction and soft tissue involvement. CT reveals evidence of tumor in the jugular fossa (Fig. 7.19), middle ear, and neck (Fig. 7.20) including the nasopharynx and the extent of bony destruction.

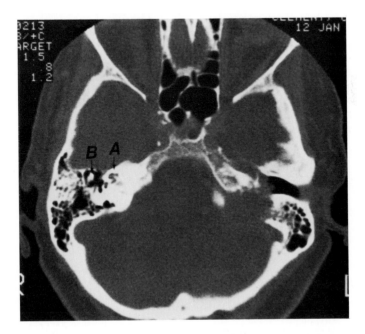

FIG. 7.19. Left glomus jugular tumor, axial section. Destruction of the posteroinferior aspect of the left petrous pyramid is present, with extension of the glomus tumor into the hypotympanum. (A) cochlea, (B) malleus.

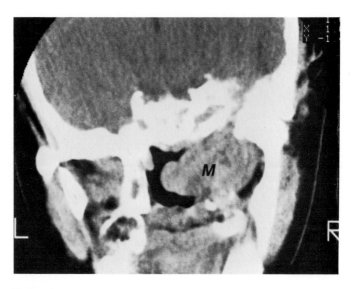

FIG. 7.20. Right glomus jugulare tumor. This coronal section obtained after infusion of contrast material shows a large mass in the right parapharyngeal space protruding into the nasopharynx.

Invasion of the posterior cranial fossa, cerebellum, and brainstem; associated hydrocephalus; involvement of the middle cranial fossa, extension along the carotid artery, and cavernous sinus (Fig. 7.21) are all best demonstrated by computed tomography.

Sometimes an extensive glomus jugulare tumor may be seen without signifi-

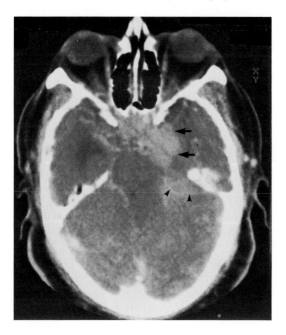

FIG. 7.21. Left glomus jugular tumor, axial section. The tumor extends into the posterior and middle cranial fossae. Notice the enhanced soft tissue mass in the left cerebellopontine angle (arrowheads) and along the left parasellar region (arrows).

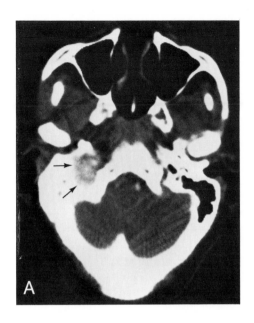

7.22. Right glomus jugulare tumor. (A) This postinfusion axial section demonstrates a moderately enhanced soft tissue mass in the region of the right enlarged and eroded jugular fossa. (B) Dynamic study of the same patient at the level of the enlarged jugular fossa (arrows). Note the marked enhancement in the region of the enlarged jugular fossa, which is best seen in section 3.

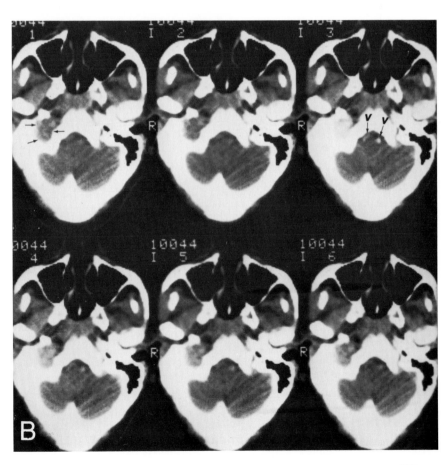

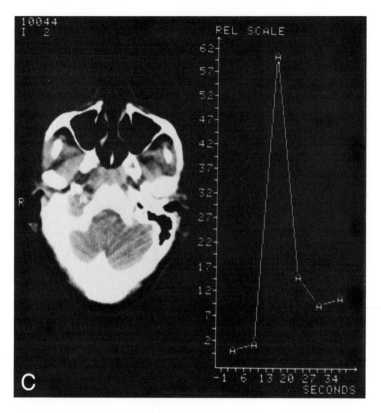

FIG. 7.22 (*Cont.*). (C) The density–time curve demonstrates high peak with rapid wash-in and wash-out phases characteristic for glomus tumor.

cant middle ear or intracranial involvement (mainly intratemporal extension). Routine infusion CT in such a case may show no significant enhancement, but dynamic CT studies will demonstrate the vascular nature of the lesion.[3,4]

High resolution CT of temporal bone coupled with dynamic CT performed at the level of the tympanic cavity is the diagnostic method of choice to demonstrate the glomus tympanicum, or any extension of glomus jugulare tumor into the tympanic cavity. With this technique, glomus tumors demonstrate an intense contrast enhancement and the computer-generated density–time curves demonstrate a high arterial peak with rapid wash-in (up slope) and wash-out (down slope) phases (Fig. 7.22).

ACOUSTIC NEUROMA

Computed tomography with infusion of iodinated contrast material and CT combined with pneumocisternography are the procedures of choice for the diagnosis of acoustic neuromas and other lesions of the cerebellopontine angle.[2] We perform the entire procedure in one sitting on an outpatient basis. The intravenous infusion of contrast material is performed while the patient sits or lies down in the waiting area. Approximately 15 to 20 min. later the patient is taken to the scan room and 1.5-mm axial sections are obtained through the internal auditory canal and cerebellopontine cistern. Since the maximal enhancement of an acoustic neuroma is usually delayed, this time sequence is optimal in our opinion. If a tumor is recognized, the study is completed with 1.5-mm coronal sections (Figs. 7.23, 7.24). Otherwise a spinal puncture is immediately performed and 3 cc of air are injected into the subarachnoid space while the patient lies on his or her normal side or on the side opposite

FIG. 7.23. Left acoustic neuroma. (A) Axial section, (B) coronal section. The enhanced tumor mass (arrows) fills the slightly dilated left internal auditory canal and protrudes into the adjacent cerebellopontine cistern.

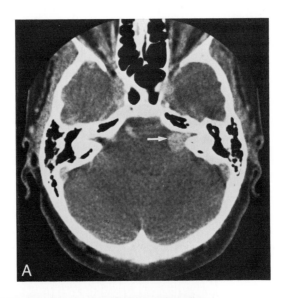

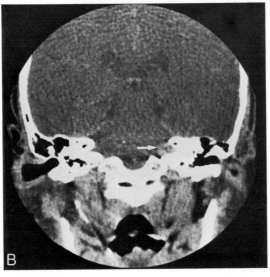

to the one being examined. The patient is then asked to lift his back and head while resting on his elbow for 15 to 30 sec. At the same time the head is slightly overextended and rotated upward. As soon as the air enters the posterior cranial fossa and cerebellopontine cistern, the patient will complain of sudden pressure and pain in the region of the ear. The head is then lowered and following scout view centering, four to eight 1.5-mm sections are obtained. In a normal case the cerebellopontine cistern and internal auditory canal appear filled with air and the seventh and eighth cranial nerves are visualized as they course from the brainstem through the cistern into the internal auditory canal (Fig. 7.25). If a tumor is present, air will reveal the complete or partial block

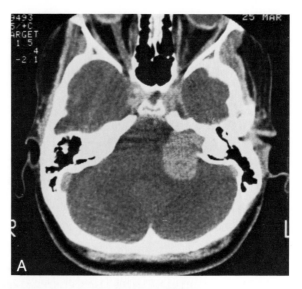

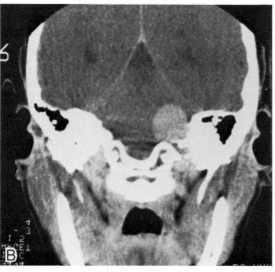

FIG. 7.24. Left acoustic neuroma. (A) Axial section, (B) coronal section. A large enhanced mass in the left cerebellopontine angle is present. Notice the large erosion of the posterior aspect of the petrous pyramid with gross enlargement of the internal auditory canal.

FIG. 7.25. Normal left cerebellopontine pneumocisternogram. Air fills the left cerebellopontine cistern and internal auditory canal and outlines the seventh and eighth cranial nerves. Notice the splitting of the nerves at the fundus of the canal.

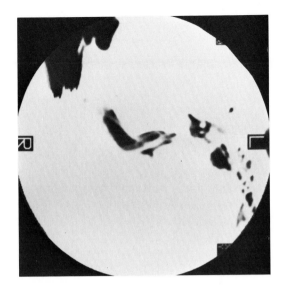

of the internal auditory canal and outline the contour of the mass (Figs. 7.26–7.28). By this technique intracanalicular tumors as small as 2 mm are well demonstrated. The patient is then rapidly rotated on the opposite side and after waiting 1 or 2 min. to allow the air to ascend into the other and now higher cerebellopontine cistern, the scan is repeated using the same modalities.

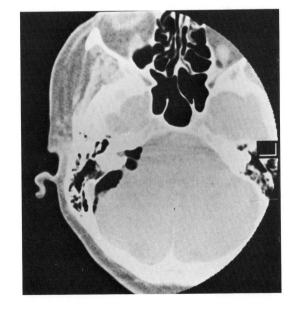

FIG. 7.26. Right acoustic neuroma. The cerebellopontine pneumocisternogram demonstrates a small tumor filling the fundus of the internal auditory canal. The cisternal portion of the eighth cranial nerve is normal.

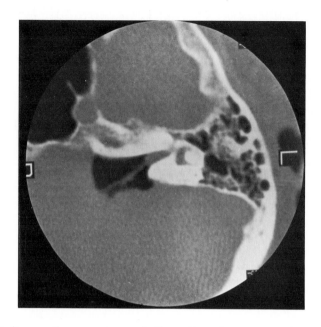

FIG. 7.27. Left acoustic neuroma, cerebellopontine cisternogram. A tumor mass fills the internal auditory canal. The cerebellopontine cistern and cisternal portion of the eighth cranial nerve are normal.

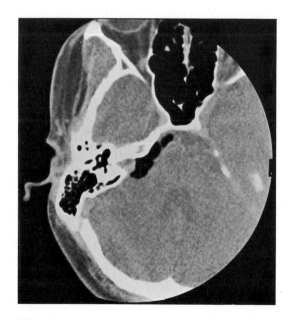

FIG. 7.28. Right acoustic neuroma, cerebellopontine pneumocisternogram. A tumor mass fills the dilated right internal auditory canal and protrudes slightly into the cerebellopontine cistern.

PRIMARY MALIGNANT NEOPLASMS OF THE TEMPORAL BONE

Whenever a soft tissue mass is seen within the external auditory canal or middle ear, associated with bleeding and radiographic findings of irregular bone destruction, carcinoma or adenocarcinoma should be considered. These tumors spread by local invasion. When the middle ear is primarily or secondarily involved, the tumor can spread from the protympanum into the eustachian tube and nasopharynx. Involvement of the temporomandibular joint, parotid gland, and facial nerve canal due to direct extension is not uncommon. Malignant (necrotizing) external otitis can clinically and radiographically simulate carcinoma of the ear. This condition is usually seen in elderly patients with uncontrolled diabetes and is secondary to infection by *Pseudomonas aeruginosa*. CT is the best method for accurately assessing the extent of malignant tumors of the ear and temporal bone. With CT it is now possible to identify subtle erosion of the external auditory canal, facial nerve canal, middle ear (Fig. 7.29), and otic capsule.[14] If sugery is contemplated, CT is mandatory to rule out extratemporal extension of the tumor and to define the planes of surgical resection. If radiation therapy is employed, CT is extremely useful in planning the treatment.

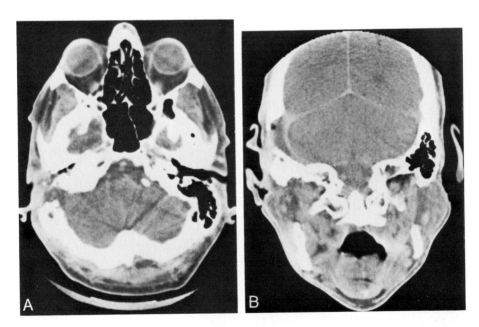

FIG. 7.29.   Carcinoma of the right ear. (A) Axial section, (B) coronal section. The tumor mass fills the external auditory canal and extends into the middle ear. Notice the large destruction of the canal walls and mastoid. The lesion exposes the dura but does not extend intracranially.

OTOSCLEROSIS

Otosclerosis is a primary focal disease of the labyrinthine capsule.[15] The otosclerotic foci may be single or multiple and undergo periods of resorption and redeposition of bone at variable intervals. The most common site of a focus is the labyrinthine capsule just anterior to the oval window. This focus tends to extend posteriorly to fix and then invade the stapes footplate, which becomes thickened. Similar foci may occur in other areas of the labyrinthine capsule, particularly in the cochlea. Involvement of the oval window with fixation of the stapes causes conductive deafness. Cochlear foci produce sensorineural hearing deafness by an unknown mechanism.

Fenestral Otosclerosis

Coronal and axial CT sections at 1-mm increment should be obtained. The oval window is best seen in the coronal sections, as a well-defined bony dehiscence in the lateral wall of the vestibule below the ampullated limb of the horizontal semicircular canal. In contrast, the round window is more satisfactorily visualized in the axial sections through the lower portion of the promontory. The window appears as a gap or indentation in the contour of the posterior aspect of the basal turn.

The CT findings of fenestral otosclerosis vary with the severity and extent of the process.[1] The changes range from loss of definition due to demineralization of the margin of the window, to narrowing (Fig. 7.30A), and finally to complete obliteration of the oval window opening and niche. CT is particularly helpful in determining the cause of poststapedectomy vertigo and hearing loss. The CT study may disclose protrusion of the prosthesis into the vestibule,

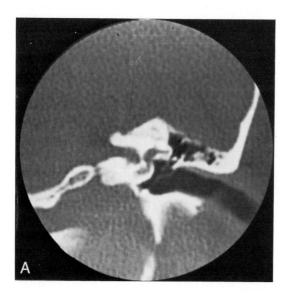

FIG. 7.30 Left otosclerosis. (A) Coronal section showing marginal thickening of the footplate of the stapes.

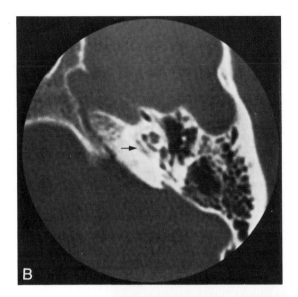

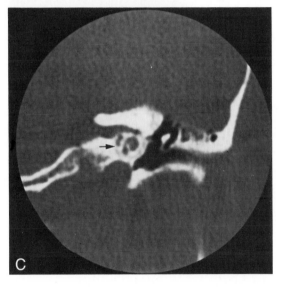

FIG. 7.30 (*Cont.*). (B) Axial and (C) coronal sections showing severe demineralization of the cochlear capsule with formation of a double ring effect (arrows).

separation of the lateral end of the prosthesis from the incus, dislocation of the medial end of the strut from the oval window, and reobliteration of the window with fixation or dislocation of the prosthesis.

Cochlear Otosclerosis

Otosclerotic foci arise in the enchondral layer of the capsule. An active focus is characterized by a loose and irregular network of bony trabeculae with numerous blood vessels, osteoblasts, and osteoclasts. In a mature focus, a dense

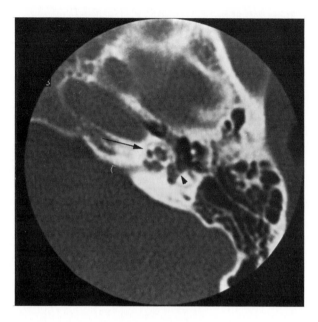

FIG. 7.31. Left otosclerosis, axial section. Notice the thickening of the footplate of the stapes (arrowhead) and the demineralization of the anterior aspect of the cochlear capsule (arrows).

type of bone that is relatively avascular and acellular is present. These foci may progressively enlarge and extend to the periosteal and endosteal layers of the labyrinthine capsule. Active otosclerotic foci appear as single, multiple, or confluent areas of demineralization in the thickness of the capsule (Figs. 7.30B, C, 7.31). Mature foci are only recognizable if their density differs from that of the normal otic capsule. Localized or diffuse areas of thickening and scalloping of the capsule due to apposition of new otosclerotic bone are observed.[16]

REFERENCES

1. Valvassori GE, Potter GD, Hanafee WN, et al.: Radiology of the Ear, Nose and Throat. WB Saunders, Philadelphia, 1982.
2. Valvassori GE, Mafee MF, Dobben GD: Computerized tomography of the temporal bone. Laryngoscope 92:562–565, 1982.
3. Mafee MF, Valvassori GE, Shugar MA, et al: High resolution and dynamic sequential computerized tomography in the evaluation of glomus complex tumors. Arch Otolaryngol 109:691–696, 1983.
4. Mafee MF: Dynamic CT and its application to otolaryngology—head and neck surgery. Otolaryngol 11:5:307–318, 1982.
5. Proctor B: Attic–aditus block and the tympanic diaphragm. Ann Otol Rhinol Laryngol 80:371–375, 1971.

6. Mafee MF, Kumar A, Yannias DA, et al.: Computed tomography of the middle ear in the evaluation of cholesteatoma and other soft tissue masses: comparison with pluridirectional tomography. Radiology 148:465–472, 1983.

7. Swartz JD, Goodman RS, Russel KB, et al.: High-resolution computed tomography of the middle ear and mastoid. Radiology 148:455–459, 1983.

8. Johnson OW, Voorhees RL, Lufkin RB, et al.: Cholesteatoma of the temporal bone: role of computed tomography. Radiology 148:733–737, 1983.

9. Mafee MF, Valvassori GE, Dobben GD: The role of radiology in surgery of the ear and skull base. Otolaryng Clin North Am 15:723–753, 1982.

10. Yanagihara N, Matsumoto Y: Cholesteatoma in the petrous apex. Laryngoscope 91:272–278, 1981.

11. Davis KR, Roberson GH, Taveras JM, et al.: Diagnosis of epidermoid tumor by computed tomography. Radiology 119:347–353, 1976.

12. Kinney SE: Glomus jugulare tumors with intracranial extension. Am J Otol 1:67–71, 1979.

13. Spector GJ, Maisel RH, Ogura JH: Glomus tumors in the middle ear. 1. An analysis of 46 patients. Laryngoscope 83:1652–1672, 1973.

14. Bird CR, Hasso AN, Stewart CE, et al.: Malignant primary neoplasms of the ear and temporal bone studied by high-resolution computed tomography. Radiology 149:171–174, 1983.

15. Shambaugh GE Jr, Glasscock ME III: Surgery of the ear. WB Saunders, Philadelphia, 1982.

16. Valvassori GE: The interpretation of the radiographic findings in cochlear otosclerosis. Ann Otol Rhinol Laryngol 75:572, 1966.

8 The Salivary Glands

MARK S. BANKOFF
BARBARA L. CARTER

INTRODUCTION

As with other areas of the body, and other organ systems, computed tomography has proven useful in evaluating many disease processes involving the salivary glands.[1-4] The ability of cross-sectional imaging to display complex anatomy is used to great advantage in demonstrating pathology in and around the major and minor salivary glands. The superb density discrimination of CT is utilized in many ways to aid in making diagnoses. For example, a small mass may often be identified, even in an unenhanced parotid gland, by the ability of CT to discriminate subtle differences in density. Likewise, specific diagnoses can occasionally be made when the absolute density measurement is characteristic of one tissue or another, as in the case of a lipoma. Mainly, the discussion will center on diseases of the parotid and submandibular glands although the other salivary glands will also be considered.

The indications for performing CT of the salivary glands are many. Often a patient presents with a suspected mass in a salivary gland. In this instance, CT can be performed to confirm or deny the presence of a mass. In a patient with a definitely palpable mass it may be impossible to determine clinically whether the mass is intrinsic or extrinsic to a salivary gland. CT is then frequently helpful in accurately differentiating the two possibilities and thus changing the differential diagnosis.

The question of total extent of a lesion is often best answered with CT. In the instance of tumor, total extent often dictates whether surgery or perhaps radiotherapy or chemotherapy will be the treatment of choice, depending on whether or not vital surrounding structures are shown to be involved. Accurate localization and delineation of extent are likewise important in directing either the surgical or the radiotherapy approach in the actual treatment. Once therapy, particularly nonsurgical therapy, has been instituted, CT proves very useful in assessing response. Finally, CT proves most advantageous in monitoring patients following therapy to assess the possible recurrence of disease.

SCANNING METHODS

With these major indications for CT in mind, one must consider how to acquire the optimal images of the salivary glands in order to make accurate and clinically useful diagnostic judgements. CT scanning of the minor salivary glands amounts to obtaining relatively thin (4–5-mm) contiguous slices through the areas in which they are located, mainly the buccal cavity, palate, and tongue, but also to a lesser extent the paranasal sinuses, nasopharynx, and nasal cavity.[5] Since the minor salivary glands are located at many sites, more detailed descriptions of scanning techniques can be found under the specific anatomic regions in which they are located. Of prime interest here are the major salivary glands: the parotid, submandibular, and sublingual glands. Since the sublingual gland can very rarely be opacified for sialography, images must be obtained without gland opacification.

The parotid glands are scanned in axial and/or coronal planes with contiguous sections (4–5-mm thick). The axial images are generally performed parallel to the orbitomeatal line but the angle can be varied to avoid dental fillings, which may cause significant artifact. Choosing an angle to avoid dental fillings can easily be done with a lateral "topogram" or scout view. Coronal views often help define the relationship of a parotid mass to the skull base and to the parapharyngeal space.

Since the parotid gland is most frequently lower in density than muscle, as a result of variable amounts of intercellular fat deposits, scanning may frequently be performed without sialography. When it is thought necessary to differentiate vascular structures from surrounding lymph nodes, intravenous contrast should be employed (such as a rapid infusion of 300 cc of Reno-M-DIP). (Fig. 8.1).

When the parotid gland is atypically dense or a relatively low density mass is suspected, sialography may be necessary prior to scanning. Cannulation of Stenson's duct is performed following gentle dilation of the orifice with dilators, either metal or Teflon. A snug fit is then possible with an appropriate size cannula. These cannulas have a closed end and a side hole. Injection of contrast material (water soluble such as Sinografin or oily such as Ethiodol) should ideally be made under fluoroscopic control to help obtain adequate small duct filling while avoiding extravasation. The end point of injection is determined by fluoroscopic visualization of the filling ducts and/or pain secondary to duct distention. The total volume is usually 0.3 to 0.5 cc. Water soluble material will resorb quickly and thus filming must be performed as quickly as possible. Plain films are obtained and then the CT scan is performed, leaving the cannula in position to help avoid emptying of contrast from the duct system. If emptying does occur after the patient has left the fluoroscopic area, he/she is carefully reinjected, with pain as the end point.

Since the submandibular gland is generally denser than the parotid glands,

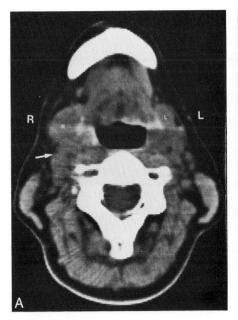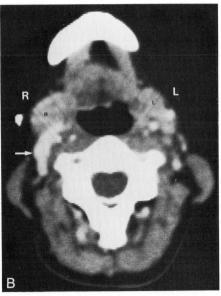

FIG. 8.1.   (A) Submandibular glands, axial. Right (R) and left (L) submandibular glands are visualized. No tumor is differentiated from normal gland tissue. Soft tissue masses (arrow) raise the possibility of enlarged lymph nodes on scan without IV contrast. (B) Submandibular glands, axial. During IV contrast administration, soft tissue masses (arrow) enhance, as do vessels, excluding possibility of adenopathy.

the CT evaluation for mass lesions is generally performed following sialography. Again, Wharton's duct is dilated and cannulated, water soluble or oily contrast is injected under fluoroscopic control, and plain films are taken. Axial and coronal CT images (4–5-mm thick) are obtained. Intravenous contrast is again used if it is deemed necessary to differentiate vessels from lymph nodes (Fig. 8.1). It should also be mentioned at this time that IV contrast may be helpful in identifying certain tumors and metastatic lymph nodes that enhance to various degrees.

ANATOMIC RELATIONSHIPS

Parotid Gland

The parotid gland lies in front of and below the external auditory canal (Figs. 8.2, 8.3). The gland extends anteriorly a variable distance to wrap around the masseter muscle, and the deep portion of the gland extends posterior to the mandible toward the lateral pharyngeal space. This deep portion of the gland is generally separated from the pharyngeal musculature by a fat plane. The

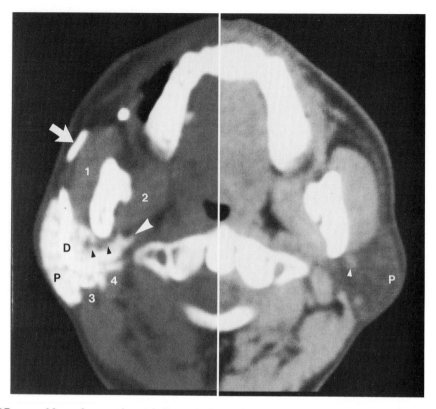

FIG. 8.2. Normal parotid, axial. Parotid glands (P), following sialography on the right, without contrast on left. Left gland is of lower density than muscle, secondary to presence of fat. Stensen's duct (D) is opacified on right side and arrow marks the duct passing over masseter muscle (1). Medial pterygoid muscle (2) is adjacent to deep portion of parotid (large arrowhead). Posterior surface of parotid is indented by sterno-cleidomastoid (3) and posterior belly of digastric (4) muscle. Small arrowheads mark the vessels passing through parotid in retromandibular area.

cephalad extent of the parotid gland is the under surface of the temporal bone. The inferior, more narrowed portion of the gland, called the tail, is triangular in shape in the axial plane, convex laterally. The posteroinferior surface is grooved by the sternocleidomastoid muscle and the posteromedial surface by the posterior belly of the digastric muscle. The facial nerve is not visible on CT but enters the gland posteriorly adjacent to the superior border of the posterior belly of the digastric muscle. The deep and superficial portions of the parotid gland lie medial and lateral, respectively, to the facial nerve as it courses anteriorly through the parotid gland. The facial nerve exits the skull base through the stylomastoid foramen and then passes lateral to the base of the styloid process before entering the posterior aspect of the gland. Shortly after entering the gland, the nerve divides into two major trunks, which then branch further.

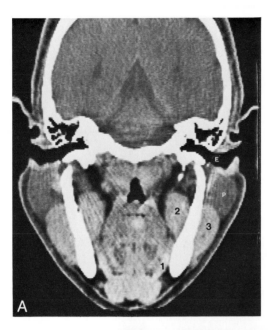

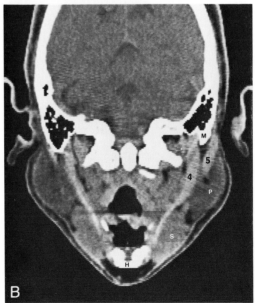

FIG. 8.3. (A) Normal parotid (coronal). On the section through the external auditory canal (E) the parotid gland (P) is visualized and is of lower density than surrounding muscles: medial pterygoid (2), masseter (3), mylohyoid (1). (B) Normal parotid (coronal). Section through mastoid tip (M) and hyoid bone (H) shows close proximity of parotid (P) and submandibular glands. The sternocleidomastoid (5) and posterior belly of the digastric (4) muscles are well visualized.

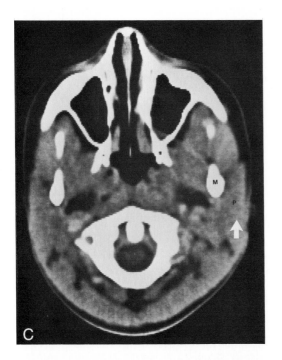

FIG. 8.3 (*Cont.*). (C) Normal parotid, axial. The density of the parotid glands (P) is higher than usual, about isodense with muscle. Border between sternocleidomastoid muscle and left parotid (arrow) is therefore difficult to distinguish.

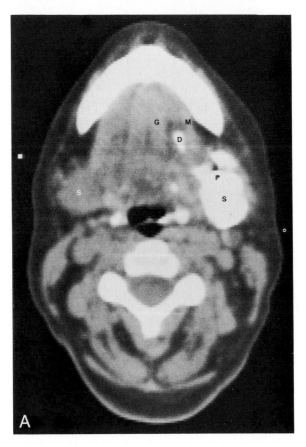

FIG. 8.4. (A) Normal submandibular gland, axial. Following sialography the left submandibular gland (S) is opacified; the right submandibular is not. Wharton's duct (D) is seen in part. The geniohyoid (G) and mylohyoid (M) muscles are well visualized.

The external carotid artery and the posterior facial vein are visualized within the gland just posterior to the ramus of the mandible, and the facial nerve lies just lateral to them. Lymph nodes are present within the parotid fascia (the superficial layer of deep cervical fascia divides to encase the gland). Other lymph nodes lie within the substance of the gland and occasionally a normal sized node may be seen within the gland on CT images. Stensen's duct extends forward from the hilum of the gland, overlies the masseter muscle, and enters the oral cavity opposite the second maxillary molar tooth. The orifice is located at the apex of a small papilla.

Submandibular Gland

The second largest salivary gland is essentially oval in shape but appears round when cut in the axial plane. It lies just below and anterior to the angle of the mandible. One portion of the gland extends superior or deep to the mylohyoid muscle, wrapping around the free margin, and the major portion lies inferior or superficial to the mylohyoid muscle (Fig. 8.4). Posteriorly, the sub-

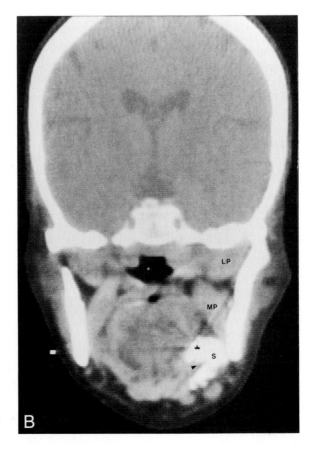

FIG. 8.4 (*Cont.*)   (B) Normal submandibular, coronal. On the coronal view the superior (deep) and inferior portions of the submandibular gland (S) are seen to wrap around the mylohyoid muscle (arrowhead). The lateral pterygoid (LP) and medial pterygoid (MP) muscles are well seen.

mandibular gland is separated from the parotid gland by a fascial layer (Fig. 8.3B). The submandibular gland duct (Wharton's) empties via a papilla on the anterior aspect of the floor of the mouth, beside the frenulum. The duct originates from the small, superior portion of the gland and extends forward from this point.

Sublingual Gland

The smallest of the three major salivary glands, the sublingual gland, is located superior to the mylohyoid muscle, lateral to the geniohyoid muscle, and medial to the mandibular body. It is covered superiorly by the mucosa of the floor of the mouth. This gland is not always well defined on CT scans but can sometimes be identified in this location as a slightly lower density area. The gland usually empties via multiple small ducts into the floor of the mouth but may occasionally join Wharton's duct or even have a dominant, separate orifice just posterior to the orifice of Wharton's duct. This ductal anatomy explains the reason that sialography of the sublingual gland cannot be routinely performed.

TUMORS OF THE SALIVARY GLANDS

The details of the classification of salivary gland tumors are rather complex and are beyond the scope of this chapter. An excellent review of tumor histology and clinical behavior is found in Batsakis,[6] from which Tables 8.1 and 8.2 are reproduced. Table 8.1 outlines the benign and malignant tumors that involve the salivary glands as classified by the author. Table 8.2 represents the W.H.O. classification of salivary gland tumors by Thackray and Sobin in 1972. This is the more widely known classification scheme. Knowledge of the basic histology of the salivary gland explains the cellular origin of the majority of the neoplasms encountered. Serous or mucinous acini lead to an intercalated duct, which connects to a striated duct, which then empties into an extralobular excretory duct. Surrounding the periphery of the acini and the intercalated ducts are myoepithelial cells. Parotid acinar cells are mainly or totally serous in type, whereas those in the submandibular and sublingual glands are seromucous. Knowledge of the cell of origin of these various tumors is not very important in the direct interpretation of CT scans, since the appearance of these tumors is generally nonspecific. However, one must at least have some familiarity with the nomenclature of the tumors encountered and gain appreciation of the various clinical presentations so that the implications of CT findings will be more apparent.

Tumors of the salivary glands comprise less than 3 percent of all head and neck neoplasms.[7] Tumors of the parotid glands are 12 times more common than those of the submandibular gland. A solitary tumor mass in the parotid gland has proved to be a pleomorphic adenoma (benign mixed tumor) in about 60 to 80 percent of cases in various series. This tumor accounts for between

TABLE 8.1 Classification of Epithelial Salivary Gland Tumors

Type of lesion	Variations
Benign	Mixed tumor (pleomorphic adenoma)
	Papillary cystadenoma lymphomatosum (Wharthin's tumor)
	Oncocytoma (oncocytosis)
	Monomorphic tumors
	Basal cell adenoma
	Glycogen rich adenoma
	Clear cell adenoma
	Membranous adenoma
	Myoepithelioma
	Sebaceous tumors
	Adenoma
	Lymphadenoma
	Papillary ductal adenoma (papilloma)
	Benign lymphoepithelial lesion
	Unclassified
Malignant	Carcinoma ex pleomorphic adenoma (carcinoma arising in a mixed tumor)
	Malignant mixed tumor (biphasic malignancy)
	Mucoepidermoid carcinoma
	Low grade
	Intermediate grade
	High grade
	Adenoid cystic carcinoma
	Acinous cell (acinic) carcinoma
	Adenocarcinoma
	Mucus-producing adenopapillary and nonpapillary carcinoma
	Salivary duct carcinoma (ductal carcinoma)
	Other adenocarcinomas
	Oncocytic carcinoma (malignant oncocytoma)
	Clear cell carcinoma (nonmucinous and glycogen-containing or non-glycogen-containing)
	Primary squamous cell carcinoma
	Hybrid basal cell adenoma/adenoid cystic carcinoma
	Undifferentiated carcinoma
	Epithelial–myoepithelial carcinoma of intercalated ducts
	Miscellaneous (includes sebaceous, Stensen's duct, melanoma, and carcinoma ex lymphoepithelial lesion)
	Metastatic
	Unclassified

From Batsakis JG: Tumors of the Head and Neck: Clinical and Pathological Considerations, 2nd Ed. © 1979, the Williams & Wilkins Co., Baltimore.

TABLE 8.2 W.H.O. Classification of Salivary Gland Tumors

Epithelial tumors
  Adenomas
  Pleomorphic adenoma (mixed tumor)
Monomorphic adenomas
  Adenolymphoma
  Oxyphilic adenoma
  Other types
Mucoepidermoid tumor
Acinic cell tumor
Carcinomas
  Adenoid cystic
  Adenocarcinoma
  Epidermoid carcinoma
  Undifferentiated
  Carcinoma in pleomorphic adenoma (malignant
    mixed tumor)
Nonepithelial tumors
Unclassified tumors
Alied conditions
  Benign lymphoepithelial lesion
  Sialosis
  Oncocytosis

From Batsakis JG: Tumors of the Head and Neck: Clinical and Pathological Considerations, 2nd Ed. © 1979, the Williams & Wilkins Co., Baltimore.

35 and 60 percent of submandibular gland tumors.[8,9] The tumor is composed of a mixture of epithelial and myoepithelial cells. A varying degree and type of stroma is also present.

The CT appearance of this prototype of the benign lesion is as follows: The mass is typically well circumscribed, lying in an otherwise normal gland. When in the parotid, it is most often found in the tail of the gland, and since the mass is usually of higher denisity than the typically low density parotid gland, it may often be seen without ductal opacification. This point has been stressed by at least one author (Fig. 8.5).[4] However, as noted above, some parotid glands are relatively dense and the mass may be isodense with gland tissue. Identification may then depend on CT sialography to outline the tumor mass (Fig. 8.6). The mass in Fig. 8.6 happens to be a lymphomatous lesion, having a typically benign appearance.

Masses in the submandibular gland have similar CT appearances to those in the parotid. However, as noted, the normally high density of the subman-

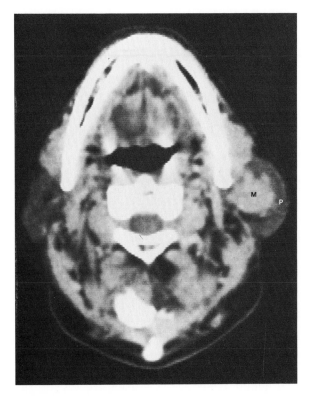

FIG. 8.5. Parotid glands, axial. Mass (M) is of higher density than normal parotid gland (P). The mass is sharply marginated.

dibular gland often necessitates sialography prior to obtaining the CT images in order to reliably identify tumors that may be relatively isodense with the gland.

Most pleomorphic adenomas behave like benign masses clinically but will recur if total excision has not been performed. In the parotid, this necessitates a superficial parotidectomy for tumors that lie superficial to the facial nerve and a total conservative parotidectomy with preservation of the facial nerve for tumors lying in the deep portion of the gland.[6] The tumors are very rarely multicentric. When pleomorphic adenomas are located in either the submandibular or the sublingual gland, total removal of the gland is the procedure of choice. A small percentage of these benign tumors show malignant degeneration, another reason that necessitates their complete removal.

The second most frequently occurring benign tumor in the parotid gland is Warthin's tumor or papillary cystadenoma lymphomatosum. This tumor makes up approximately 8 percent of all parotid gland tumors. It represents a neoplasm arising from ductal epithelial elements that are interspersed among lymphoid tissue usually found in or around the parotid gland.[6] With this combination of cellular elements involved, it can be understood why true Warthin's

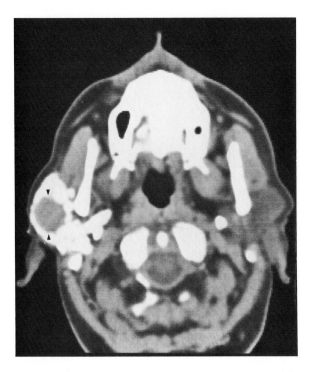

FIG. 8.6. Parotid glands, axial. Mass (arrowheads) within contrast-filled parotid gland.

tumors occur extremely rarely outside of the parotid gland, where lymphoid tissue is normally located. The CT appearance of a Warthin's tumor is nonspecific, usually appearing as a well-circumscribed mass within or on the surface of the parotid gland. Though histologically these tumors often have cystic components and some mucoid fluid within, the CT characteristics are not specific since the cystic spaces are very small. Note the sharply defined mass outlined by contrast in Fig. 8.7.

As seen in Tables 8.1 and 8.2, there is a long list of benign neoplasms that involve the salivary glands. CT is often nonspecific in identification of these tumors. However, in evaluating suspected or known tumor patients, CT has many other uses beyond its generally limited aid to diagnostic specificity. One valuable role of CT in relationship to parotid gland tumors is the ability of CT to accurately differentiate tumors originating in the deep portion of the parotid gland from those arising within the lateral pharyngeal space, such as minor salivary gland neoplasms, and from tumors arising from other tissues. Most tumors of the parotid are found superficial to the facial nerve, and hence resection involves a surgical approach through the overlying skin with careful dissection of tumor to avoid the facial nerve. The deep portion of the parotid gland makes up a small percentage of the gland by weight and tumors are thus less frequent in this part of the gland. When tumors do occur here, they are of the same tissue types as superficial portion tumors. Deep portion tumors

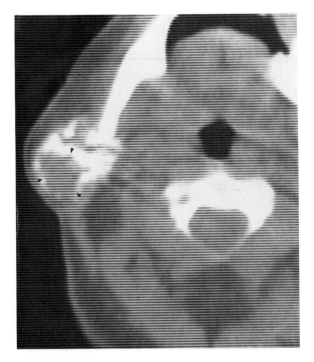

FIG. 8.7. Parotid gland, axial. Mass (arrowheads) outlined by contrast-filled parotid gland represents Warthin's tumor.

are likewise generally resected through a conventional parotidectomy incision, and often the facial nerve can be spared. However, the clinical presentation of these tumors is often very similar to that of a tumor originating in the lateral pharyngeal space.[6] Since removal of the latter type of tumor requires a different (intraoral) operative approach, it is important to define the point of origin of these masses. It is here that CT can frequently be very helpful. A deep portion parotid mass is generally easy to define as originating in the parotid gland, as in Fig. 8.8. In addition, the fat normally present in the lateral pharyngeal space, adjacent to the pharyngeal musculature, will usually be preserved to mark the boundary between the deep parotid mass and normal tissue.

A mass originating in the lateral pharyngeal space is easily differentiated from the above case. A tumor arising in the lateral pharyngeal space will enlarge and extend laterally toward the deep portion of the parotid gland. The normal fat around the pharyngeal musculature is replaced, but a fat plane may be visible separating tumor from the deep portion of the parotid gland, which may be compressed. These points are well demonstrated in Fig. 8.9, which shows scans from a woman with a recurrence of a previously removed pleomorphic adenoma of a minor salivary gland in the tonsilar region.

Another example of the ability of CT to provide precise localization of a mass in the parotid region is provided by the patient whose scan is shown

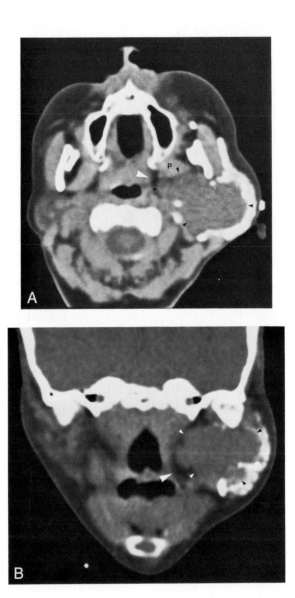

FIG. 8.8. (A) Parotid glands, axial. Note large parotid mass (pleomorphic adenoma) outlined by small arrowheads extending into deep portion of parotid gland, displacing pterygoid muscle (P) anteriorly. Large arrowhead marks normal fat adjacent to pharyngeal wall. (B) Parotid glands, coronal. Small arrowhead defines margins of parotid tumor on coronal view. Again large arrowhead identifies normal fat adjacent to pharynx wall.

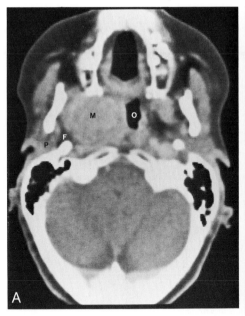

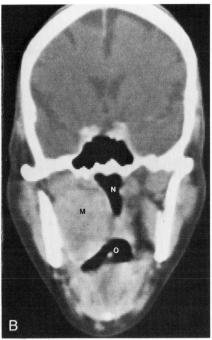

FIG. 8.9. (A) Pleomorphic adenoma, minor salivary gland, axial. Large mass (M) in right parapharyngeal space distorts oropharynx (O). Fat plane (F) is clearly seen between mass and deep portion of parotid (P). (B) Mass (M) is again seen on coronal view showing cephalocaudal extent and distortion of oropharynx (O) and nasopharynx (N).

in Figure 8.10. In this patient, a mass was palpated in the region of the parotid tail and was considered to be a benign parotid tumor on clinical grounds. The CT sialogram revealed a small extrinsic mass of fat density adjacent to the parotid gland, compatible with a lipoma (Fig. 8.10). By demonstrating the extrinsic nature of the mass the scan helped in the differential diagnosis. Secondly, the absolute attenuation number helped make a specific tissue diagnosis.

In other uncommon instances CT can help make a tissue-specific diagnosis. In most neoplasms involving the salivary glands, enhancement of tumor following IV contrast administration is nonspecific and not of any help in forming a differential diagnosis. However, the vascular tumors (most notably the capillary hemangioma) demonstrate a typical diffuse enhancement. These tumors will become essentially as dense as normal vascular structures become with intravenous contrast, unlike most neoplasms, which may or may not enhance at all. This rather specific type of enhancement can aid in making the diagnoses with such lesions, which in fact are not rare tumors. For example, in children under 1 year of age, the capillary hemangioma is the most common salivary gland tumor encountered. It usually occurs in the parotid gland and blue discoloration of the overlying skin or true vascular lesions involving the skin often

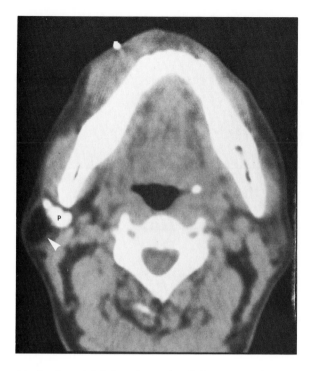

FIG. 8.10. Parotid glands, axial. Mass (arrowhead) lies posterolateral to the enhanced portion of the parotid gland (P). The fat density mass is clearly extrinsic to the parotid and represents a lipoma.

aid in making a clinical diagnosis.[6] However, when confirmation is necessary, CT can make a contribution by demonstrating the characteristic appearance of the lesion, as seen in Figure 8.11. The cavernous hemangioma is seen less frequently in children after infancy and in adults and may demonstrate enhancement patterns similar to those ocurring in the liver.

Cystic lesions represent some of the other uncommon masses that may involve the salivary glands. Any malignant neoplasm in a salivary gland has the potential to undergo hemorrhage and subsequent necrosis, but to recognize such a phenomenon on CT is rare. Cysts that involve the salivary glands involve mainly the parotid gland. They are a mixture of true epithelial cysts and branchial cleft cysts that are congenital in origin and acquired cysts that develop secondary to ductal obstruction.[10] The clinical importance of cysts is that they most often simulate tumor by palpation. The CT appearance of cysts in the salivary glands is similar to that of cysts in other organs of the body. Generally, cysts have thin walls, are well circumscribed, and contain water-density material (though this can vary depending on cyst contents). The branchial cleft cysts are particularly interesting because of their embryological etiology. The cysts that may involve the parotid arise from the first or second branchial clefts. Those arising from the first branchial cleft occur in the preauricular region

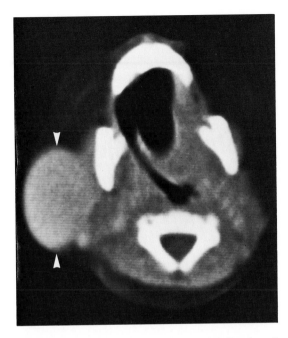

FIG. 8.11.   Parotid gland, axial. Marked enhancement of diffusely enlarged right parotid gland (arrowheads) secondary to capillary hemangioma.

of the parotid and those from the second cleft may involve the lower portion of the gland.[6] An example of a branchial cleft cyst is shown in Figure 8.12. The patient presented with a 4-month history of swelling in the tail of the parotid gland and a benign tumor such as Warthin's tumor was suspected clinically. CT demonstrated a cystic mass compatible with a branchial cleft cyst, which was removed and confirmed pathologically. It should be noted that branchial cleft cysts may appear in the region of the parotid gland or may actually lie within the gland.

Another example of the clinical utility of CT is seen in certain patients in whom a mass is suspected by palpation. In such instances CT can be performed to confirm or deny the clinical impression of a mass lesion. In the patient whose scan is shown in Figure 8.13, a firm mass was palpated in the region of the parotid gland and was thought to represent the lateral mass of C_1. Figure 8.13 demonstrates that a parotid mass is in fact present. However, it should be noted that the lateral mass of C_1 is in close proximity to this portion of the parotid gland, which harbored a benign pleomorphic adenoma in this patient. In some patients, it may be difficult to palpate the parotid gland accurately and occasionally the lateral mass of C_1 can be palpated and suspected of being a parotid gland mass. In such cases, CT can define a nomal gland and explain precisely the unclear physical findings.

Concerning the malignant neoplasms that involve the salivary glands, a glance at Tables 8.1 and 8.2 will reveal the wide range of cell types that appear at

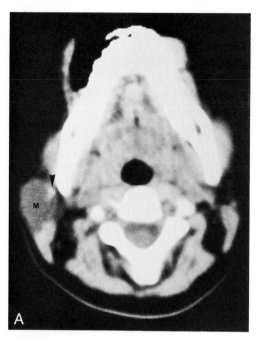

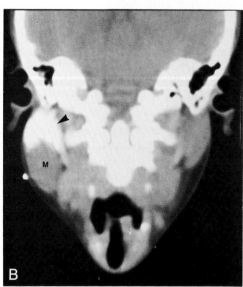

FIG. 8.12. (A) Branchial cleft cyst. Water density mass (M) is seen adjacent to small area of enhanced parotid gland (arrowhead) following sialography. (B) Coronal view reveals intrinsic nature of branchial cleft cyst (M) within the parotid gland (arrowhead).

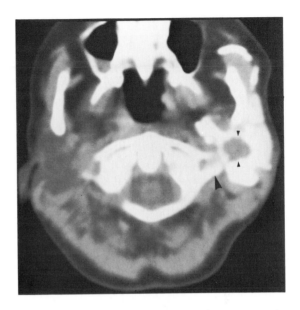

FIG. 8.13. Pleomorphic adenoma. Well circumscribed mass (small arrowheads) within enhanced parotid gland. Note proximity of lateral mass of C1 (large arrowhead) to mass.

these sites. Although benign tumors often have a CT appearance that suggests benignity, as demonstrated above, the rules are frequently broken and benign-appearing masses may prove to be malignant. Likewise, malignant lesions often have an appearance suggesting their agressive nature, i.e., the margins are less distinct and it is more difficult to define the border between normal gland and tumor mass. This fact is exemplified in Figure 8.14. Here, in a parotid gland that is of relatively low density, tumor can be seen without sialographic contrast, and the margins of the tumor are seen to be rather indistinct, suggesting malignancy. However, differentiating benign from malignant lesions is not the primary goal of CT. Rather, CT becomes important in demonstrating total extent of disease—direct extension, local lymph node involvement, and distant metastasis.

A malignant tumor in a salivary gland may be removed successfully when the tumor is still maintained within the confines of the gland. As local extension to surrounding structures occurs, surgical removal may or may not be feasible. For example, tumors deeply invading the carotid sheath or the base of the skull may need nonsurgical treatment. Thus, the ability of CT to demonstrate the local extent of tumor growth is useful in identifying those patients who are likely to be surgically resectable and those who need other forms of therapy. In the patient presented in Figure 8.14, the squamous cell carcinoma extended locally from the primary parotid lesion along the course of the facial nerve, into the middle ear, internal auditory canal, and cerebellopontine angle. Surgical cure in this patient was deemed impossible and radiation therapy was instituted. The ability of CT to define areas of complex anatomy and to demonstrate tumor extension into areas that could previously only be studied by indirect and less sensitive methods is dramatically represented in this case.

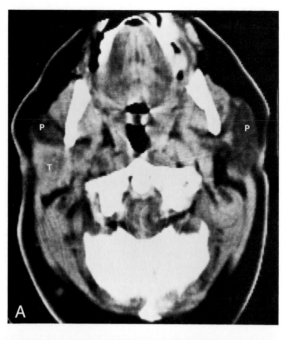

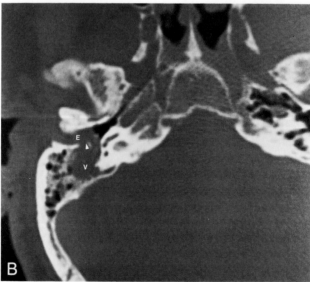

FIG. 8.14. (A) Poorly differentiated squamous cell carcinoma. Tumor (T) is seen within posterior aspect of right parotid gland (P). Left parotid gland (P) is also marked for comparison. (B) Two axial sections through temporal bone reveal tumor within external auditory canal (E), destroying its posterior wall (arrowhead), and around vertical position (V) of facial nerve canal, which is enlarged by tumor.

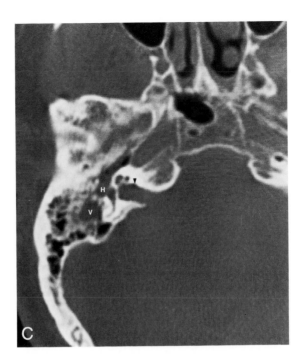

FIG. 8.14 (*Cont.*). (C) Slightly higher level shows erosion of anterior wall of IAC by tumor (arrowhead) in region of horizontal (H) and vertical (V) course of facial nerve.

The various malignant salivary tumors have different propensities to spread to lymph nodes, either by contiguous growth or by normal lymphatic channels. The clinical significance of lymph node involvement varies depending on the tumor type, and varying opinions exist as to whether neck node dissection need be performed in the absence of involved nodes. Suffice it to say that CT is quite sensitive in identifying enlarged lymph nodes in the neck and can thus be useful in directing clinical management by identifying areas of pathology that may not be palpable. As in other areas of the body, CT cannot identify microscopic tumor involvement and thus tumor can exist in small lymph nodes and go undetected by CT. On the other hand, enlarged nodes may be related to infection or other cause and may not be secondary to neoplasm. As outlined by Biorklund and Eneroth,[9] radical neck dissection should be performed for all tumors of the parotid except for the benign tumors and low-grade mucoepidermoid and acinic cell carcinoma. Whether or not a given surgeon adheres to this treatment principle, the utility of CT becomes apparent. Specifically, in patients in whom node dissection would not normally be performed, unsuspected tumor-related lymphadenopathy discovered by CT could greatly alter a given patient's therapy.

In those patients in whom radiation therapy is indicated as the primary treatment modality, CT can provide extremely useful information concerning the total extent of tumor. Such information is quite helpful to the radiotherapist in attempting to define accurate radiation portals. Nonpalpable tumor left untreated could lead to a treatment failure.

Distant metastases from salivary gland tumors are to the lungs, bones, and, less commonly, other sites. The sensitivity of CT in demonstrating small lung lesions is well documented. In this regard CT can help uncover patients who need more than local therapy for their salivary gland neoplasm.

Similar utility has been demonstrated for CT in evaluating malignant neoplasms whether they occur in the major or in the minor salivary glands. Evaluating the local extent of tumor and a search for unsuspected lymphadenopathy as well as evaluation of possible distant metastases are equally important in patients presenting with minor salivary gland neoplasms. Since the majority of minor salivary gland tumors are malignant and since many of these tumors arise in areas that are difficult to examine clinically, the use of CT to define these lesions can be very helpful.

Figure 8.15 is from a patient who presented with an opaque maxillary sinus, presumably secondary to a known oral antral fistula resulting from a dental extraction. Osteomyelitis of the maxilla, causing bony destruction, was presumed to be present. A biopsy revealed an adenoid cystic carcinoma in the sinus and the CT revealed quite accurately the full extent of tumor and presumably the site of origin. The major mass on CT is in the soft palate, likely the original site of this minor salivary gland tumor. CT also showed extension of tumor cephalad into the pterygopalatine fossa and through the inferior orbital fissure to the apex of the orbit. With this information at hand, radiotherapy

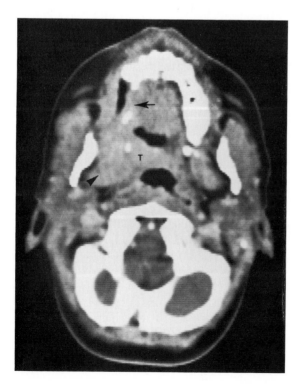

FIG. 8.15. Adenoid cystic carcinoma. Soft tissue mass (T) in soft palate is well visualized. Tumor extends laterally into parapharyngeal space (arrowhead). The destroyed alveolar bone is also noted (arrow).

was chosen as the treatment of choice and accurate portals, including all tumor bearing sites, could be planned.

It should also be noted that occult neoplasms occurring in the minor salivary glands can often be identified by CT. Many such patients present either with focal symptoms or signs, lymphadenopathy in the neck, or perhaps distant metastases that might be associated with a small primary neoplasm. In such patients, CT is often useful in uncovering the primary tumor.

Once surgery has been performed in a patient with a malignant salivary gland tumor or a benign tumor that tends to recur (i.e., pleomorphic adenoma), CT can aid in assessing possible recurrence (Fig. 8.16). CT is also successful in assessing the results of nonsurgical therapy for malignant lesions. Since surgery and radiation therapy can produce their own changes in local anatomy (i.e., soft tissue scarring, loss of fat planes, and bony dissolution or sclerosis), care must be taken when trying to determine if recurrent tumor is present. Therefore, a baseline scan should be performed following surgery or radiation therapy in order to assess subsequent recurrence.

Other malignant tumors that can present as mass lesions in the salivary glands include lymphoma and metastatic tumors of various types. Regarding lymphoma, the incidence of primary salivary gland involvement is very low, representing well under 1 percent of primary parotid neoplasms. The parotid, with its intraglandular lymph nodes, is the most common salivary gland to be involved with lymphoma. Less commonly, lymphoma occurs in the submandibular gland. The CT appearance of lymphoma is that of a mass lesion or lesions within the parotid, or more infrequently, the submandibular gland.

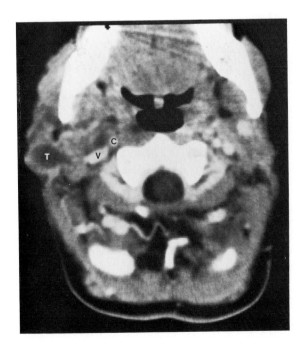

FIG. 8.16. Recurrent pleomorphic adenoma (T) is revealed in the bed of the previously resected right parotid gland. Internal jugular vein (V) and carotid artery (C) are well visualized.

As seen in the parotid gland, most lymphomatous masses have been well-circumscribed, relatively high density lesions resembling other typically benign masses.[2,4] This appearance is what might be expected, since primary lymphoma of the parotid gland is mainly a neoplasm of the intraparotid lymph nodes. If a lymphomatous mass lesion is very eccentric, appearing to have invaded the parotid gland from without, it may very well represent lymphoma that has spread into the parotid gland from surrounding nodes and not represent a true primary salivary gland lymphoma. Alternatively, eccentric lesions that do clearly lie within the parotid gland may have arisen in any of the clumps of lymphoid tissue that exist within the normal parotid gland. An example of a typical lymphomatous lesion within the parotid gland has been seen in Figure 8.6. Lymphoma may also occur in a salivary gland already involved with one of the disorders that produce a nonspecific lymphocytic infiltration, such as may be seen in chronic recurrent parotitis and in Sjogren's syndrome. In any event, lymphoma developing in an already diseased gland is more difficult to identify since it is superimposed on an already abnormal background.

Finally, metastasis should be considered in the list of malignant lesions involving the salivary glands. Concerning the parotid gland, most metastases occur via the lymphatic route, originating in tumors that occur in locations that drain to the parotid region lymph nodes. These areas include the nasopharyngeal, oropharyngeal, and sinonasal cavities but also include the scalp, face, external portion of the nose, pinna, eyelids, and lacrimal glands. Melanoma and squamous cell carcinoma from these sites make up 80 percent of parotid metastases. Of the more distant primary tumors to metastasize to the parotid gland, the lung is the most common site. The same is true for the submandibular

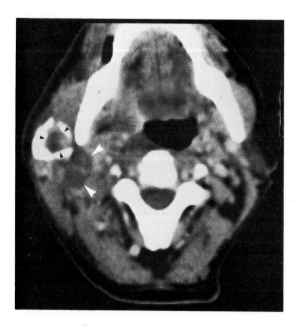

FIG. 8.17. Metastasis to parotid gland, axial. Low density mass (small arrowheads) is well defined in contrast-filled right parotid gland. Two low density masses (large arrowheads) represent necrotic tumor in lymph nodes.

gland. The CT appearance of metastatic tumor in the parotid or submandibular glands is nonspecific and may appear either well circumscribed, as with most benign primary salivary gland tumors, or may have poorly defined margins, more suggestive of a malignant neoplasm. An example of a metastatic lesion in the parotid gland is provided in Figure 8.17. The mass is relatively well circumscribed and represents a metastatic lesion from a primary tumor probably in the oropharynx.

OTHER DISEASE ENTITIES

Up to this point, the contribution of CT to the evaluation of focal masses of the salivary glands, has been the major concern. There are, however, numerous other disease entities that may involve the salivary glands. Although CT can play some role in evaluating such disorders, one should understand that routine sialography still has a major role in the diagnosis of certain diseases that affect the parotid and submandibular glands, namely those diseases that affect ductal caliber. For example, chronic infectious sialadenitis, sialadenitis associated with rheumatological diseases, and sarcoidosis may alter ductal anatomy to various degrees. These alterations are best diagnosed by conventional sialography. Similarly, asymptomatic salivary gland hyperplasia is a diagnosis made by history and by exclusion of ductal abnormalities on sialography. Also, calculi and complications of calculi, such as ductal strictures, are best evaluated with routine sialography. However, one should be aware of the appearance of such entities when they are encountered on CT.

For example, calculi, which are radiopaque on plain x-rays approximately 80 percent of the time, are easily seen on CT. In fact, as with urinary tract calculi, even those stones that are radiolucent on plain films should be dense enough to be easily seen on CT.[12] Hence, CT could serve as an adjunct to plain films in evaluating suspected radiolucent calculi if sialography fails for some reason to demonstrate such stones. An example of a submandibular calculus is demonstrated in Figure 8.18A, B. This case is typical of salivary gland calculi. The great majority (90 percent) occur in the submandibular gland, often near the hilum, and very few stones are found in the parotid gland. In the patient presented here, CT was performed to evaluate an atypical right-sided facial pain of 2 years duration. The calculus in Wharton's duct and marked atrophy of the submandibular gland were unsuspected findings that retrospectively could explain the patient's symptoms. Most likely, plain films or a sialogram could have made the diagnosis in this patient, but such findings should not be missed on CT examinations.

Whether or not the complication of calculi is present, infections in and around the salivary glands may be advantageously evaluated with CT. Well-defined abscesses may occur in the submandibular and parotid glands. The typical appearance of an abscess is that of a water density (or slightly higher) mass with a wall of variable thickness that probably enhances with intravenous contrast. In the appropriate clinical setting a definite diagnosis of abscess can often be made. Abscesses in the submandibular gland are usually found in

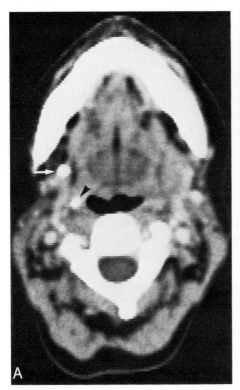

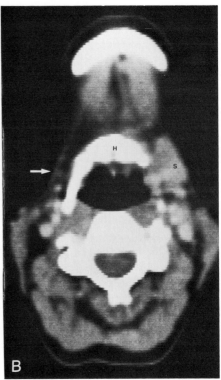

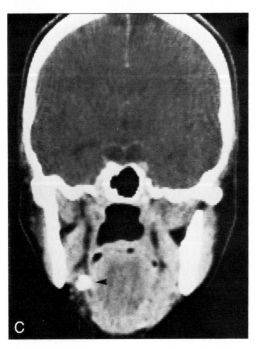

FIG. 8.18. (A) Calculus (arrow) is shown in the region of the right submandibular gland. Second density (arrowhead) is calcified stylohyoid ligament. (B) Normal left submandibular gland (S) is shown. The region of the right submandibular gland (arrow) reveals atrophic gland. (C) Calculus (arrowhead) in hilum of atrophic gland seen on coronal view.

younger patients and are most often secondary to ductal obstruction from stone or stricture. The typical parotid gland abscess occurs in an elderly, debilitated patient with poor oral hygiene.

When the institution of antibiotic therapy and the relief of any ductal obstruction are prompt, most salivary gland infections should respond well. In the early stages, the infection produces either a focal or a diffuse inflammatory process comparable with a cellulitis. It should be noted that the CT appearance of focal sialadenitis, infections or not, can mimic that of malignant tumors. As one author points out, focal sialadenitis will appear as a poorly marginated mass and hence be indistinquishable from malignant tumors.[4]

When true abscess forms, with or without spread beyond the confines of the salivary gland, drainage is generally necessary. Here, CT is useful in defining the full extent of an abscess that may not be apparent clinically. An example of an abscess with widespread involvement is presented in Figure 8.19A. In fact, this patient had a parotid cyst and chronic sialadenitis with superimposed abscess involving many of the surrounding tissues. The precise anatomic information that CT provides in a case such as this can be invaluable to the physician who must drain all purulent fluid collections.

Generally, the appearance of the salivary gland, when affected by a chronic sialadenitis such as occurs with various types of rheumatological disease, in the context of Sjögren's syndrome or not, is usually recognizable. In the normally low density parotid glands, a diffuse inflammatory process would be expected to raise the density in areas of cellular infiltrate, scarring, or edema, producing an enlarged gland with heterogeneously increased density. The process may or may not be bilateral and can involve the other salivary glands as well. In the submandibular glands the density changes may not be as easily appreciated. Diffuse enlargement might be the only abnormality, though heterogeneous density might be seen. Since the histological changes of chronic sialadenitis run a spectrum from simple lymphocytic infiltration and ductal destruction to complete replacement by lymphoid and epithelial elements, which may or may not have mass effect, the varied appearance of glands involved with Sjögren's syndrome can be understood. In Figure 8.20A, from a patient with Sjögren's syndrome, both salivary glands are enlarged (right greater than left). The lack of filling ducts in a large area of the parotid gland is compatible with a tumor mass, proved in this patient to represent a true "lymphoepithelial" lesion, or a mass composed of combinations of lymphoid tissue and islands of metaplastic ductal epithelium.[6] Figure 8.20B is from the plain sialogram in this patient. The sialectatic changes of the ducts are well seen and the mass is also noted. This case demonstrates one end of the spectrum of changes that may be seen in Sjogren's syndrome (or other forms of chronic sialadenitis).

Another inflammatory disease that can involve the salivary glands is sarcoidosis. It seems appropriate to mention this disorder at this time, since the clinical presentation of sarcoid in the salivary gland may be similar to that of the autoimmune diseases as they affect these glands. One or both glands may be involved, as in the rheumatological diseases. The point has been emphasized that typically, sarcoidosis is a disease that produces multiple small masses in

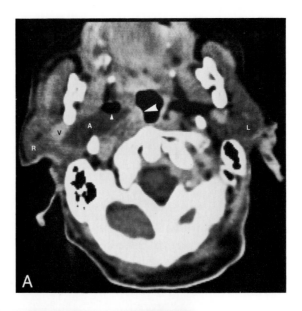

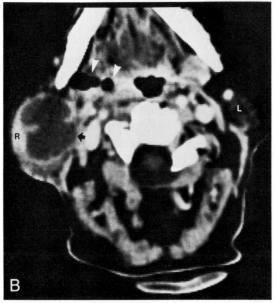

FIG. 8.19. (A) Fluid collection represents abscess (A) in parapharyngeal space with bulging into pharynx (large arrowhead). Note air–fluid level (small arrowhead). V, retromandibular vessels. Right parotid gland (R) is of higher density than left gland (L), since it was involved with chronic sialadenitis. (B) Arrow points to the branchial cleft cyst within the right parotid gland (R). Arrowheads point to air within parapharyngeal space. (L) is left parotid gland.

salivary glands secondary to multiple noncaseating granulomas.[13] These may involve gland parenchyma or intraparotid lymph nodes. As discussed above, CT is more sensitive than routine sialography in detecting small mass lesions. Thus, in patients with a history of sarcoidosis the CT diagnosis of multiple benign appearing masses should be considered typical, and a search for other diseases that can produce multiple masses can be delayed. As mentioned earlier,

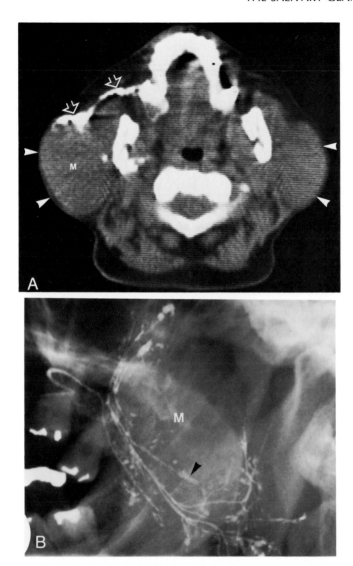

FIG. 8.20. (A) Sjögren's syndrome with "lymphoepithelial" lesion. Bilaterally enlarged parotid glands (arrowheads). Parotid gland partially filled with contrast and duct on the right side (open arrows) are draped over a mass (M) representing the "lymphoepithelial" lesion. (B) Ducts are draped around the mass (M) in this parotid gland. Areas of ductal dilatation are seen (arrowhead).

metastatic carcinomas and lymphoma can produce multiple salivary gland masses. Tuberculosis, atypical mycobacterial infections, actinomycosis, cat scratch fever, and rarely some of the benign salivary gland tumors may also produce multiple small masses. Such diseases must be excluded clinically if salivary gland abnormalities do not improve along with resolution of the other manifestations of sarcoidosis in a given patient.

CONCLUSION

An attempt has been made to outline the important contributions that CT can make in evaluating patients with various diseases of the salivary glands. As in other areas of the body, the accurate density discrimination of CT is useful in helping to detect small mass lesions within the salivary glands, and occasionally the absolute density measurement can make a specific diagnosis. The ability of CT to image areas of complex anatomy makes CT ideal for defining the extent of both neoplasms and inflammatory processes that involve the salivary glands and their surroundings. Although plain film sialography still has a primary role in evaluating certain disease states, we have tried to show how CT can add information in certain of these patients. Likewise, it is important that these diseases be recognized on CT and not be confused with other similarly appearing processes. As in other areas of the body, the contribution of CT to patient care can be great, but only when the CT study is coupled with an adequate knowledge of the history and clinical findings can its true potential be reached.

REFERENCES

1. Som BM, Biller HF: The combined CT–sialogram. Radiology 135:387, 1980.
2. Carter BL, Karmody CS, Blickman JR, Panders AK: Computed tomography and sialography: 1 & 2. J Comput Assist Tomogr 1:42–53, 1981.
3. Mancuso A, Rice D, Hanafee W: Computed tomography of the parotid gland during contrast sialography. Radiology 132:211, 1979.
4. Bryan NR, Miller RH, Ferreyro RI, Sessions RB: Computed tomography of the major salivary glands. AJR 139:547, 1982.
5. Gates GA, Jones ME: Embryology and anatomy of the salivary glands. In Paparella MM, Shumrick DA (eds): Otolaryngology. WB Saunders, Philadelphia, 1980.
6. Batsakis JG: Tumors of the Head and Neck: Clinical and Pathological Considerations, 2nd Ed. Williams & Wilkins, Baltimore, 1979, pp. 9–10.
7. Leegaard T, Lindeman H: Salivary gland tumors: clinical picture and treatment. Acta Otolaryngol 263:155, 1970.
8. Work WP, Hecht DW: Tumors and cysts of major salivary glands. In Paparella MM, Shumrick DA (eds): Otolaryngology. WB Saunders, Philadelphia, 1980.
9. Biorklund A, Eneroth CM: Management of parotid gland neoplasms. Am J Otolaryngol 1:2, 1980.
10. Shaheen NA, Harboyan GT, Nassif RI: Cysts of the parotid gland. Review and report of two unusual cases. J Otolaryngol 89:439, 1975.
11. Stone DN, Mancuso AM, Rice D, et al: Parotid CT sialography. Radiology 138:393, 1981.
12. Mitcheson HD, Zamenhof RG, Bankoff MS, Prien EL: Determination of the chemical composition of urinary tract calculi by CT. J Urol (In press).
13. Som PM, Shugar J, and Biller HF: Parotid gland sarcoidosis and the CT sialogram. J Comput Assist Tomogr 5:674, 1981.

9 Head and Neck Lesions in Children

ROY G. K. McCAULEY
LUCIUS F. SINKS
BARBARA L. CARTER

INTRODUCTION

Before computed tomography became readily available, radiographic diagnosis of diseases of the head and neck in children centered on plain radiography, tomography, and angiography. Dynamic changes in the airway were, and still are, often best evaluated by fluoroscopy. However, for delineation of anatomic and pathological processes at the base of the skull, in the bony and soft tissues of the neck, in the sinuses, orbits, and temporal bone, CT combines the advantages of the earlier methods, especially if enhancement of vessels and tissues is performed by using bolus injections of intravenous contrast material (2–3 ml/kg). Plain radiographs are still used primarily to diagnose the more common everyday pediatric head and neck disorders such as croup, epiglottitis, retropharyngeal inflammation, suspected dislocation or fracture, and anomalies of the cervical spine, trauma to the facial bones, sinusitis, and mastoiditis. Plain radiographs are also often used initially to investigate the cause of a mass or swelling in the head and neck region or to delineate the source of pain. Conventional tomography has been replaced largely by CT in those centers where modern equipment can give high resolution images, though hypocycloidal tomography will still give excellent bony detail in many situations if required.

The decision to perform head and neck CT in a child should not be taken lightly, and a clear understanding of its advantages and limitations should be presented to the referring clinician. In general, CT should not be performed if a simpler method can give the same answer. Many referring clinicians still have too high expectations of what computed tomography can do. They should also be made aware that when lesions are shown, sometimes the histology of the tissue cannot be confidently determined without a biopsy. Despite these limitations, CT is still the best method for diagnosing and following many of these disorders. It is of the greatest importance that the physician supervising the CT studies be thoroughly familiar with the disorders of the pediatric head and neck.

Disadvantages of CT in pediatric practice include the use of absorbed ionizing radiation, the occasional need for sedation (chloral hydrate, 75 mg/kg to a maximum of 2 g) particularly in younger patients, and the usual potential allergic reaction to intravenous contrast materials. Also, the tissue planes are somewhat less well delineated than in adult patients because of the relatively small amount of fat between the planes, but this is less of a problem than it would be in abdominal studies.

RADIATION

Use of radiation is of concern, particularly in those instances when the eye or thyroid gland is in the field to be studied. The differences between pediatric and adult CT radiation dose exposure are discussed by Brasch and Cann,[1] Berger et al.,[2] and Schmidt and Stieve.[3] They state that "the surface dose at radiation entrance is higher in children because of a smaller body diameter for the same dose rate at the tube. . . . however, the absorbed energy, i.e., integral dose, is lower in children than in adults because of lesser volume of tissue." Multidirectional tomography delivers an even larger dose to the area being examined. Use of CT can reduce this dose by up to 50 percent in some instances while giving the same information.[4] Technological advances can be expected to further reduce patient dose, but the radiologist and technologist can substantially reduce exposure at present by carefully screening requests for examination, by carefully tailoring those that are performed to the clinical problem, and by modifying the technical factors used, i.e., lower kV and mAs.

DISEASES

As in the adult, the pediatric head and neck can be divided into different anatomic areas, such as the orbit, sinuses and facial bones, temporal bones, base of skull and upper neck, pharynx and larynx, and neck. Some disease processes are unique to particular areas, but often they may affect multiple areas and may spread across boundaries, e.g., sinus infection spreading to the orbit or intracranially, or tumor in the skull base spreading up or down to involve the brain or infratemporal fossa and parapharyngeal area. The remainder of this chapter will discuss the basic disease processes (i.e., neoplastic, inflammatory, traumatic, and congenital) that involve the different areas. The temporal bone is not discussed in depth as it is covered in Chapter 7.

NEOPLASIA

These lesions may be considered as benign or malignant (primary or secondary). Of interest is a paper by Schramm[5] in which he has abstracted the relative incidence of benign and malignant tumors of the nasal cavity and paranasal sinuses from the records of the University of Pittsburgh and the AFIP Otolar-yngic–Pathology Registry, where a total of 376 cases were reviewed. The entire subject of diseases in the head and neck area in children is completely covered by Bluestone and Stool.[6]

Malignant Tumors

These include lymphoma, rhabdomyosarcoma, other sarcomas, carcinomas, neuroblastoma, and metastases.

Rhabdomyosarcoma

Apart from lymphoma, this is the most common malignant tumor of the head and neck in children and this area is the most common site of involvement in this age group.[7] It occurs as frequently as neuroblastoma and Wilms' tumor.[8] The peak age of incidence is 8 years. The tumor originates in striated muscle and there are five common histological types: (1) embryonal, (2) pleomorphic, (3) alveolar, (4) embryonal–pleomorphic, and (5) botryoid. There are no specific signs or presenting symptoms that would allow a definitive clinical diagnosis to be made, and the presentation is often related to the size of the tumor and the size and extent of involvement of adjacent tissues. Within the head and neck region the two most common sites are the pharynx and orbit.[8] The staging of rhabdomyosarcoma has been defined by the Intergroup Rhabdomyo-sarcoma Study[9] and is based on clinical stage groups I to IV depending on the extent of disease and resectability of the tumor at the time of surgery. Group I includes localized disease (1) confined to muscle or organ of origin that is completely resected (regional nodes not involved) and (2) contiguous involvement-infiltration outside the muscle or organ of origin as through fascial planes. Group II includes (1) grossly resected tumor with microscopic residual disease (nodes negative), (2) regional disease completely resected (nodes positive or negative), and (3) regional disease with involved nodes, grossly resected but with evidence of microscopic residual disease. Group III includes those patients with incomplete resection or a biopsy specimen with gross residual disease. Group IV includes all patients with metastatic disease present at the time of onset. CT is currently the best method for showing the size and extent and distant spread of these tumors, though other modalities are also used in this staging process (Fig. 9.1).

Scotti and Harwood-Nash[10] have described the value of CT in rhabdomyosar-comas of the skull base in children. They point out that the CT picture is nonspecific and, prior to biopsy, the differential diagnosis must include other aggressive lesions involving the base of the skull such as other sarcomas, histio-cytosis X, neuroblastoma, and lymphoma. In these cases CT clearly shows the extent of bony involvement, including the margins of the lesion and the extent of spread into the intra- and extracranial compartments. Because of spread from one compartment to another, the primary site of origin of an

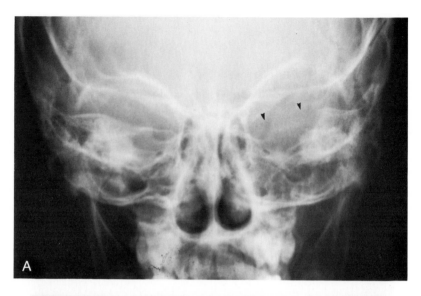

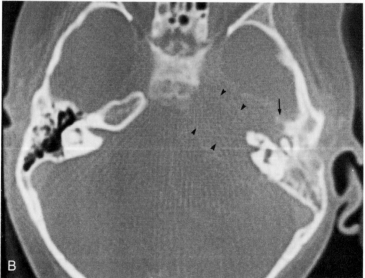

FIG. 9.1 This 5-year-old girl was noted by her parents to have a lazy eye followed by a left facial palsy and ataxia. Within 24 hours she changed from alert to drowsy and was admitted for evaluation. She had a draining left ear and neurological involvement of the left fifth through tenth cranial nerves. Plain film (A) shows destruction of the left petrous apex (arrow). An emergency CT scan (B) confirmed destruction of the petrous apex (open arrow heads) and middle ear cavity (arrow).

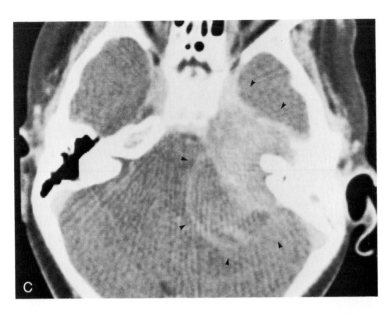

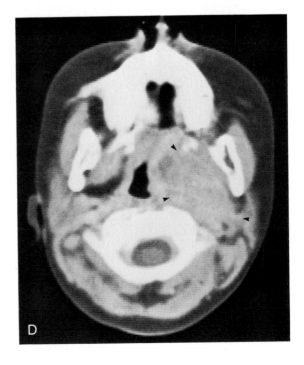

FIG. 9.1 (*Cont.*). Contrast enhancement revealed the soft tissue extent of the tumor (C) intracranially (arrowheads) in the middle and posterior cranial fossae. The tumor was also demonstrated inferiorly (D) in the parapharyngeal space (arrowheads) encroaching on the airway. Biopsy revealed this to be rhabdomyosarcoma. The findings were consistent with a rhabdomyosarcoma. A left suboccipital craniectomy with subtotal excision of the tumor was performed. Chemotherapy and radiation therapy were instituted. Follow-up of the operative site showed regression in the size of the residual tumor, but recurrence took place and the patient eventually succumbed.

extensive tumor may be impossible to determine. Intracranial extension, if present, is usually initially extradural, although the tumor may erode through the dura as it encroaches on the brain. If meningeal involvement is noted, the prognosis is relatively poor.[11,12] Rhabdomyosarcomas arising primarily in the petrous bone manifest initially as a nonspecific loss of pneumatization of the mastoid air cells. Later destruction of the petrous bone with soft tissue extension can be seen. CT is an ideal way to follow the efficacy of chemotherapy and radiotherapy; and, often, total regression of soft tissue mass with partial or total reossification of bone can be documented.

Danziger et al.[13] and Littman et al.[14] have also specifically studied the contribution of CT to the diagnosis and staging of these patients. They have shown from their experience that CT adds significant complementary information to conventional radiography and tomography, particularly after intravenous contrast enhancement. They also stress that it is often only after biopsy that the true nature of the tumor is known.

Incidence and significance of metastatic spread of rhabdomyosarcoma: The most common sites of distant metastases are lung, followed by bone, subcutaneous tissues, central nervous system, and liver.[15] Although approximately one-third of the cases show localized bone erosion at the time of presentation,[7] the incidence of distant bony metastasis at the time of diagnosis is low. This is in contradistinction to rhabdomyosarcoma in other areas of the body. In the past the overall prognosis of head and neck rhabdomyosarcoma was worse than in other parts of the body, but recently there has been dramatic improvement in the 2-year, disease-free survival rate.

Lymphatic spread: The records of 264 patients entered in the Intergroup Rhabdomyosarcoma Study revealed incidences of lymphatic metatasses of 19 percent for genitourinary sites, 17 percent for the extremities, 10 percent for the trunk, but only 3 percent for the head and neck and 0 percent for the orbit.[16] In most cases, therefore, a radical neck dissection may not be necessary unless palpable lymph nodes are felt or involved nodes are found at biopsy.[17] Orbital rhabdomyosarcoma has a better prognosis than rhabdomyosarcoma in other head and neck sites, possibly because (1) the tumor is relatively well contained within the bony confines of the orbit and (2) these tumors present early since small lesions produce prominent physical signs (Fig. 9.2). The histological type of the tumor and the initial extent of disease have not been shown to correlate well with prognosis as judged by comparable survivals in patients with stage I and stage III disease.[7,8,15] However, most workers have shown a decreasing survival with increasing stage of tumor.

The importance of demonstrating meningeal involvement when rhabdomyosarcoma of the ear is diagnosed is emphasized also by Raney and colleagues.[18] They reported 24 children with rhabdomyosarcoma of the ear treated with the IRS-1 protocol and showed that 47 percent of children were alive without recurrence at a median of 3.6 years after diagnosis. Of the 13 who had died, the outcome was most influenced by whether or not signs of meningeal extension were present. The death rates were five of five with intracranial tumor,

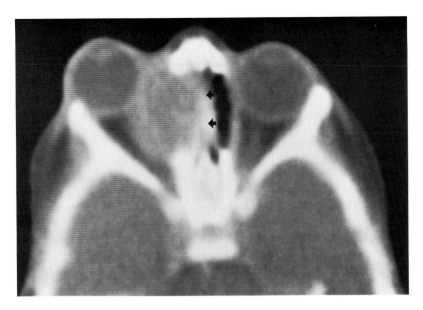

FIG. 9.2.   This 1-year-old baby girl presented with proptosis of the right eye of 2 weeks duration. CT scan shows a mass in the medial aspect of the right orbit involving the right ethmoid sinuses (the right globe is displaced inferolaterally and anteriorly). A coronal view (not included) showed the mass to extend into the cranial cavity superiorly and into the maxillary sinus inferiorly. Electron microscopy diagnosis was undifferentiated sarcoma, most likely rhabdomyosarcoma.

three of four with petrous bone erosion, two of six with facial nerve palsy, and three of nine without evidence of meningeal extension. This report confirms an earlier one[11] in which poor prognosis of patients with meningeal involvement was also pointed out. In that series, 57 of 141 cases had parameningeal sites of tumor and 20 of these 57 developed direct meningeal extension. Of those 20, 18 (90 percent) died of this complication. These results clearly dictated that a more aggressive therapeutic plan be instituted. The IRS-2 protocol included radiation to the entire cranium plus intrathecal triple chemotherapy and adjuvant systemic chemotherapy. One group also received craniospinal axis radiation, but this has been discontinued because the results with intrathecal chemotherapy are similar and the toxicity is less. Since then a further 68 patients with parameningeal sarcomas were treated using the above recommendations. The relapse rate was reduced from 28 percent in IRS-1 to 6 percent in the more intensively treated group, and the overall relapse free survival rate increased from 33 percent to 68 percent.[18]

Thus it is of the utmost importance that these parameningeal lesions be clearly outlined and meningeal involvement documented. Computed tomography is the best way of showing such extension.

Lymphoma

In childhood, lymphomas and sarcomas are the most common malignancies of the head and neck, with carcinomas being rare. Malignant lymphomas account for half of pediatric head and neck malignancy and are three times as common as rhabdomyosarcoma.[19] They present as nodal or extranodal disease. Extranodal disease involves the tonsils, nasopharynx, salivary glands, maxilla, maxillary sinus, or tongue, and the nodal variety involves the cervical lymph nodes. In children, Hodgkin's lymphoma presents most commonly around 10 years of age and in over 80 percent of patients presents as unilateral cervical or supraclavicular adenopathy. The Ann Arbor Clinical Staging classification is the one most widely used. After initial histological diagnosis, which is generally based on node biopsy, the extent of disease is assessed by a variety of clinical and diagnostic methods. Staging laparotomy has been found to be the most accurate method of assessing spread of disease, but radionuclide bone scans, liver–spleen scans, lymphangiograms, and CT scans are all helpful in showing spread of disease. In the head and neck the node masses that have

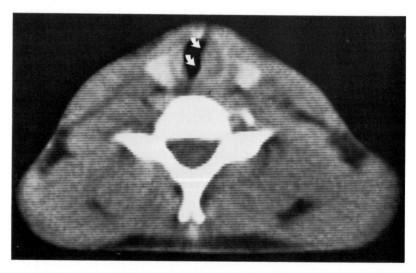

FIG. 9.3.   This 16-year-old boy developed painful swelling of the left axilla with a temperature of 102°F that was unresponsive to antibiotics. Lymph node biopsy was equivocal for lymphoma. He shortly developed progressive hoarseness with eventual loss of voice and he lost 18 lb in weight. Because of increasing stridor, a lateral neck x-ray was performed and showed a subglottic mass. CT scan of the neck shows a definite soft tissue mass within the larynx (arrows), causing encroachment on the airway with subglottic extension of the soft tissue tumor. The left lobe of the thyroid gland is somewhat flattened and displaced, implying extrinsic as well as intrinsic involvement of the larynx. The laryngeal mass was considered to be part of the patient's generalized lymphadenopathy, which was subsequently shown to be histiocytic lymphoma. His adenopathy and stridor resolved following chemotherapy.

soft tissue attenuation are clearly shown to displace various adjacent structures such as muscle planes. The soft tissue mass has no specific CT characteristics that allow a diagnosis of lymphoma, but CT is of great help in showing the degree of local extension in the initial staging of the disease (1) in the neck and (2) elsewhere in the body. Once a histological diagnosis has been made, the response to therapy is often best monitored by CT. Non-Hodgkin's lymphoma also commonly presents as cervical adenopathy. It has a more rapid onset and poorer prognosis than in adults. As in Hodgkin's disease, non-Hodgkin's lymphoma is more than twice as common in boys as in girls. Initial evaluation of tumor mass relies heavily on CT to show the extent of nonpalpable lesions in the neck, thorax, and abdomen (Fig. 9.3).

Nasopharyngeal Carcinoma

Vita et al.[20] reviewed clinical findings and treatment of 27 patients with naso-pharyngeal carcinoma in the second decade of life. The histological diagnosis was poorly differentiated carcinoma in 18 patients and undifferentiated carcinoma in nine patients. The overall survival was 64 percent at 5 years and 57 percent at 10 years. Although nasopharyngeal carcinoma is a rare tumor in childhood, this report of 27 cases emphasizes that such malignancy must be considered in the differential diagnosis of mass lesions in the nasopharyngeal area, particularly when associated bone destruction is noted or a condition that has been or is considered to be sinusitis fails to respond to therapy. In adults, CT assessment of these tumors has been shown to advance the TNM stage of disease in 57 percent of patients.[21] CT is therefore of prime importance in evaluating this type of malignancy in children as well as adults. CT shows the size of tumor, any adjacent bony destruction, and particularly the extent of soft tissue spread (Fig. 9.4).

Metastatic Disease

Metastatic involvement of the head and neck is seen in neuroblastoma, Ewing's sarcoma, and the leukemias, particularly the myelomonocytic variety. The most common of these is neuroblastoma (Fig. 9.5). The lesions from metastatic neuroblastoma may be localized to the orbit or any part of the facial bones or vault. Occasionally, advanced tumor will cause widening of the diploic space of the vault and meningeal extension may give rise to local spreading of the sutures as a sign of pseudo-raised intracranial pressure.

Benign Tumors

These include nasopharyngeal angiofibroma, histiocytosis X, hemangioma, lipoma, cystic hygroma, and glomus jugulare tumor.

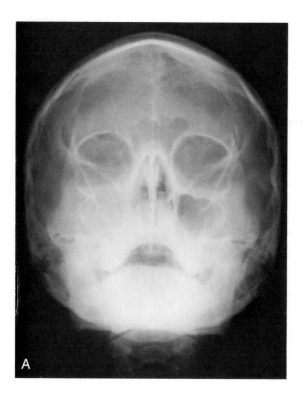

FIG. 9.4. This 14-year-old girl developed right temporal headaches, a blocked nose on the right side, and tearing from the right eye. A Water's view (A) shows opacification of the right maxillary sinus. She was initially treated with antibiotics with the presumed diagnosis of sinusitis. After failure of this medical therapy, a transnasal sinus biopsy was performed and the histological diagnosis of osteogenic sarcoma resulted.

Nasopharyngeal Angiofibroma

This tumor (Fig. 9.6), which most commonly arises in the vault of the nasopharynx of adolescent boys, is a benign tumor, but because of its locally destructive nature may become life threatening. It is rarely if ever seen in girls and often presents with epistaxis or obstructive nasal symptoms; it may be discovered at the time of proposed adenoidectomy when the tumor is felt as a hard mass rather then the expected soft adenoid tissue. Evaluation of these tumors prior to surgery or embolization is extremely important. CT can clearly show the extent of spread and document the amount of extension into the nearby recesses and intracranial space. It can also demonstrate the degree of bone destruction caused by this tumor. The highly vascular nature of the tumor is seen after intravenous contrast enhancement. Angiography of the vessels supplying the tumor is often performed and, in some cases, embolization may be done to control the tumor mass either as a primary form of treatment prior to surgical removal or as a definitive method of ablating the tumor. Radiographic staging of juvenile angiofibroma based on CT and determined by the extension of the tumor from the site of origin has been proposed.[22] This staging system is based on CT findings in 12 consecutive patients. Scans were obtained in coronal and axial projections with contrast. The stages are (IA) tumor enters into the posterior nares and/or nasopharyngeal vault, no paranasal sinus extension, (IB) same as IA, but with extension into one or more paranasal sinuses, (IIA)

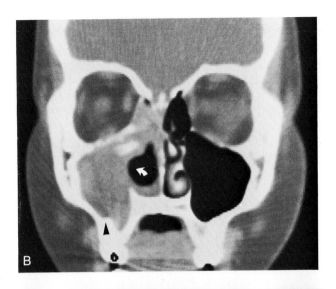

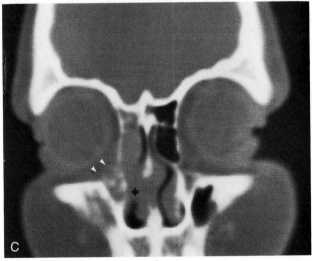

FIG. 9.4 (*Cont.*). Computed tomography (B) shows opacification of the right maxillary sinus, with postoperative changes of the medial wall (arrow). There is extension into the right ethmoid air cells and nasal cavity. The tumor extends inferiorly to the right alveolar region in contact with the roots of several teeth (arrowhead). The roof of the ethmoid air cells and the cribriform plate are intact. Minimal soft tissue density in the anteromedial corner of the orbit (C) (white arrowheads) is tumor extension into the orbit via the nasolacrimal duct (black arrow). The orbit and globe were resected along with the right maxilla and ethmoid sinuses.

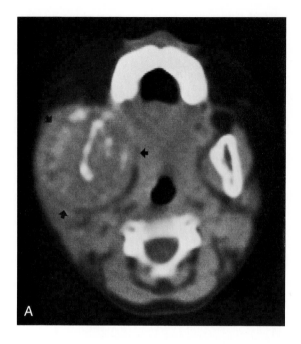

FIG. 9.5. This 18-month-old girl had fever with right jaw swelling. Initial radiographs and bone scan were considered compatible with osteomyelitis. Failure to respond to intravenous antibiotics and increase in size of the swelling led to biopsy, which could not rule out the possibility of malignancy. After referral, a second bone scan revealed increased uptake over the mandible and a lower rib. CT of the mandible (A) showed extensive destruction of the mandible with a large soft tissue mass containing calcification. CT of the lower ribs (B) revealed a right adrenal mass containing calcific density consistent with neuroblastoma. The mandibular lesion was metastatic neuroblastoma.

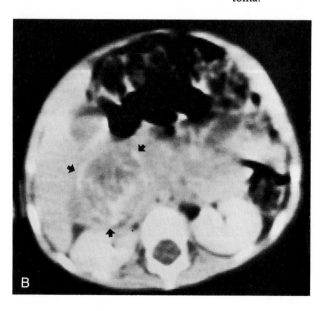

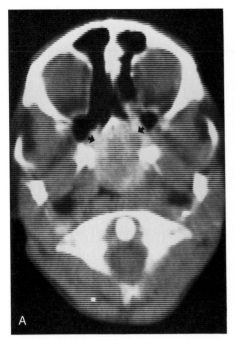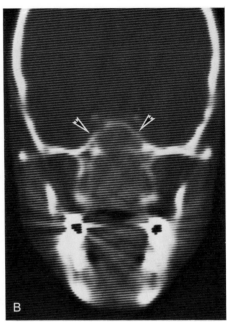

FIG. 9.6. This 13-year-old boy had symptoms of nasal obstruction for over a year before he sought treatment. He was scheduled for tonsillectomy and adenoidectomy. Examination under anesthesia showed a pink fleshy mass obstructing the choanae. An axial CT scan (A) with intravenous contrast enhancement reveals a highly vascular mass arising from the roof of the nasopharynx, extending anteriorly into the nasal cavity (arrows) between the maxillary sinuses and back to the region of the pterygoid plates. Superiorly (B) a coronal view shows the tumor to extend into the sphenoid sinus and left posterior ethmoid sinuses. This proved to be an angiofibroma.

minimal lateral extension through the sphenopalatine foramen into and including a minimal part of the most medial part of the pterygopalatine fossa (PPF), (IIB) full occupation of the PPF with displacement of the posterior wall of the maxillary antrum forward, a lateral and/or anterior displacement of the branches of the maxillary artery, and possible superior extension eroding the orbital bones, (IIC) extension through the PPF to the cheek and temporal fossa, (III) intracranial extension. As the tumor becomes more extensive, the treatment plan changes accordingly.

Histiocytosis X

Histiocytosis X describes an entity that has variable clinical and pathological features and that, although not neoplastic in the classical sense, is viewed as a malignant disorder. The term first suggested by Lichtenstein[23] includes the previously described syndromes of eosinophilic granuloma, Hand-Schuller-

Christian disease, and Letterer-Siwe disease. In all probability these have a common etiological factor, although this has not been proven. Granulomatous lesions are particularly prone to develop in bone. These destructive changes often involve the hypothalamus. Other bones such as the skull and mandible can be involved, and in the latter case the so called "floating teeth" appearance may be seen radiologically when the mandible becomes severely demineralized locally.

Lipoma

Occasionally lipomas present as a mass in the neck in childhood and their nature is not fully appreciated prior to surgery. CT will often show that these are in the subcutaneous soft tissues; they most commonly are fairly well contained in tissue planes but rarely may infiltrate the surrounding structures. Because of their fatty nature, they have a characteristic low attenuation number.

Glomus Jugulare Tumor

These rare tumors are also histologically benign but locally invasive and potentially life threatening. These chemodectomas may be found in the tympanic cavity, jugular fossa, carotid sheath along the course of the vagus nerve to the aortic arch, and at the carotid bifurcation. A typical case is discussed in Figure 9.7.

Fibrous Dysplasia

Fibrous dysplasia occasionally involves the skull and facial bones and may also selectively involve the temporal bone.[24,25] Sites of involvement of the craniofacial bones include the skull base, mandible, sphenoid, and maxilla.[26,27] Clinically, patients with fibrous dysplasia present with pain or swelling or asymmetry of the face. It commonly presents in late childhood and early adolescence. In children the lesion will tend to slow or cease growing after puberty.

FIG. 9.7. This 17-year-old boy has had headaches, recently becoming worse and more intense. He has also noted pulsations in his right ear and has had two episodes of documented hypertension lasting 5 to 10 min. Examination revealed a mass in the hypotympanum but no bruit and no neurological deficit. Clinical diagnosis of right glomus jugulare or intravagale tumor was made. CT of the neck and skull base with intravenous contrast enhancement (A) shows destruction of the carotid canal and jugular foramen (arrowheads) by tumor that also extended into the hypotympanum. This enhancing mass (arrowhead) extends inferiorly in the vascular space to the level of the superior cornu of the hyoid bone. It lies deep to the posterior belly of the digastric muscle (asterisk) as seen in (B). Angiography showed tumor with blood supply derived from the right external carotid and right vertebral artery. The proximal right internal jugular vein was completely obstructed. Surgical removal of the tumor was performed after initial biopsy. Histology was nonchromaffin paraganglioma (glomus jugulare tumor).

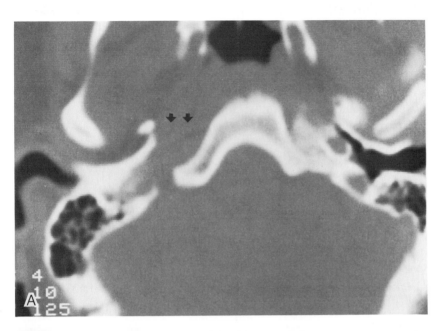

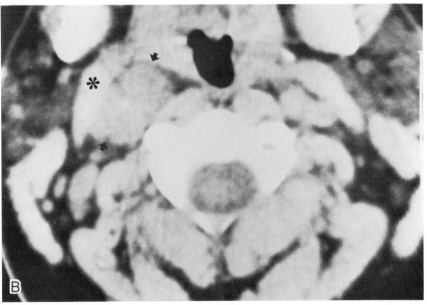

Three forms of fibrous dysplasia are described. (1) The sclerotic type is evidenced by a diffuse, uniform, homogeneous dense area that follows the contour of the bone and expands it. (2) The cystic form is characterized by a radiolucent area with a sharp, often sclerotic border that causes cortical thinning and expansion with small flecks of irregular calcification seen within the lesion; it is most commonly found in the mandible. (3) In the pagetoid form bone is markedly expanded, with alternating areas of radiolucency and radiodensity; this type is most common in older patients.[26] Periosteal reaction and soft tissue masses are uncommon with this lesion.

Temporal bone involvement by fibrous dysplasia is uncommon in the monostotic form, very rare in the polyostotic form, and unknown in McCune-Albright syndrome. Twenty-three cases of monostotic and four cases of polyostotic fibrous dysplasia of the temporal bone are reported. Hearing loss and increased volume of the temporal region were the most common symptoms, with hearing loss caused by obstruction of the external auditory canal and involvement of the middle ear by proliferation of the tumor. Secondary cholesteatoma may occur medial to the blocked external canal and facial paralysis may ensue if the facial nerve is entrapped. The squamous portion of the temporal bone is less affected than the mastoid or petrous portion. The volume of the mastoid area is increased, with thinning of the mastoid cortex. Air cells may be preserved or obliterated. The labyrinth was not involved in the cases described.[25] The authors describe three clinical stages: (1) radiological bone changes without symptoms, (2) a symptomatic phase, and (3) a phase associated with complications of the tumor. An example of this lesion is seen in Figure 9.8.

Giant Cell Lesions

Giant cell lesions of the facial bones may occur in childhood.[28] These lesions include giant cell reparative granuloma, the brown tumor of hypoparathyroidism, true giant cell tumor, cherubism, and aneurysmal bone cyst. The radiographic features of giant cell granuloma of the sinuses are nonspecific but the tumor tends to be less invasive than carcinoma. Ossification in these lesions can be demonstrated by CT and may indicate a benign lesion.[29]

Gorham's Disease

A rare, destructive, tumor-like lesion of bone is described in Figure 9.9. Osteolysis or vanishing bone disease, first described by Gorham,[30] usually presents in childhood or early adulthood.[31] Angiomatosis or lymphangiomatosis is found in the bone at the site of the disease. Initial radiological signs include localized osteoporosis in one or more sites; it progresses to partial or complete bone resorption. The lesions may be painful, may cross joints, and may give rise to pathological fracture with resulting physical deformity. The ^{99m}Tc pyrophosphate bone scan usually shows decreased uptake but may rarely show increased uptake. The lesions may be fairly localized or widespread and can

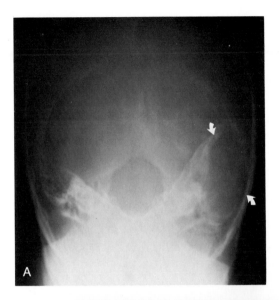
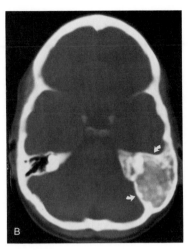
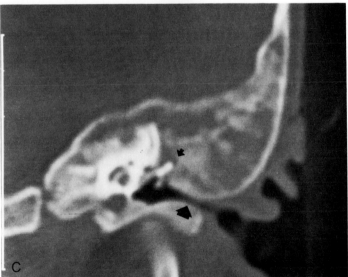

FIG. 9.8. This 5-year-old girl had repeated episodes of bilateral acute otitis media, with the left ear more involved than the right. Audiograms showed a left conductive hearing loss. Attempted left myringotomy and tube insertion failed, as the external canal was too narrow. Mastoid films (A) showed an abnormal expanded left temporal bone (arrows). CT of the temporal bone (B) showed marked expansion of the temporal bone. The mastoid air cells have been replaced by mottled tissue of intermediate and high density. A coronal scan (C) shows narrowing of the external canal (black arrowhead) with bony encroachment upon the left epitympanic recess and middle ear cavity (arrow). Subsequent biopsy of the mastoid process showed appearances of fibrous dysplasia.

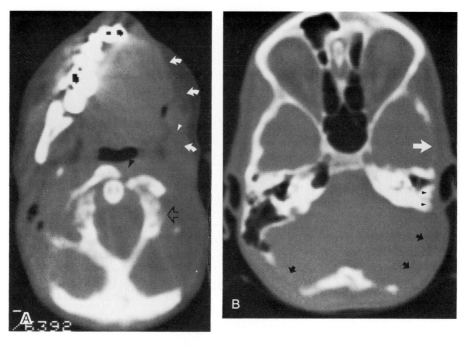

FIG. 9.9. A loose molar tooth led to dental films on this 12-year-old boy. A sharply defined cyst-like defect was found, which later progressed to complete destruction (arrows) of the left mandible (A). Subsequent studies over the next 2 to 3 years revealed progressive lysis of other bones of the head and neck, including the occipital bone around the foramen magnum (open arrow). A more cephalad section (B) reveals more lysis of the occipital bone (arrows), temporal bone (arrowhead) and greater wing of the sphenoid (white arrow). Biopsy revealed angiomatosis replacing the bone consistent with Gorham's disease.

cause death from thoracic cage involvement. Partial remission may occur. Radiotherapy has been shown to be of value in some cases.

Tumors of the Orbit

Tumors of the orbit present a special area in head and neck oncology and the following section includes a discussion of some of the masses that are found within the orbit. Lallemand et al.[32] have described and discussed the differential diagnosis and incidence of 40 pediatric orbital tumors, 13 of which were ocular and 27 extraocular. They were found in the following incidence: retinoblastoma, 13; optic nerve glioma, six; rhabdomyosarcoma, four; neuroblastoma, three; lymphangioma, three; hemangioma, three; leukemia, two; Burkitt's lymphoma, one; histiocytosis X, one; dermoid cyst, one; osteoma, one; malignant nevus, one; and hemangiopericytoma, one. Based on the location in the orbit, extent of spread, involvement of bone and muscle, periorbital sinuses and neural structures, presence of calcification, attenuation coefficient, contrast enhancement, and patient age they were able to suggest a confident diagnosis in many instances. Kennerdell and Goshhajro[33] have presented their experience of CT and orbital tumors. Their experience includes the following tumors.

Retinoblastoma

This tumor arises from the retina. It nearly always contains calcium. The incidence of calcium on plain films has varied from 20 to 75 percent. Of 18 eyes examined by CT 17 contained calcium.[34] The noncalcified area of tumor enhanced with contrast. Very small tumors less than 3 discs in diameter may not be shown even with very thin CT slices. However, if calcium is present in the tumor, even small lesions of 1 disc diameter may be visible. Retinal detachments associated with retinoblastoma were not routinely shown even with contrast enhancement, as abnormal permeability of tissues in that region of the retina allowed leakage of contrast into the subretinal fluid making it difficult to differentiate the fluid from solid tissue.[33]

Neurofibromatosis

This may occur in any area of the body including the orbital region. Zimmerman et al.[35] have classified the orbital lesions of neurofibromatosis (NF) into orbital neoplasms, plexiform neurofibromatosis (PNF), orbital osseous dysplasia, and congenital glaucoma (buphthalmos). They have shown that successful treatment is based on CT evaluation of the extent of each of these entities. Orbital tumors that have been found in association with NF include optic gliomas, neurofibromas, neurofibrosarcoma, and perioptic meningioma. Approximately one-third of Zimmerman's patients had plexiform neurofibromas. Most commonly this entity involves the choroid, ciliary body, conjunctiva, iris, eyelids, and limbus.[36] A high incidence of enlargement of the cavernous sinus may reflect PNF involvement of either the third, fourth, fifth, or sixth cranial nerves.[35] CT demonstrates the poorly circumscribed tortuous tumor as a contrast-enhanced irregular soft tissue mass with planes that enlarge and deform the muscular anatomy of the temporalis fossa, eyelid, and recti of the orbit.

Buphthalmos is shown as a uniform enlargement of the globe and was most commonly seen with PNF on the same side.

The most common orbital osseous dysplasia with NF is hypoplasia of the greater wing of the sphenoid, with the lesser wing of the sphenoid the next most commonly involved. Occasionally, the temporal lobe of the brain displaces the posterior contents of the orbit forward, giving rise to the classical appearance of pulsating exophthalmos.

Osteomas

Osteomas are benign ossific bone tumors that may arise from the orbital wall and may be lobulated and intrude into the sinuses or orbits, particularly the frontal and ethmoid sinuses. They contain very dense bone and generally have smooth margins.

Dermoid Cysts

Dermoid cysts are commonly found in the sutures around the orbit. They are usually oval or rounded, are well circumscribed, and may be seen clearly by plain radiography. CT shows a low attenuation of the central fluid, which does not enhance with contrast.

Hemangiopericytoma

Hemangiopericytoma is a highly vascular tumor consisting of scattered capillary-like spaces surrounded by proliferating pericytes. These tumors enhance intensely with intravenous contrast. Their margins may be hazy as they attempt to spread into the extraocular muscles.[33]

HEAD AND NECK TRAUMA

The basic principles of diagnosis of bone and soft tissue trauma to the head and neck in children are similar to that in adults. Knowledge of the different appearances of various structures in the growing pediatric head and neck is important. In particular, one must be aware of the relatively small size of the sinuses and facial bones in relation to the size of the skull vault in children as compared with that in adults. Also, the sutures are relatively more prominent in the pediatric patient.

Plain radiography is performed initially when there is a question of fracture in the head and neck area. If the fracture is relatively minor and the symptoms are clear cut, the patient may not need other radiographic studies. Often, however, the full extent of the fracture is not shown by plain films and conventional tomography is performed. The superb detail afforded by thin section, high resolution CT scans in the axial and coronal planes has all but replaced conventional tomography in the evaluation of facial and other head and neck injuries.[37] Advantages of CT include the ability to show the extent of soft tissue injury adjacent to a bony fracture. In many cases of severe trauma CT images of the vault and brain may be performed at the same time to see if there is associated intracranial pathology such as subdural or epidural hematoma, intracranial bleed, cerebral damage, evidence of increased intracranial pressure, or pneumocephalus. Also the radiation dose is 50% less when CT is used instead of polytomography.[38] A further advantage is the ability to perform accurate studies quickly with minimal disturbance to the patient.

Although coronal views can usually be performed in these patients, they may not be advisable if damage to the cervical spine or cord is present. This position may be uncomfortable for adult patients but is rarely a problem for younger pediatric patients, particularly if they are heavily sedated or anesthetized.

Carter and Bankoff[37] and Rowe et al.[38] have compared multidirectional tomography with CT in a series of patients with maxillofacial trauma and found that CT added useful information in nearly every case—mainly concerning the extent of associated soft tissue injury and displacement.

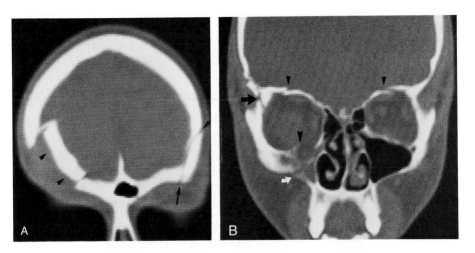

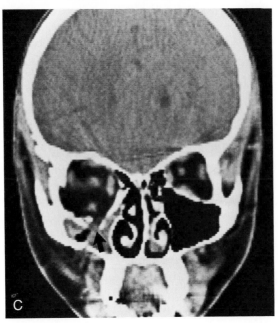

FIG. 9.10. This 16-year-old girl was transferred for further evaluation 10 days after a motor vehicle accident where she had sustained multiple facial and skull fractures. On examination she had bilateral conjunctival hemorrhage, significant enophthalmos of the right eye, with restricted upgaze and downgaze in the right eye. (A) Coronal section through frontal region reveals a large depressed fragment of the frontal bone (arrowheads). A nondisplaced fracture through the left lateral portion of the frontal bone is noted (arrows). (B) Coronal view through midorbit shows bilateral orbital fractures (arrowheads), fracture through the right superolateral orbital margin (arrow), a fracture through the inferior orbital rim with opacification of the maxillary sinus (black arrowhead), and a fracture of the inferior margin of the right maxillary sinus (white arrow). (C) Coronal section through posterior orbit clearly shows the rectus muscles, with the inferior rectus slightly depressed inferiorly, depression of the floor of the right orbit (arrow), and opacification of the maxillary sinus. The patient also had brain contusion and edema secondary to the local trauma. In this type of injury computed tomography allows good evaluation of the soft tissues around the fracture site that are not so well delineated by conventional tomography.

The ability of CT to show associated hematoma and entrapped ocular muscles not seen by conventional tomography in cases of maxillofacial trauma has also been described in a series of patients that included some in the pediatric age group.[39] Complex fractures with displacement of small and large fragments are easier to visualize three-dimensionally using axial and coronal CT and this is of great help to the surgeon planning operative treatment.

Figure 9.10 shows an example of the wide range of fractures that may be shown clearly by CT, including complications such as muscle entrapment in a blow-out fracture and associated intracranial and brain injury.

Fractures of the skull base, particularly those involving the temporal bone, are shown by CT and this may be the only method of demonstrating the site of a cerebrospinal fluid leak. Fracture of the cervical spine with associated soft tissue injury either inside or outside the spinal canal is clearly shown by computed tomography. Bony encroachment into the spinal canal, particularly associated with crush fractures of the vertebrae, are clearly shown by CT, and compression of the spinal cord may be demonstrated using water soluble contrast material in the subarachnoid space.

Soft tissue damage to the larynx including fractures of the laryngeal and hyoid cartilages are shown well by computed tomography.[40]

A further use of this modality is shown in Figure 9.11 where rotary subluxation of C1 on C2 is clearly demonstrated. In this instance the cause was probably retropharyngeal inflammation and muscle spasm, but a similar appearance may be seen as an idiopathic cause of acute torticollis or secondary to trauma. Plain films of the atlantoaxial junction, including right and left oblique views, possibly followed by fluoroscopy may also give this diagnosis, but in an uncooperative patient the results are sometimes equivocal.

Foreign bodies in the soft tissues, including injuries from high velocity missiles, are well shown by CT. Figure 9.12 describes a case that shows the value of CT in locating soft tissue foreign bodies in the orbit. Prior to CT, uncomfortable, sometimes slightly dangerous radiological procedures were performed to locate such foreign bodies, and the full extent of injury was often not appreciated despite these studies. Sometimes unnecessary surgical exploration of the orbit and globe was performed. The CT diagnosis of ruptured eye has been described by Sevel and colleagues.[41] Scleral perforation of the globe following ocular trauma may be obvious on physical examination but occult perforations occur. CT of the orbit may suggest occult scleral rupture with posterior collapse of the sclera and flattening of the posterior contour of the globe, giving the "flat tire" sign. Other findings include intraocular foreign body or gas, thickening of the sclera posteriorly, and a blood–vitreous fluid level. Serration of the posterior sclera may also be present.

Some intraorbital foreign bodies such as wooden fragments are easily missed by conventional radiography but have been demonstrated by CT. Glass and plastic foreign bodies are also better shown by CT.[42] Foreign bodies that are located far forward in the globe under the iris may not be visible with gonioscopy or indirect ophthalmoscopy. CT can precisely determine their location relative to the lens–iris diaphragm.[43]

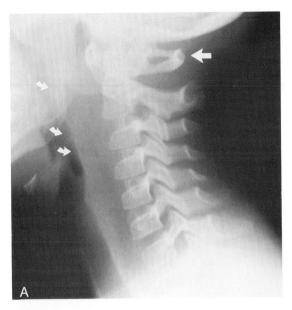

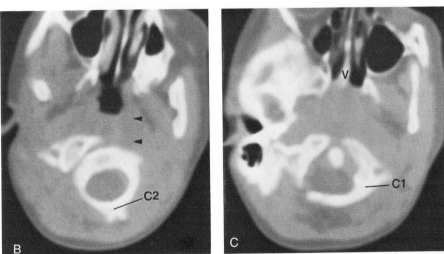

FIG. 9.11. This 7-year-old girl was treated for a sore throat using amoxicillin without success. Her sore throat progressed to a stiff neck and dysphagia. Her white cell count was 13,600 and her sedimentation rate was 110 mm/hr. Plain lateral radiograph of the neck (A) shows widening of the retropharyngeal space (curved arrows), suggesting the presence of significant soft tissue thickening probably due to inflammation. Note is also made of tilting of the ring of C-1 (arrow) consistent with mild torticollis. Despite what was considered appropriate antibiotic therapy, she remained afebrile and her white cell count continued to rise. A retropharyngeal abscess was thought to be present and a CT scan was performed. The CT scan (B) shows increased soft tissue thickening in the retropharyngeal area (arrowheads) without evidence of abscess formation. Note is made of malalignment of the facial bones and vomer with the body and arch of C-2, whereas in (C) the first cervical vertebra (C-1) is noted to be normally aligned with the vomer (V). This appearance is consistent with rotary subluxation of C-1 on C-2, which in this instance is probably caused by muscle spasm in association with retropharyngeal inflammation (Grisel's syndrome).

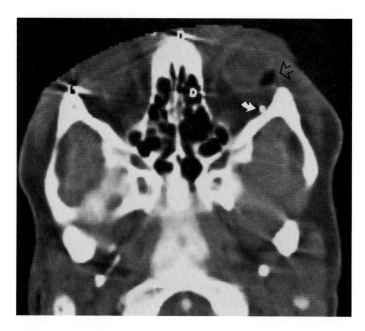

FIG. 9.12. This 17-year-old youth received a shotgun blast in the face from a passing car. On examination, multiple pellet entrance wounds were noted over the face. He did not lose consciousness. He was noted to have markedly decreased visual acuity in the left eye and had hyphema in the anterior chamber with probable scleral laceration and vitreous hemorrhage with retinal damage. CT of the head and orbits revealed a pellet in the retro-orbital soft tissues just adjacent to the posterolateral bony margin of the orbit (arrow). Air was also noted in the soft tissues adjacent to the lateral rim of the orbit (open arrowhead). The figure also shows metallic foreign bodies in the left ethmoid air cells, in the soft tissues anterior to the nose, and just adjacent to the left lateral orbital rim.

INFLAMMATORY LESIONS OF THE HEAD AND NECK

Uncomplicated inflammatory lesions of the head and neck soft tissues such as sinusitis, epiglottitis, and retropharyngeal abscess are often diagnosed and monitored either clinically or by plain radiography. When a clear diagnosis is not established by these methods or if the lesions fail to respond adequately to medical or surgical therapy, CT is used to help delineate the area of pathology.

Inflammatory Lesions of the Orbit

CT scans of the orbit are currently of great value in that they may often distinguish between inflammatory and neoplastic lesions, thereby obviating surgical exploration and allowing medical therapy for certain diseases. Trokel[44] has classified inflammations of the orbit into (1) specific orbital infections and

(2) orbital pseudotumor (idiopathic inflammations). Specific infections include those secondary to sinus disease, foreign bodies, and infestations. Orbital pseudotumor in children presents in four ways.

1. In dacryoadenitis (infection of the lacrimal apparatus), patients typically present with a tender swelling of the upper outer quadrant with lateral upper lid swelling. CT shows that the lacrimal gland in the superolateral area of the orbit is enlarged, with pooling of fluid under Tenon's capsule.

2. Orbital myositis is characterized by rapid onset of exophthalmos with redness and congestion over the extraocular muscle insertions. CT shows that one or more of these extraocular muscles are thickened.

3. In perineuritis, edema fluid, which may be seen by CT, is concentrated around the optic nerve.

4. Fasciitis is evidenced by diffuse, poorly localized inflammation in the orbit. Edema fluid may pool in Tenon's space. Orbital fasciitis is suggested when inflammation is not localized to a specific structure and edema is diffuse with an irregular patchy border. These pseudotumors of the orbit often respond well to steroid therapy and such improvement can be monitored by CT.

Preseptal versus Postseptal Cellulitis and Abscess

The periorbita is a tough fibrous lining of the orbit that extends anteriorly into the upper and lower tarsal plates of the eyelids. Preseptal infection is usually a cellulitis of the superficial soft tissues around the eye that responds well to oral antibiotics and is not commonly associated with complications, though abscess may occasionally form. Postseptal infection, on the other hand, is a more serious condition and is difficult to distinguish clinically from more superficial inflammation, as both may present together and may present with markedly swollen eyelids. If preseptal inflammation fails to respond to treatment within 24 to 48 hr, abscess of that area or infection in the postseptal space should be suspected and CT performed.[45] Postseptal infection most commonly is due to spread from sinusitis.[46] The infection may spread directly through the thin lamina papyracea or may travel through the valveless venous plexus that interconnects the sinus and orbital areas. The resulting inflammatory process may be contained beneath the periorbita as an abscess or may break through into the postseptal orbital space. A rare but serious complication of orbital infections is cavernous sinus thrombosis, which may be diagnosed by a bolus injection of intravenous contrast with sequential scanning of the cavernous sinus.

Inflammatory Lesions of the Paranasal Sinuses

Plain radiography is routinely used to define infection of the sinuses in children, although it is sometimes difficult to make this diagnosis in the younger child because of the small size of the sinuses. The ethmoid sinuses in particular are difficult to define, and this may be of great importance in the diagnosis

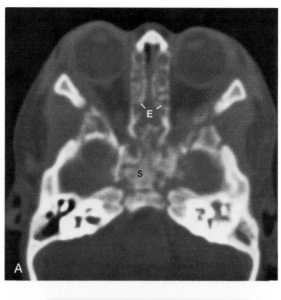

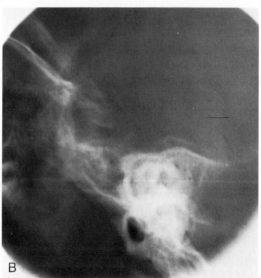

FIG. 9.13. This 1½-year-old girl developed fever and irritability 3 weeks prior to admission. *Hemophilus influenzae* meningitis was diagnosed by lumbar puncture. After initial improvement the eyelids became more swollen and purulent drainage from the back of the throat developed. Examination showed soft tissue swelling over the temporal areas, left more than right. Right eye proptosis with normal conjunctivae and bilateral swollen, boggy soft palate with foul smelling odor were noted. Pharyngeal and retroton-sillar abscesses were diagnosed. Culture revealed probable *Acinetobacter anitratum* involvement. CT scan showed osteomyelitis of the sphenoid bone with abscesses deep to the temporalis muscles and a nasopharyngeal abscess. (A) The ethmoiditis (E) was followed by osteomyelitis of the entire sphenoid bone (S), the latter verified by plain film study (B).

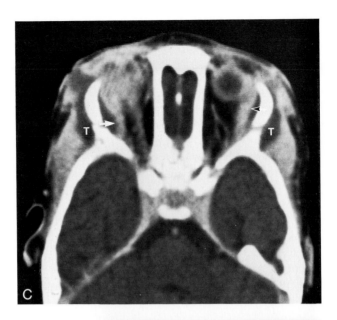

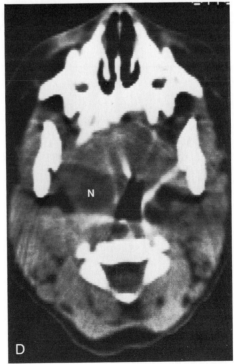

FIG. 9.13 (*Cont.*). In (C) periorbital cellulitis is seen with subtemporal abscesses (T) extending into the orbit lateral to the lateral rectus muscles (arrows). (D) A large nasopharyngeal abscess (N) extends along the parapharyngeal area to the palate.

of retro-orbital inflammation. Carter et al.[47] have shown that CT may be invaluable in rapidly diagnosing the cause of these patients' symptoms. They showed examples where unsuspected sinusitis was responsible for serious intracranial and extracranial infections in a series that included seven pediatric patients and discussed routes of spread, which include contiguous spread directly through the thin bony walls of the sinuses, perivenous spread, spread along the perineural spaces of the olfactory nerves; spread via the various canals such as the semicanalis ethmoidalis or the craniopharyngeal canal; dehiscence of bone due to infection, trauma, or tumor; and congenital openings in the lamina papyracea and in the sphenoid bone. Venous spread occurs along the diploic veins of Breschet, the ethmoid veins to the dura, the ophthalmic vein to the cavernous sinus, the veins from the nasal cavity via the foramen cecum, the veins through the cribriform plate to the dural veins, the sphenopalatine veins in the pterygoid plexus to the ophthalmic veins, the sphenoid sinus veins to the cavernous sinus, and the pterygoid plexus to the cavernous sinus.

Prompt treatment of sinusitis is essential to minimize the morbidity and mortality associated with such complications as brain abscess, meningitis, or-

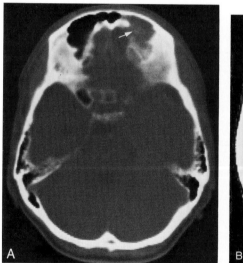 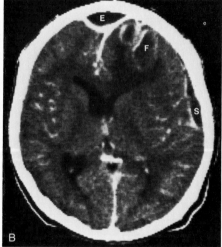

FIG. 9.14. This 13-year-old Vietnamese boy had 10 days of headache, a fever, and vomiting of varying severity. His headache was frontal and he was lethargic and confused on admission. Physical examination suggested meningitis, which was confirmed by lumbar puncture. Two days after treatment started, he developed a seizure, which resulted in an emergency CT scan of the head. This shows (A) left frontal sinus opacification with destruction of the posterior wall of the left frontal sinus (arrow) and (B) large epidural (E), subdural (S), and frontal lobe (F) abscesses, the latter displacing the ventricles to the right. Surgery was performed to drain the abscesses and trephine the left frontal sinus. (From Carter BL, Bankoff MS, Fisk JD: Computed tomographic detection of sinusitis responsible for intracranial and extracranial infections. Radiology 147:739–742, 1983.)

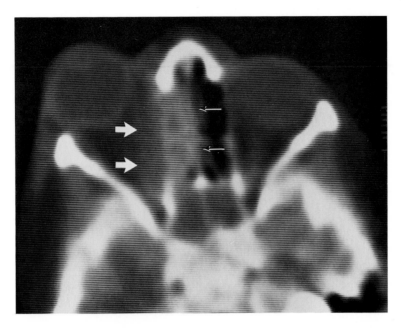

FIG. 9.15. This 2-year-old girl developed a runny nose, cough, and fever 6 days prior to admission. Two days later she developed a runny right eye with clear liquid. The following day her right eye began to swell. This was considered to be an allergy. She was treated with Benadryl compresses and neomycin eyedrops. Showing no improvement, she was referred to an ENT surgeon for treatment for orbital cellulitis. There was no history of purulent nasal discharge and she was afebrile with the right eye swollen shut. Sinus radiographs showed cloudy ethmoid sinuses, and the white blood cell count was 20,000/cu mm. She was initially treated with intravenous oxacillin for periorbital cellulitis secondary to ethmoid sinus infection. However, a CT scan of the area revealed right proptosis. The right ethmoid sinus is opacified (thin arrows), with demineralization of the bony septae. Soft tissue density along the medial aspect of the right orbit displacing the medial rectus muscle (thick arrows) is present. Appearances were most consistent with intraorbital infection. Surgical exploration of the right orbit was performed and a medial subperiosteal abscess was evacuated. The lamina papyracea and periosteum in the area were intact. She recovered uneventfully.

bital cellulitis, osteomyelitis, and cavernous sinus thrombosis. Examples of these diseases are shown in Figures 9.13 to 9.15.

Infection of the soft tissues of the lower neck region often originates in lymph nodes and may progress to abscess formation that becomes clinically obvious with pain or swelling that may compress adjacent structures. Spread of neck infections may occur, and this is particularly serious in the retropharyngeal area if inflammation spreads down the prevertebral planes into the mediastinum, causing mediastinitis. Plain lateral films often show inflammation in the retropharyngeal area; but downward extension, if suspected, is better shown by computed tomography. An example of such abscess which probably originated in lymph nodes is shown in Figure 9.16.

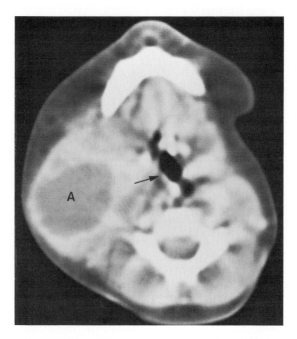

FIG. 9.16. This 16-month-old girl was well until 15 days prior to admission when her parents noted a firm mass in the region of the right parotid gland. Mumps titer was low at the time. On examination the neck had a firm, rubbery, fixed, somewhat tender mass over the right angle of the mandible in the region of the parotid. There was a central soft area that was nonpulsatile. Cranial nerves were intact. A CT scan was performed to evaluate the mass. The scan shows a very large mass just below the level of the parotid gland lateral to the submandibular gland. The mass has an irregular margin with a large low density center A. The mass is deep to the sternocleido-mastoid muscle, which is distended and distorted. There is associated soft tissue swelling with encroachment on the airway (arrow). The findings are consistent with an abscess with central liquefaction. Needle aspirate showed many gram positive cocci. The abscess cavity was then drained of 20 cc of purulent material. Culture grew out group A beta hemolytic streptococci. Biopsy of the capsule showed chronic inflammation without evidence of neoplasm.

CONGENITAL LESIONS OF THE HEAD AND NECK

Congenital malformations may occur in any compartment of the head and neck. They may be solitary lesions localized to one area or may be part of a more generalized dysplasia. Often, physical examination and plain radiographs will delineate the defects enough to give a firm diagnosis and allow definitive management and counselling; but in certain circumstances CT is the most effective and simple technique to fully outline complex bony and soft tissue abnormalities. In particular, if associated brain abnormality is suspected, a CT study can quickly show whether this is present or not. For example, an infant with hypotelorism may have underlying holoprosencephaly.

Craniofacial Malformations

In head and neck syndromes such as mandibulofacial dysostosis, a CT study will show the degree of hypoplasia of the zygomatic arches and other facial and temporal bone structures quickly and accurately. At the present time, plain radiographs of the skull and facial structures with cephalometric measurements are still relied on heavily for planning craniofacial surgery, but CT is complementary in showing the involved areas and has begun to replace pluridirectional tomography in some instances.

Meningoencephalocele

Protusion of meninges with or without associated brain substance through the bony cranium or skull base occurs most commonly in the midline but may also present as a more lateral mass. The most common areas of protrusion are in the occipital region or more anteriorly between the sutures around the nose, orbit, ethmoid, and sphenoid bones. Depending on the size and site, they may cause visible deformities such as a bulging mass as associated with hypertelorism in nasofrontal encephalocele or with exophthalmos due to naso-orbital protrusion. Embryologically, the encephaloceles in frontal areas may be related to failure of complete closure of the bony cranium with incomplete medial ingrowth of the mesoderm from each side leaving a bony defect through which glial tissue remains attached to the skin. In the occipital area, anomalies of migration of the neural crest are thought to be a more likely cause of these lesions.[48]

When a central mass is detected either clinically or radiologically, the differential diagnosis may be quite wide. Neurogenic masses include true encephaloceles, nasal gliomas, meningoceles, and neurofibromas. Masses of ectodermal origin include dermoid cysts, epidermoid inclusion cysts, sebaceous cysts, nasal polyps, lacrimal duct cysts, ethmoidal cysts, abscesses, and papillomas. Mesodermal masses include hemangioma, lymphangioma, lipoma, and angiofibroma.[48] Malignant tumors may also cause similar central masses. Many of the above lesions require CT evaluation to show their size and possible intracranial extension. A carotid angiogram or CT metrizamide study may eventually be necessary to distinguish a true encephalocele from a meningocele. The case discussed in Figure 9.17 is an example in which CT was the only diagnostic modality able to suggest the cause of the patient's symptoms. Diagnosis of encephalocele was thus invaluable in allowing prompt and successful treatment for what could have been future life-threatening intracranial infections.

Although encephaloceles may occur as isolated malformations, they may also present as part of various syndromes or associations. Cohen and Lemire[49] have pointed out that encephaloceles may be found in (1) aberrant tissue band syndrome, (2) Chemke syndrome, (3) cryptophthalmos syndrome, (4) dyssegmental dwarfism, (5) frontonasal dysplasia, (6) Knoploch syndrome, (7) Meckel syndrome, (8) pseudo-Meckel syndrome, (9) vonVoss syndrome, and (10) war-

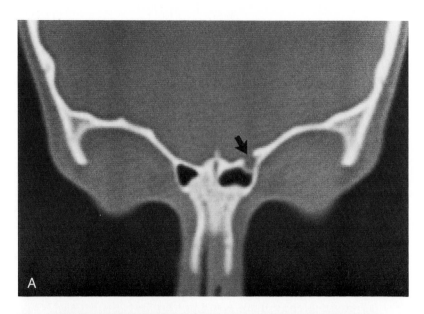

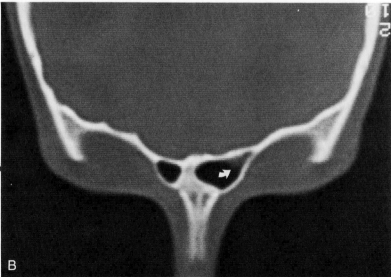

FIG. 9.17. An 8-year-old boy had three separate episodes of bacterial meningitis, twice due to pneumococcus and once to *Hemophilus influenzae*. A radionuclide cisternogram failed to show any leakage of cerebrospinal fluid. A CT scan of the sinuses shows (A) a small bony defect superiorly in the posterior aspect of the left frontal sinus (arrow) which is associated with (B) a soft tissue mass in the superior aspect of the left frontal sinus. The question of an encephalocele was raised. Surgical exploration of the anterior fossa revealed herniation of brain through the left frontal floor and just anterolateral to the cribriform plate. The defect was repaired with a facial graft and the patient had an uncomplicated recovery.

When other methods had failed to demonstrate the cause of the persistent meningitis, CT scan in this instance was able to suggest a correct diagnosis and allow treatment for what might have become serious repeated meningeal infections.

farin syndrome. Associated anomalies include absent corpus callosum, orofacial clefting, craniostenosis, Dandy-Walker defect, Arnold-Chiari defect, ectrodactyly, hemifacial microsomia, hypothalamic–pituitary dysfunction, Klippel-Feil deformity, and myelomeningocele.

Choanal Atresia

Before diagnosis of this condition by CT was possible (Fig. 9.18), radiopaque contrast was instilled into the affected nasal cavity with the head in the supine position and a cross-table lateral film taken to show the level of hold-up of contrast in the posterior nasopharynx. Shirkoda and Biggers[50] have described a case of bilateral choanal atresia diagnosed by CT and have shown that this will outline the level, type, and thickness of the obstructing septum better than the traditional method. Asymmetry of the nasal cavities and any associated anomalies of the hard palate or adjacent structures will be seen. Knowledge of this level and extent of obstruction is of great help to the surgeon. In the past, occasionally a blind surgical approach to perforate the septum was used, thereby placing the patient at risk of damage to the spinal cord through the

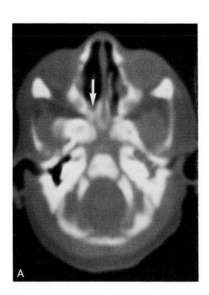
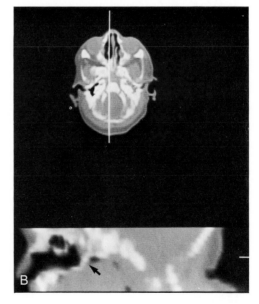

FIG. 9.18. This baby girl was born with multiple congenital anomalies including esophageal atresia, microcephaly, and abnormal facies. CT evaluation of the skull and temporal bones for microcephaly shows that (A) the left nasal cavity is patent but narrower than normal. The posterior right nasal cavity is severely stenosed (arrows) and a bony septum is visualized at the level of the choana with air posterior and anterior to it consistent with choanal atresia. (B) Sagittal reconstruction views confirm the diagnosis.

atlanto-occipital joint. With good delineation of the nature of the surgical problems, such risks now are not necessary.

Choanal atresia is due to the presence of an obstructing membrane (10 percent of cases) or bony septum (90 percent of cases) in the posterior nasal cavity just anterior to the back of the hard palate. The membraneous type occurs a little more posteriorly than the bony type. The atresia is unilateral in two-thirds of cases and bilateral in one-third. The bilateral type presents shortly after birth. Infants with this condition exhibit signs of suffocation; like all neonates they are obligatory nasal breathers, since they do not learn to breathe through their mouths for several weeks. Unilateral choanal atresia may not be diagnosed for several years but is usually associated with longstanding nasal discharge on the affected side. Embryologically, choanal atresia occurs when the aperture between the buccal and nasal cavities remains obstructed by the nasobuccal membrane or associated mesodermal tissue.

Craniosynostosis

When craniosynostosis is part of a malformation (i.e., Apert's syndrome), CT has been shown to be of great help diagnostically. Carmel and colleagues[51] have used CT in 24 children with craniosynostosis to evaluate the skull base, calvarium and underlying brain structures. Bone window settings show thickening of the affected sutures with thinning of the adjacent surrounding bone. Deformities are measured and postoperative progress is monitored by axial CT scans.

Basal Cell Nevus Syndrome

Figure 9.19 is a good example of the ability of CT to demonstrate the extent of involvement of the maxilla and mandible by the dentigerous cysts associated with this syndrome. The cysts, which are present in 65 to 75 percent of patients, present clinically with swelling and pain in the jaw, with secondary infection, and with pathological fractures. They are lined by stratified keratinizing squamous epithelium that occasionally exhibits buds resembling embryonal skin. Associated skeletal anomalies, which occur in 75 percent of cases, include anomalous ribs and nonsegmented cervical and upper thoracic vertebrae. Frontal and parietal bossing are present and a characteristic lamellar pattern of intracranial calcifications is seen in the falx in more than 90 percent of patients over 40 years of age. Mild mental retardation and hydrocephalus are common and epilepsy has been reported.[52] The basal carcinomas that occur are typically numerous and occur most commonly as small brownish papules, nodules, or plaques scattered over the face, neck, back, thorax, and abdomen. These carcinomas, which are indolent until puberty, then tend to enlarge and ulcerate.

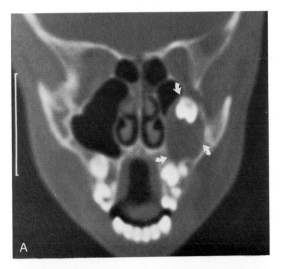

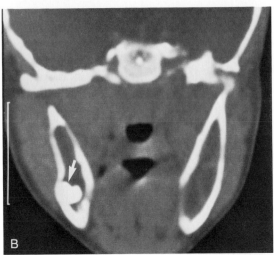

FIG. 9.19. A 12-year-old boy had progressive pain and felt pressure in his upper right jaw in the month prior to admission. A dental consultation led to routine jaw radiographs, which showed multiple dentigerous cysts. A diagnosis of basal cell nevus syndrome was made. A skeletal survey revealed confirmatory evidence of this syndrome including malformations of the spine, bifid ribs, Sprengel's deformity, and a short fourth metacarpal. (A) Axial view through maxilla shows partial opacification of the left maxillary sinus by a large oval cyst containing a tooth. The cyst expands laterally into the zygomatic process. It involves the roots of the second molars on the left side. (B) Coronal view through posterior mandible demonstrates marked cystic expansion of the medulla of the mandibular rami, with a tooth in the right dentigerous cyst (arrow).

Delineation of the cysts was extremely useful in planning dental surgery. Histology of the cyst lining was attentuated stratified squamous epithelium, consistent with odontogenic keratocyst. Four cysts had been identified by plain film; six were shown by CT scan.

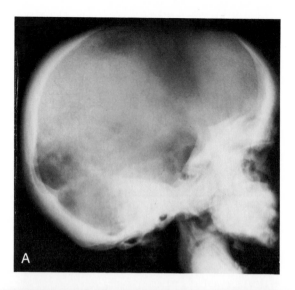

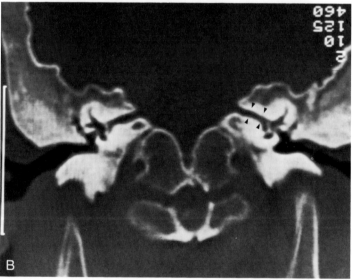

FIG. 9.20. This 15-year-old boy with craniometaphyseal dysplasia has many of the stigmata of the disease, including hypertelorism, prognathism, glabellar prominence, and decreased visual acuity and hearing. He was noted to have bilateral partial facial nerve paralysis and bilateral sensorineural hearing loss. Funduscopic examination of the retina showed bilateral optic atrophy. A plain lateral skull film (A) shows marked thickening of the frontal and occipital bony cortex with considerable thickening and sclerosis of the bones at the skull base. (B) CT performed to evaluate the acoustic, optic, and facial nerve pathways with the objective of possible decompression of narrowed canals if necessary, shows narrowed internal auditory canals bilaterally in the cephalocaudad dimension (arrowheads). Small tympanic cavities and extremely small mastoid antra were noted bilaterally in other sections. The vertical portion of the facial nerve canal was patent but bony hyperostosis in the region of the horizontal portions of the facial nerve canals was noted.

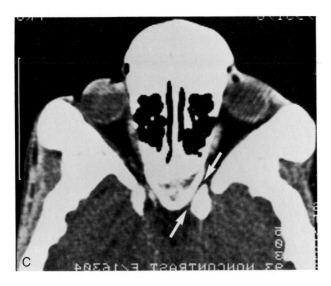

FIG. 9.20 (*Cont.*). (C) Axial view of orbits shows massive thickening of the bony orbit and vault with severe narrowing of the optic nerve canal by thickened bone (between arrows). Decompression of the optic canals was subsequently performed.

Craniometaphyseal Dysplasia

The major features of this disease include a large head with hypertelorism, frontal bossing, and a wide nasal root. The mandible is often large with dentition and there may be noisy nasal breathing because of an obstructed nasal cavity. Neurological manifestations include optic atrophy (Fig. 9.20), progressive deafness and facial nerve paralysis, hemiplegia, and medullary compression.[53] Mental and motor retardation are present. Radiological studies demonstrate progressive thickening and sclerosis of the bony skull base and facial bones which cause nerve and vascular compression. The sinuses and mastoids may be obliterated. Hypertelorism is present and modeling of the metaphyses of the tubular bones is absent. This condition should be distinguished from metaphyseal dysplasia (Pyle's disease), in which the skull bones are much less affected.[54]

Orbital Teratoma and Ocular Coloboma

Congenital lesions of the orbit, other than those described above, include congenital orbital teratoma[55] and ocular colobomas.[56] Ocular colobomas and associated orbital cysts are relatively common malformations that result from defective fusion of the fetal optic fissure. The ability of high-resolution CT to show the location and extent of these defects and their associated abnormalities has been discussed by Simmons and colleagues.[56] They point out that those colobomas classified as typical occur in the region of the fetal optic fissure in the inferonasal portion of the optic nerve and globe (atypical colobomas occur in the iris and are considered a separate condition). The CT features include the following: (1) the globe is malformed and may be elongated or conal in shape; (2) the mass effect caused by the coloboma differs from other masses by its continuity with the low density vitreous cavity and by surrounding thin, dense sclera; (3) cysts containing fluid of density similar to CSF are present; (4) the orbit may be expanded; (5) microphthalmos with displacement of the globe may be present; and (6) there may be associated optic nerve atrophy.

Congenital Cystic Masses of the Neck

These include branchial cleft cysts, cystic hygroma, thyroglossal duct cyst, and hemangioma.

Branchial Cleft Cyst

Branchial cleft cysts are due to failure of the cervical sinus to obliterate, resulting in persistence of a cystic space lined by squamous epithelium. These cysts present most commonly in childhood but may present in adult life. These second-groove cysts are formed most commonly high in the lateral neck with their posterior segment deep to the sternocleidomastoid muscle. They often present because of infection and CT may be useful in distinguishing between these masses and other similar clinical lesions such as cystic hygroma, hemangioma, carotid artery aneurysm, Warthin tumor of the parotid or submandibular salivary glands, and lymphadenopathy. The cysts are sharply marginated and contain fluid that is usually low in attenuation but may be relatively high with an increased protein content. Cysts of the first branchial cleft present in the periauricular area.

Cystic Hygroma

This lesion presents in the neck in 80 percent of cases and is present at birth in two-thirds of patients, with most of the remainder appearing by the 2nd year of life. Embryologically they develop when the primitive lymph spaces fail to connect with the rest of the lymphatic system. The sequestered segments continue to grow as soft cystic masses and often are intimately involved with other structures of the neck such as the tongue, vessels, larynx, and pharynx. Rarely, these masses cause respiratory obstruction. Approximately 3 to 10 percent will extend into the mediastinum and may be associated with chylothorax and chylopericardium. CT demonstrates a characteristic homogeneous water-density cystic mass and shows the extent of involvement of adjacent tissues. Ultrasound also shows the cystic nature of such masses but does not show regional extension as well. The main reason for performing CT is to show mediastinal extension, since this would alter the surgical approach.[57]

Thyroglossal Duct Cyst

Thyroglossal duct cysts are found most commonly in the midline at the base of the tongue in the path of the duct from the foramen cecum to the thyroid gland. They may appear more superiorly or inferiorly or laterally from this common central site. They result from the failure of the duct to regress and are most common below the hyoid bone, presenting more often in children than in adults. They may be seen by CT as cystic or mass lesions in the areas described and are subject to recurrent infections.

Hemangioma

Hemangiomas may occur in any location in the head and neck and may present in many different ways depending on their size and site. Their size ranges from tiny to huge. When present in the orbit, for example, a relatively small lesion may cause prominent symptoms.[58] Occasionally, a hemangioma in the neck may be so large that during birth, cervical dystocia occurs and, after birth, tracheal compression interferes with respiration.

Histologically, these hemangiomas may be classified as (1) capillary, (2) cavernous and (3) other types.[59] Capillary hemangiomas may present as masses in the parotid in infancy. The cavernous type, seen most commonly in childhood, consists of large blood spaces or sinusoids lined by endothelium or compact masses of endothelial cells. They often grow rapidly during the first 3 to 6 months of life, after which they grow in proportion to the overall body growth. In general, they then tend to undergo spontaneous regression. However, surgical removal may be necessary for cosmetic reasons or because of symptoms produced by the tumor. The more superficial the lesion, the greater the likelihood of spontaneous regression. CT is an excellent method for defining the extent of hemangiomas. The mass effect is seen to displace or infiltrate normal tissues. Occasionally, phleboliths will be present as small calcific densities. Contrast enhancement confirms the vascular nature of the lesion and allows even more precise delineation of its margins. The hemangioma may opacify evenly after bolus injection or may take up the contrast peripherally at first and more centrally after a few seconds. The intensity of opacification is usually enough to allow a confident distinction between these and other tumor masses. Hemangiomas may be combined with other soft tissues such as fibromas, lipomas, lymphangiomas, and neurofibromas, in which case spontaneous regression does not occur.

Hemangioma in the subglottic region of the trachea is usually suggested by symptoms of stridor, which become worse on crying. Plain films of the area may show the lesion well, but CT also shows encroachment on the tracheal lumen. CT determination of tracheal dimensions in children and adolescents have been made by Griscom[60] and Effman et al.[61] Large series have not yet been performed, but the technique shows promise in being able to show whether or not the tracheal diameter is decreased.

Hypoplasia of the Maxillary Antrum

This is an uncommon congenital lesion, but plain films may give the impression that chronic sinusitis is present when the underlying lesion is really hypoplasia of the antrum. Occasionally, the orbit on the affected side may be a little larger, and this should not be mistaken for the presence of an intraorbital mass. CT is better than plain film for showing the antral hypoplasia and any associated mucosal thickening.[62]

REFERENCES

1. Brasch RC, Cann CE: Computed tomographic scanning in children. II. An updated comparison of radiation dose and resolving power of commercial scanners. AJR 138:127–133, 1982.
2. Berger TE, Kuhn JP, Bruseharber J: Techniques for computed tomography in infants and children. Radiol Clin North Am 19:399–408, 1981.
3. Schmidt TH, Stieve FE: Radiation exposure of infants and children in computed tomography. Ann Radiol 23:143–149, 1980.
4. Rowe LD, Miller E, Brandt-Zawadski M: Computerized tomography in maxillo-facial trauma. Laryngoscope 91:745–757, 1981.
5. Schramm VL Jr: Inflammatory neoplastic masses of the nose and paranasal sinuses in children. Laryngoscope 89:1887–1898, 1979.
6. Bluestone CD, Stool SE: Pediatric Otolaryngology. W.B. Saunders, Philadelphia, 1983.
7. Kilman JW, Clatworthy HW, Newton WA, et al.: Reasonable surgery for rhabdomyosarcoma: a study of 67 cases. Ann Surg 78:346–350, 1973.
8. Sutow WW, Sullivan MP, Ried HI, et al.: Prognosis in childhood rhabdomyosarcoma. Cancer 25:1384–1390, 1970.
9. Maurer HM, Moon T, Donaldson M, et al.: The Intergroup Rhabdomyosarcoma Study: a preliminary report. Cancer 40:2015–2026, 1977.
10. Scotti G, Harwood-Nash DC: Computed tomography of rhabdomyosarcomas of the skull base in children. J Comput Assist Tomogr 6:33–39, 1982.
11. Tefft M, Fernandez C, Donaldson M, et al.: A report of the Intergroup Rhabdomyosarcoma Study (IRS). Cancer 42:253–258, 1978.
12. Raney RB Jr, Lawrence W Jr, Maurer HM, et al.: Rhabdomyosarcoma of the ear in childhood—a report from the Intergroup Rhabdomyosarcoma Study–I. Cancer 51:2356–2361, 1983.
13. Danziger J, Handell SF, Bao-Shan J, Wallace S: Computerized tomography in rhabdomyosarcoma of the head and neck. Cancer 44:463–467, 1979.
14. Littman P, Raney B, Zimmerman R, et al.: Soft tissue scans of the head and neck in children. Int J Radiat Oncol Biol Phys 9:1367–1371, 1983.
15. Schuller DE, Lawrence TL, Newton WA Jr: Childhood rhabdomyosarcomas of the head and neck. Arch Otolaryngol 105:689–694, 1979.
16. Lawrence W Jr, Hays DM, Moon TE: Lymphatic metastasis with childhood rhabdomyosarcoma. Cancer 39:556–559, 1977.
17. Maurer EM, Donaldson M, Gehan EA, et al.: Rhabdomyosarcoma in childhood and adolescence. Curr Probl Cancer 2:3–36, 1978.
18. Raney BR Jr, Tefft M, Newton WA, et al.: Intensive treatment of children with cranial parameningeal sarcoma. A report from the Intergroup Rhabdomyosarcoma Study (IRS) presented in part to the 73rd meeting of the American Association for Cancer Research. St. Louis, Missouri, April 28, 1982.

19. Myers EN, Skolnick KB: Tumors of the neck. pp. 1425–1438. In Bluestone CD and Stool SE (eds): Pediatric Otolaryngology. W.B. Saunders Philadelphia, 1983.

20. Vita HC, Mendiono OA, Shaw DL, et al.: Nasopharyngeal carcinoma in the second decade of life. Radiology 148:253–256, 1983.

21. Jeans WD, Gilani S, Bullimore J: The affect of CT scanning on staging of tumors of the paranasal sinuses. Clin Radiol 33:173–179, 1982.

22. Sessions RB, Bryan N, Nacleiro RM, et al.: Radiographic staging of juvenile angiofibroma. Head Neck Surg 3:279–283, 1981.

23. Lichtenstein L: Histiocytosis X. Arch Pathol 56:84, 1953.

24. Sherman NH, Rao VM, Brennan RE, Edeiken J: Fibrous dysplasia of the facial bones and mandible. Skeletal Radiol 8:141–143, 1982.

25. Barrionuevo CE, Marcallo FA, Coelho A, et al.: Fibrous dysplasia and the temporal bone. Arch Otolaryngol 106:298–301, 1980.

26. Fries JW: The roentgen features of fibrous dysplasia of the skull and facial bones. AJR 77:71, 1957.

27. Zimmerman DC, Dahlin DC, Stafne EC: Fibrous dysplasia of the maxilla and mandible. Oral Surg 11:55, 1958.

28. Som PM, Lawson W, Cohen BA: Giant cell lesions of the facial bones. Radiology 147:129–134, 1983.

29. Rhea JT, Weber AL: Giant cell granuloma of the sinuses. Radiology 147:135–137, 1983.

30. Ross JL, Schinella R, Stenkman L: Massive osteolysis: an unusual case of bone destruction. Am J Med 65:367, 1978.

31. Taybi H: Osteolysis. p. 294. In Gorham (ed): Radiology of Syndromes and Metabolic Disorders, 2nd Ed. Year Book Medical Publishers, Chicago, London, 1983.

32. Lallemand DP, Brasch RC, Normal D, Newton TH: Orbital tumors in children: a differential diagnostic approach based on computed tomography. AJR (abs) 141:851, 1983.

33. Kennerdell JS, Ghoshhajra K: Computed tomographic scanning of orbital tumors. Int Ophthalmol Clin 22:99–131, 1982.

34. Harris GL, Williams AL, Reiser FH, Abrams TW: Intraocular evaluation by computed tomography. Int Ophthalmol Clin 22:1972, 1972.

35. Zimmerman RA, Bilaniuk LT, Metzger RA, et al.: Computed tomography of orbital–facial neurofibromatosis. Radiology 146:113–116, 1983.

36. Kobrin JL, Block SC, Weingiest TA: Ocular and orbital manifestations of neurofibromatosis. Surg Ophthalmol 24:45–51, 1979.

37. Carter BL, Bankoff MS: Facial Trauma: computed versus conventional tomography. p. 319. In Littleton JT, Durizch M (eds): Sectional Imaging Methods: A Comparison. University Park Press, Baltimore, 1983.

38. Rowe LD, Miller E, Brandt-Zawadski M: Computerized tomography in maxillo-facial trauma. Laryngoscope 91:745–757, 1981.

39. Zilkha A: Computed tomography in facial trauma. Radiology 144:545–548, 1982.

40. Mancuso AA, Hanafee WN: Computed tomography of the injured larynx. Radiology 133:139–144, 1979.

41. Sevel E, Kraus ZH, Ponder T, Centeno R: Value of computed tomography for the diagnosis of a ruptured eye. Comput Assist Tomogr 7:870–875, 1983.

42. Grove AS Jr: Orbital trauma evaluation by computed tomography. Int Ophthalmol Clin 22:133–153, 1982.

43. Lobes LA Jr: Computed tomography in the detection of intraocular foreign bodies. Int Ophthalmol Clin, 22:219–234, 1982.

44. Trokel SL, Hilal SK: Recognition and differential diagnosis of enlarged extraocular muscles in computed tomography. Am J Ophthalmol 87:503, 1979.

45. Fernbach SK, Naidich TP: CT diagnosis of orbital inflammation in children. Neuroradiology 22:7–13, 1981.

46. Chandler JR, Langenbrunner DJ, Stevens ER: Pathogenesis of orbital complications in acute sinusitis. Laryngoscope 80:1414–1428, 1970.

47. Carter BL, Bankoff MS, Fisk JD: Computed tomographic detection of sinusitis responsible for intracranial and extracranial infections. Radiology 147:739–742, 1983.

48. Sprinkle PM, Sporck FT: Congenital malformations of the nose and paranasal sinuses, pp. 769–780. In Bluestone CD and Stool SE (eds): Pediatric Otolaryngology. W.B. Saunders, Philadelphia, 1983.

49. Cohen NM Jr, Lemire RJ: Syndromes with cephaloceles. Teratology 25:161–172, 1982.

50. Shirkhoda A, Biggers WP: Choanal atresia. Radiology 142:93, 1982.

51. Carmel BW, Luken MG, Ashcherl GF Jr: Craniosynostosis: Computed tomographic evaluation of skull base and calvarial deformities and associated jaw cranial changes. J Neurosurg 9:366–372, 1981.

52. Murphy MJ, Tensor RV: The nevoid basal cell carcinoma syndrome and epilepsy. Ann Neurol 11:372–376, 1982.

53. Taybi H: Radiology of Syndromes and Metabolic Disorders, 2nd Ed. Yearbook Medical Publishers, Chicago, 1983, p. 82.

54. Carlson DH, Harris GBC: Craniometaphysial dysplasia. Radiology 103:147–151, 1972.

55. Plonsky L, Virapongse C, Markowitz RI: Congenital orbital teratoma. J Comput Assist Tomogr 7:367–369, 1983.

56. Simmons JD, La Masters D, Devron C: Computed tomography of ocular colobumas. AJNR 4:1049–1052, 1983.

57. Silverman PM, Korobkin M, Moore AV: CT diagnosis of cystic hygroma of the neck. J Comput Assist Tomogr 7:519–520, 1983.

58. Savoiardo M, Strada L, Passerini A, et al.: Cavernous hemangiomas of the orbit: value of CT angiography and phlebography. *AJNR* 4:741, 1983.

59. Lindsay WK: Neoplasms. p. 1490. In Ravitch MM, Welch KJ, Benson CD, et al (eds): Pediatric Surgery, 3rd Ed. Yearbook Medical Publishers, Chicago, 1979.

60. Griscom NT: Computed tomographic detection of tracheal dimensions in children and adolescents. Radiology 145:361–364, 1982.

61. Effman EL, Fram EK, Vock P, Kirks DR: Tracheal crosssectional area in children CT determination. Radiology 149:137–140, 1983.

62. Mendelsohn DB, Hertzmann Y: Hypoplasia of the maxillary antrum. S Afr Med J 63:496–497, 1983.

10 Planning Radiotherapy for Head and Neck Tumors

OLUBUNMI K. ABAYOMI
MARK S. BANKOFF

INTRODUCTION

Cancer in the head and neck region comprises a heterogenous group of neoplasms, which have varying biological behavior and different degrees of radioresponsiveness. Accurate determination of the extent of the tumor is very important in selecting treatment. Advances in CT of the head and neck have complemented clinical examination and in some inaccessible sites have provided information that otherwise would not have been available to the physician taking care of patients with tumors in this region.[1] It is therefore the intent of this article to review the biology of head and neck tumors and the contribution of CT in their evaluation and radiotherapeutic management.

EPIDEMIOLOGY

Cancer in the head and neck is predominantly squamous cell carcinoma. It was estimated that approximately 38,000 new cases of cancer of the head and neck region would occur in 1983.[2] This figure excludes skin cancer. The epithelial tumors of the oral cavity, oropharynx, larynx, and hypopharynx have been linked to heavy use of alcohol and tobacco. Adenocarcinoma of the sinuses has been associated with prolonged exposure to wood dust. The incidence of carcinoma of the nasopharynx is higher in Southern China and in East and West Africa, and carcinoma of the postcricoid region has been associated with Plummer–Vinson syndrome.

PATHOLOGY

The common histological types of tumors found in the head and neck region include

1. Squamous cell carcinoma
2. Undifferentiated carcinoma
3. Salivary gland tumors
4. Lymphomas and plasmacytoma
5. Sarcomas (rhabdomyosarcoma is most common)

Some sites show predilection for certain types of tumors. Thus, lymphoepithelioma, which is considered to be poorly differentiated squamous carcinoma, often occurs in the nasopharynx whereas lymphoma is characteristically found in the Waldeyer's ring and, less commonly, in the maxillary sinus. Minor salivary gland tumors involve the palate, the floor of the mouth, and the maxillary sinus.

ANATOMIC GROUPINGS

From a consideration of the biological behavior, pattern of spread, and clinical presentation, the head and neck tumors can be grouped into the following categories:

1. Nasal cavity: paranasal sinuses and nasopharynx
2. Buccal cavity: anterior two-thirds of the tongue, the floor of the mouth, and the gingiva
3. Oropharynx: base of tongue, tonsil, and fauces
4. Laryngopharynx: the larynx and hypopharynx
5. Salivary glands: major and minor salivary glands.

STAGING

Proper staging of malignant tumors is very important, because it affords the physician the ability to select the appropriate treatment, to evaluate the results of treatment, and to compare results with other institutions. The American Joint Committee for Cancer Staging (AJCS) has adopted the T.N.M. (T, primary tumors; N, regional lymph nodes, M, distant metastases) staging system for most head and neck tumors (Tables 10.1–10.5).[3]

PATTERN OF SPREAD

To offer a rational treatment for head and neck tumors it is necessary to have a knowledge of the extent and the pattern of spread of the disease.

Most patients with head and neck tumors present with a primary tumor and regional node metastases. They therefore require treatment for both sites.

TABLE 10.1 Tumor (T) classification for paranasal sinuses (maxillary sinus)[a]

T1 Tumor confined to the antral mucosa of the infrastructure with no bone erosion or destruction.

T2 Tumor confined to the suprastructure mucosa without bone destruction or to the infrastructure with bone destruction of medial or inferior bony wall only.

T3 More extensive tumor invading skin or cheek, orbit, anterior ethmoid sinuses, or pterygoid muscles.

T4 Massive tumor with invasion of cribriform plate, posterior ethmoids, or sphenoid sinuses, nasopharynx, pterygoid plate, or base of skull.

[a] The maxillary sinus is divided into a posterosuperior portion, the suprastructure and anteroinferior portion, the infrastructure by a line described by Ohngren, drawn from the inner canthus to the angle of the mandible. This line serves as a useful guide to operability and prognosis.

TABLE 10.2 Tumor (T) classification for buccal cavity, nasopharynx, and oropharynx

Stage	Buccal Cavity[a]	Oropharynx[b]	Nasopharynx
T1	Tumor ≤2 cm in greatest diameter	Tumor ≤2 cm in greatest diameter	Tumor confined to one site of nasopharynx or no visible tumor (positive biopsy only)
T2	Tumor 2–4 cm in greatest diameter	Tumor 2–4 cm in greatest diameter	Tumor involving two sites [both posterosuperior and lateral walls]
T3	Tumor >4 cm in greatest diameter	Tumor >4 cm in greatest diameter	Extension of tumor into nasal cavity or oropharynx
T4	Massive tumor >4 cm in diameter, with deep invasion involving the antrum, pterygoid muscles, base of tongue, or skin of the neck	Massive tumor >4 cm in diameter, with invasion of bone, soft tissues of the neck, or root of the tongue	Tumor involving skull or cranial nerve, or both

[a] Includes lip, buccal mucosa, floor of mouth, oral tongue, hard palate, and gingiva.
[b] Includes the fauces, tonsils, pharyngeal wall, and base of tongue.

TABLE 10.3 Tumor (T) classification for larynx and hypopharynx

Stage	Larynx[a]	Hypopharynx[b]
T1	Tumor confined to site of origin with normal mobility	Tumor confined to site of origin
T2	Tumor involves adjacent supra-glottic or subglottic sites (in the case of subglottic primary, extends to the vocal cords) without fixation	Extension of tumor to adjacent region or site without fixation of hemilarynx
T3	Tumor confined to the larynx with cord fixation, or extension to involve post-cricoid area, medial wall of piriform sinus, or pre-epiglottic space	Extension of tumor to adjacent region or site with fixation of hemilarynx
T4	Massive tumor extending beyond the larynx to involve soft tissues of the neck or destruction of thyroid cartilage	Massive tumors involving bone or soft tissue of the neck

[a] Larynx subdivided into supraglottis (ventricles, arytenoids, epiglottis, and aryepiglottic folds), glottis (true vocal cord), and subglottis (inferior to the true cords).
[b] Region includes the pyriform sinus, posterior surface of the larynx (post-cricoid area), and lower posterior pharyngeal wall.

TABLE 10.4 Nodal (N) classification

N0	No clinically positive nodes
N1	Single clinically positive homolateral node ≤3 cm in diameter
N2	Single clinically positive node >3 cm but ≤6 cm in diameter
N2a	Single clinically positive node >3 cm but ≤6 cm in diameter
N2b	Multiple clinically positive homolateral nodes, none >6 cm in diameter
N3	Massive homolateral, bilateral, or contralateral node(s)
N3a	Clinically positive homolateral node(s), one of which is >6 cm
N3b	Bilateral clinically positive nodes
N3c	Contralateral clinically positive node(s) only

TABLE 10.5 Distant metastases (M) classification

M0	No known distant metastases
M1	Distant metastases present

Because of its relevance to radiation therapy, the pattern of spread for the various anatomic sites and its impact on the choice of treatment will be discussed.

Nasopharynx

Carcinoma of the nasopharynx is characterized by the absence of symptoms referrable to the primary site in the early stage of the disease; the common presentation is metastatic neck disease, which is present in 50 to 60 percent of cases[4] and is bilateral in about 30 percent.[5] However, the primary tumor can progress and cause symptoms by invading the surrounding structures. Thus, carcinoma of the nasopharynx can spread anteriorly to involve the nasal cavity, the maxillary sinus, the ethmoids, the pterygopalatine fossa, and the orbital apex. Laterally, nasopharyngeal carcinoma can extend into the parapharyngeal space and infratemporal fossa. Superiorly, the tumor can spread to the base of the skull, where the clivus and sphenoid bone including the greater wing with the foramen ovale and spinosum may be involved. Direct invasion into the carotid sheath and cavernous sinus may result in involving cranial nerves II to VI. The most commonly affected muscle is the lateral rectus, supplied by the cranial nerve VI. Inferiorly, the tumor can spread to involve the soft palate and the oropharynx. CT scans illustrating possible routes of spread of carcinoma of the nasopharynx are shown in Figures 10.1 and 10.2.

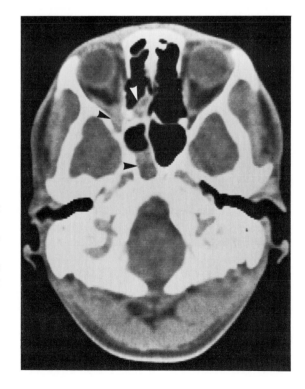

FIG. 10.1. CT of a patient with carcinoma of the nasopharynx that has extended to involve the right ethmoid sinus and apex of the right orbit (black arrowheads); the right ethmoid sinus (white arrowhead) is also involved. The extent of his disease required modification of the radiation treatment portals and techniques.

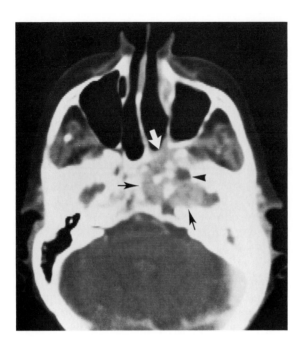

FIG. 10.2. Another patient with carcinoma of the naso-pharynx, which extended intracranially. White arrowhead shows involvement of the region of the pterygopalatine fossa. Destruction of the petrous apex and the clivus (black arrows) is shown. The foramen ovale (black arrowhead) is also involved.

Nodal metastases from nasopharyngeal carcinoma commonly involve the upper jugular nodes and the retropharyngeal node of Rouviere, which lie near the transverse process of the atlas in close relation to the jugular foramen. Involvement of this node can lead to compression of the last four cranial nerves and the cervical sympathetic nerve.

Because of the anatomic relationships of the nasopharynx and the pattern of spread of tumors in this region, it is obvious that the only modality available for primary management of these tumors is radiation therapy. However, the nasopharynx and the surrounding structures are inaccessible for adequate clinical evaluation.[1] The radiotherapist needs to know the true extent of the disease in order to plan adequate treatment fields. CT of the nasopharynx and the surrounding structures gives excellent soft tissue detail and defines the extent of bone destruction and infiltration of the various foramina. This affords the radiotherapist the means of adequately delineating the extent of disease, ensures adequate treatment fields, and thereby increases the potential for controlling the disease.[6]

Paranasal Sinuses

The maxillary sinus is the most common site for neoplasms involving the sinuses. The histological types of tumors found in the maxillary sinus include squamous cell carcinoma, adenocarcinoma, lymphomas, minor salivary gland tumors, plasmacytoma, and sarcomas.

The mucous membrane of the sinus is firmly attached to the periosteum, and this has implications for the pattern of spread and the response to radiation therapy.

The site of involvement by carcinoma of the maxillary sinus has both prognostic and therapeutic significance. Ohngren,[7] a Swedish ENT surgeon, subdivided the maxillary sinus using an imaginary line that joins the medial canthus to the angle of the mandible. The region above this line (Ohngren's line), the posterosuperior portion, is referred to as the suprastructure and the region below, the anteroinferior portion, is the infrastructure.

Early carcinoma of the maxillary sinus is usually asymptomatic. Most of the patients present with advanced disease when local extension gives rise to symptoms.[8] The maxillary sinus has three walls: anterolateral, posterolateral, and medial. Invasion of the anterolateral wall produces swelling and induration of the cheek. The infratemporal fossa is separated from the sinus by the posterolateral wall. Invasion of this wall and extension of tumor into the infratemporal fossa can cause trismus because of infiltration of the pterygoid muscles.

The medial wall is formed by the lateral boundary of the nasal cavity and contains the ostium, through which tumor can spread from the sinus into the nasal cavity.

The roof of the maxillary sinus is formed by the floor of the orbit. Therefore, tumors of the suprastructure of the maxillary sinus can invade the floor of the orbit and lead to proptosis and opthalmoplegia. The hard palate and the upper alveolus form the floor of the antrum, and tumors involving the infrastructures can extend to involve the alveolus and adjacent part of the buccal mucosa. Figures 10.3 and 10.4 demonstrate involvement of surrounding structures by maxillary sinus tumors and the use of CT for planning radiation treatment.

Lymph node metastasis is not common in carcinoma of the maxillary sinus. It occurs in about 15 percent of cases; however, another 15 percent will develop nodal metastasis during the course of the disease.[9] The lymphatics of the maxillary sinus join those of the nasal fossa and drain to the jugulodigastric node and/or pass to the lateral retropharyngeal nodes. The deep cervical nodes may also be involved.

Despite the absence of nodal metastasis in most patients, the result of treatment of carcinoma of the maxillary sinus is poor, with the 5-year survival ranging between 30 and 35 percent.[7,10] This is because most patients present with locally advanced disease. To achieve good results, these patients have to be treated by a combined modality consisting of surgery and radiation therapy. The anatomic relationships of the maxillary sinus are such that clinical evaluation and conventional radiographic studies fail to define the extent of disease adequately.[1,10] Several factors affect the response of tumors of the maxillary sinus to radiation therapy. These are

1. Invasion of surrounding structures, e.g., orbits, muscles, base of skull
2. Bone destruction
3. Adequacy of the radiation therapy fields and dose
4. Presence of dose-limiting structures, e.g., eyes, spinal cord, and brain
5. Presence of nodal metastases

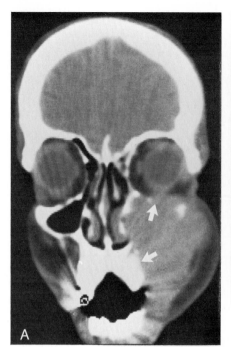
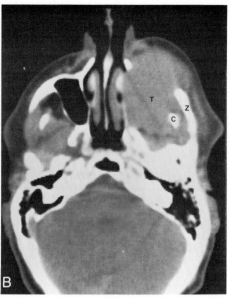
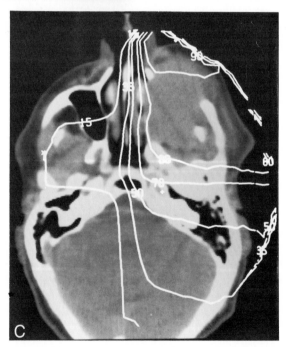

FIG. 10.3. (A) Coronal CT of a patient with diffuse histiocytic lymphoma of the left maxillary sinus. Tumor involves the floor of the orbit and left upper alveolar ridge. The soft tissues of the cheek are also involved. (B) Transverse CT of the same patient demonstrating destruction of the zygomatic arch (Z) anteriorly by the tumor (T). C is the coronoid process of the mandible. (C) The CT was used to plan treatment. The composite plan of patient's treatment is shown. He received 5000 rad to the target volume, which was encompassed by the 80 percent isodose line. The treatment field consisted of an open anterior field and two lateral opposed wedged fields.

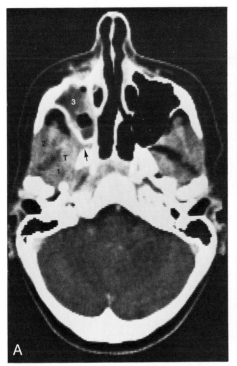 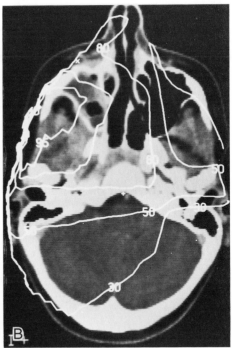

FIG. 10.4. (A) CT of a patient with adenoidcystic carcinoma of the right maxillary sinus (3). There is loss of the fat plane between the lateral pterygoid (1) and the medial pterygoid (2). The tumor has extended into the infratemporal fossa (T) and the pterygo-palatine fossa (arrow). (B) Composite treatment plan for the patient using information obtained from the CT scan. The target volume received a dose of 7000 rad using an open anterior field and wedged left lateral field.

To achieve good tumor control with radiation therapy all areas with tumor involvement must be covered by the treatment fields. The CT scan has been shown to be very valuable in defining the extent of disease, especially bony and soft tissue extension.[12,13] It has, therefore, aided the selection and arrangement of radiation therapy fields so that the areas of invasion and probable direction of spread are adequately covered. Adequate radiation therapy combined with surgery will potentially improve the results in this disease, which for the most part is a local problem, i.e., with low incidence of nodal and distant metastases.

Buccal Cavity

Tumors involving this part of the alimentary canal are predominantly squamous cell carcinoma; tumors of minor salivary glands also occur. The structures making up this segment comprise the anterior two-thirds of the tongue, the glossogingival sulci, the gingivae, the buccal mucosa, and the lips. Carcinomas arising from the various sites in the buccal cavity lend themselves very well to clinical evaluation because of their accessibility. Conventional radiographs give good information about the presence of bone invasion. The mode of spread is by local invasion or via the lymphatics. The lower jaw and the mylohyoid muscular diaphragm form a barrier to spread, which is only overcome in advanced stages. Lymph node metastases are present in 30 to 40 percent of patients with carcinoma of the anterior tongue and the floor of the mouth. Prognosis for these tumors depends on the extent of the primary lesion, on whether bone and soft tissue has been invaded, and on the presence of lymph node metastases. CT scan is useful in defining the extent of muscle and bone invasion, an important consideration in selecting treatment.

Oropharynx

This region includes the base of tongue, vallecula, fauces, tonsil, posterior and lateral walls of the pharynx, and the retromolar trigone. Squamous cell carcinoma is the predominant histological type of tumor at these sites. Lymphomas are also commonly found because of the presence of lymphoid tissue both in the base of tongue and in the tonsillar region.

The retromolar trigone is a triangular area lying between the anterior pillar and the third molar tooth. Tumors arising in this area are usually classified with tumors of the buccal cavity. In early stages, the incidence of lymph node metastases in the trigone is lower than for tumor of the oropharyx as a whole. Advanced tumors of this site can spread posteriorly to involve the anterior pillar and tonsil, medially to involve the tongue, and laterally to involve the cheek whereas inferior extension may lead to direct invasion of the submandibular salivary gland. When this occurs, as with pharyngeal involvement, the only way of demonstrating the extension is by CT scan. The radiation therapy regimen requires modification when this extension has been demonstrated.

The base of tongue is the part of the tongue posterior to the circumvallate papillae and inferior to the intrinsic muscles. Lederman[14] grouped the base-of-tongue tumors with those involving the vallecula and the linguotonsillar sulcus. This grouping is because of their similarity in prognosis and pattern of spread. Most patients with tumors involving these sites present with advanced disease. The presenting symptoms depend on the structures involved. Tumors of the base of the tongue can extend to involve the whole musculature. The pharyngeal wall can also be involved. Tumors arising from the vallecula have easy access to the pre-epiglottic space because of the poor resistance in the floor offered by the hyoepiglottic fascia. Involvement of this region is of significant prognostic and therapeutic importance. The most useful means of determining the presence of pre-epiglottic space involvement is with the CT scan. Tumors arising from the linguotonsillar sulcus can extend to involve the tonsil, the fauces, and the parapharyngeal space. Figure 10.5 demonstrates

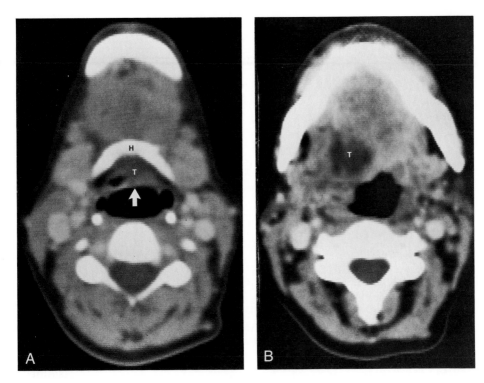

FIG. 10.5.   (A) CT scan of a patient with advanced carcinoma of the base of tongue. Tumor (T) is demonstrated in the pre-epiglottic space. The arrow shows the laryngeal surface of the epiglottis and H shows the hyoid bone. (B) The tumor (T) of the base of tongue is shown containing a necrotic component. This is significant because tumors with large necrotic areas are less radioresponsive.

pre-epiglottic space involvement and the presence of necrotic areas in a carcinoma of the base of tongue. The incidence of lymph node involvement from tumors of the base of tongue is very high, of the order of 50 to 70 percent. Bilateral neck metastases occur in about 25 percent of cases.[14] The result of treatment for tumors of the base of tongue has been poor, with survival about 25 percent at 2 years.[15] The prognostic factors include the size of the primary lesion, extent of muscular invasion, and extension into surrounding structures, e.g., pre-epiglottic space, parapharyngeal space, and lymph node metastases. These areas are difficult to assess clinically but are clearly defined by CT.[16-18] It also assists in the selection of cases with extensive disease for combined modality treatment with surgery and radiation.

The most common tumor of the tonsil is squamous cell carcinoma. Since the tonsil forms one of the components of Waldeyer's ring, lymphomas also can arise here. Tumors of the tonsil may involve both tonsillar pillars and may spread upward into the soft palate and the floor of the nasopharynx. Medially, the linguotonsilar sulcus and the adjacent base of tongue can be

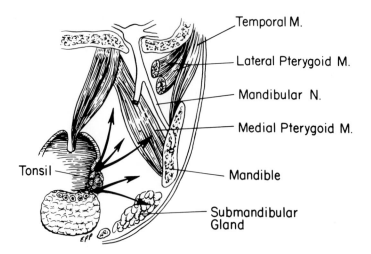

FIG. 10.6. Coronal section of the prestyloid part of the parapharyngeal space.

involved. The tumor may extend anteriorly to invade the anterior pillar and the retromolar trigone, from which invasion of the soft tissue of the neck can occur through the floor of the trigone. Extensive involvement of the tonsillar bed can lead to invasion of the parapharyngeal space, the infratemporal fossa, and the skull base. Possible routes of spread of tumors involving the tonsil, the linguotonsillar sulcus, and the retromolar trigone into the parapharyngeal space are illustrated in Figure 10.6. Metastases may involve the node of Rouvi-

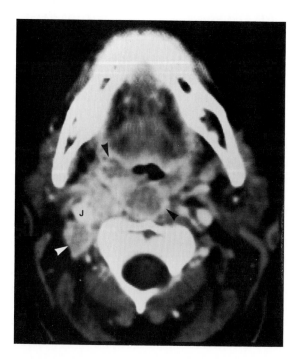

FIG. 10.7. CT of a patient with advanced squamous cell carcinoma of the right tonsillar fossa. The tumor (arrowheads) has extended into the retropharyngeal space and a metastatic node (white arrowhead) is visible adjacent to the jugular vein (J). Based on the information supplied by the CT scan and the clinical findings, the patient was not a surgical candidate. A radiation treatment field which included the retropharyngeal space in the high dose volume was chosen.

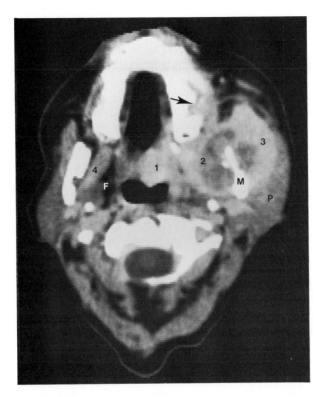

FIG. 10.8.   CT of a patient with advanced carcinoma of the left faucial arch. The tumor involved the left fauces, the tonsil and adjacent base of tongue, the soft palate (1), the retromolar trigone (2), the parapharyngeal space, and the infratemporal fossa. The mandible (M) was destroyed, the masseter muscle (3) was involved, and the parotid gland (P) displaced. Contrast the left side with the right side, where the normal anatomy of the medial pterygoid (4) and the fat (F) in the parapharyngeal space is preserved. Because of the extensive nature of his disease, this patient required treatment with both chemo- and radiation therapy.

ere, which can secondarily compress the last four cranial nerves. Figures 10.7 and 10.8 demonstrate extension of carcinoma of the tonsil to the parapharyngeal space and infratemporal fossa.

Lymph node metastases is present in 70 to 80 percent of patients with cancer of the tonsil. The most commonly involved nodal site is the subdigastric region.

Selection of treatment depends on the size and extent of involvement and on the size of nodal metastases.

Laryngopharynx

Most tumors arising in this region are laryngeal tumors. Tumors of the pyriform sinus will also be discussed under this heading. Using the true vocal cord as a landmark, it is customary to define laryngeal tumors arising above the true cord as supraglottic and those below the cord as subglottic.

Glottic Carcinomas

The superior surface of the true vocal cord forms the floor of the ventricle. Tumors arising in this region respond well to radiation therapy. Tumors extending to the anterior commisure have the potential of extending into the pre-epiglottic space. Tumors arising from the inferior surface of the cord can extend into the trachea. Carcinomas of the vocal cord are usually well differentiated and because of the minimal lymphatic supply, the incidence of lymph node metastases is very low (less than 5 percent). These tumors can, however, extend to involve the surrounding sites in the supraglottis and the piriform sinus. When this happens, the incidence of lymph node metastases increases. Poor prognostic factors in carcinoma of the cord are cord fixation, pre-epiglottic space involvement, and cartilage invasion. Under these circumstances, the response to radiation is poor, and surgical resection and radiation therapy will be required. It is difficult to determine clinically any pre-epiglottic space involvement. CT scan has been found useful for this purpose.[16]

Supraglottic Carcinomas

These tumors affect the epiglottis, pharyngoepiglottic fold, ventricles, false cords, and aryepiglottic folds. The tumors, especially those arising from the infrahyoid epiglottis, can extend to involve the pre-epiglottic space. Tumors of the ventricles and false cord may invade the piriform sinus. Extension inferiorly to involve the true cord is uncommon.[19]

The incidence of nodal metastases from supraglottic tumors is high, ranging from 50 to 60 percent. The nodes are bilateral or fixed in about 20 percent of cases.[20,21]

Factors that affect prognosis in these tumors include the size of the primary tumor, invasion of the pre-epiglottic space, extension to the base of tongue or pharyngoepiglottic fold, and lymph node metastases. Early lesions respond very well to radiation therapy alone, but extensive lesions require combined surgery–radiation management.

Piriform Sinus

The piriform sinus extends from the upper border of the pharyngoepiglottic fold to the cricopharyngeal fold below. Its medial border is formed by the aryepiglottic fold, the lateral border is partly formed by the thyroid cartilage, while the posterior pharyngeal wall lies posteriorly. Carcinoma arising from the piriform sinus can spread medially to the aryepiglottic fold, the arytenoids, and the false cord. Extension into the vallecula frequently occurs through the pharyngoepiglottic fold. Tumors of the piriform sinus can spread laterally to invade the thyroid cartilage, and posteriorly through the middle and lower pharyngeal constrictor muscles to the posterior part of the thyrohyoid membrane. Extension into the postcricoid region can result in recurrent laryngeal nerve paralysis. When the postcricoid region is involved, the radiation therapy technique has to be modified to include the upper esophagus.

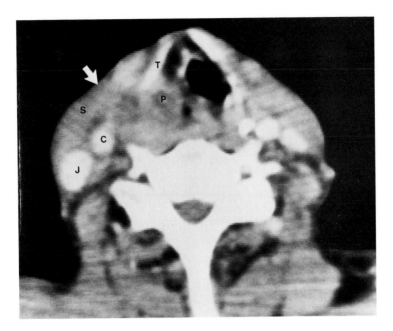

FIG. 10.9. CT of a patient with advanced carcinoma of the right piriform sinus (P). The tumor involved the aryepiglottic fold medially and invaded the thyroid cartilage (T) to extend directly into the neck (arrow). Clinically, a fixed mass was noted in the right posterior aspect of the thyroid cartilage deep to the sternocleidomastoid muscle (S). The relation to the carotid artery (C) and the jugular vein (J) is shown. Surgery in this patient was contraindicated because of the extent of his tumor. A radiation therapy technique that would treat the neck mass contiguous with the primary tumor to a high dose was employed.

Patients with carcinoma of the piriform sinus usually present with advanced disease. The incidence of lymph node metastases ranges from 60 to 80 percent.[22,23] The cure rate with either radiation therapy or surgery alone is very poor.[24,25] Therefore, combined surgery–radiation therapy is advocated for most cases.[26]

Because of its infiltrative nature, carcinoma of the piriform sinus often involves the pharyngeal musculature and the thyroid cartilage. Direct extension into the neck results in swelling, which may be confused with a metastatic node. The internal carotid artery, a close lateral relation, can be invaded. In these situations, CT aids in delineating the extent of disease so that proper selection of treatment can be made.[27] Figure 10.9 demonstrates extension to the neck by an advanced carcinoma of the piriform sinus.

MAJOR SALIVARY GLAND TUMORS

CT has been found useful in evaluating and planning treatment for major salivary gland tumors. By giving accurate three-dimensional information on the tumor's extent, CT assists the radiotherapist in choosing treatment fields

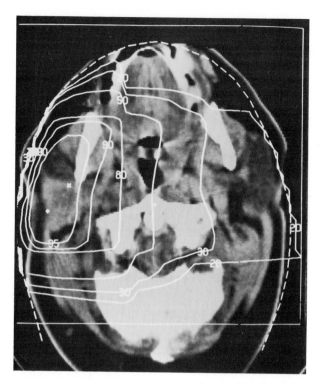

FIG. 10.10. Composite plan for the treatment of a patient with metastatic squamous cell carcinoma to the right parotid region is shown. The patient had presented with right facial paralysis and a parotid mass. CT scan demonstrated a mass in the right parotid and extension into the temporal bone along the course of the facial nerve. The CT scan was utilized in treatment planning. A mixed beam of high energy x-rays and 25 MeV electrons were used for the first part of the treatment. A final boost was given using a pair of anterior and right lateral wedged fields. He received 7000 rad to the tumor volume. The upper part of the spinal cord received 30 to 50 percent of the tumor dose and the opposite parotid gland received only 20 percent of the tumor dose. CT aided in the choice of a treatment technique that ensured adequate coverage of the tumor while sparing the spinal cord and the opposite parotid gland from receiving a high dose of radiation.

and techniques and in selecting the proper electron beam energy. This use of electrons has the advantage of limiting the volume of normal tissue treated to a high dose. Figure 10.10 shows the composite treatment plan for a patient with metastatic carcinoma to the right parotid region.

SKIN CANCER

The common tumors found in the skin of the head and neck area are basal cell carcinoma, squamous cell carcinoma, and melanoma. Most patients present with early disease and the CT scan plays no role in their evaluation. However, patients with advanced disease present with extensive invasion of the soft tissue of the head and neck. In these patients, the CT scan has been found very useful in determining the extent of disease, especially in assessing the infratemporal and intraorbital extension and the presence of bone destruction. These patients are usually not surgical candidates because of the extensive nature of their disease; they are treated with radiation therapy. The techniques and choice of fields are often based on information provided by the CT scan. A case of squamous cell carcinoma of the skin with extensive soft tissue and bone involvement is shown in Figure 10.11.

MANAGEMENT OF HEAD AND NECK TUMORS

Between 40 and 60 percent of patients with carcinoma of the head and neck region have disease both at the primary site and the neck nodes.[28] The incidence of distant metastases for all sites in the head and neck region is about 10 to 15 percent.[29] The head and neck cancer patients, therefore, present with a local and regional problem in the majority of cases.

The curative modalities available for treating carcinoma of the head and neck region are surgery and radiation therapy. Chemotherapy is employed in experimental protocols. Selection of the treatment depends on several factors including the site and extent of the primary disease, the presence of neck nodes, the age and overall condition of the patient, and the natural history of the disease. Most patients with head and neck carcinomas require radiation therapy either as the only modality of treatment or combined with surgery or chemotherapy.

Radiation Therapy

In the head and neck region, preservation of function and cosmesis are as important as the cure of the patients with carcinoma. The radiotherapist needs to deliver a dose high enough to control the tumor; however, there are several critical dose-limiting structures in the head and neck region. These include the brain, the brainstem, the spinal cord, and the eyes, ears, bone, and cartilage. The optimal dose is one that will control a high proportion of tumors without causing an unacceptable degree of morbidity. Therefore, to the radiotherapist, the therapeutic ratio (i.e., the ratio of normal tissue tolerance dose to the tumor lethal dose) is a very important parameter. The factors that affect the therapeutic ratio can be discussed under the following headings:

Dose-Related Factors

The response of tumors to radiation therapy depends on

1. The histological type: Lymphomas and plasmacytomas are more radioresponsive than epithelial tumors or sarcomas. Therefore, lymphomas can be

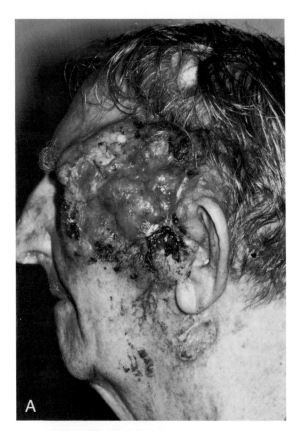

FIG. 10.11. (A) Lateral view of a patient with extensive squamous cell carcinoma of the left temporal region. (B) Anterior view of the same patient.

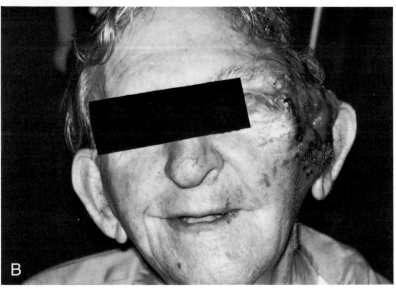

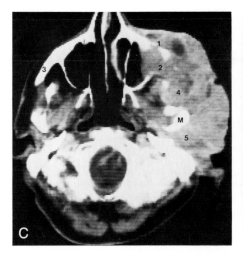 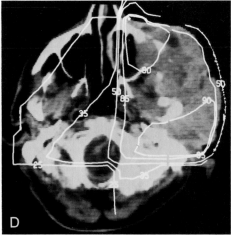

FIG. 10.11 (*Cont.*).   (C) CT scan of the patient showing the skin tumor invading underlying structures. The anterior (1) and the lateral (2) walls of the maxillary sinus have been destroyed. The zygomatic arch (3), shown on the normal side, has been destroyed on the left side. Tumor is seen in the infratemporal fossa (4) and posterior to the mandibular condyle (M), with extension to the external auditory canal. (D) Composite treatment plan using the CT to determine the tumor volume. A technique utilizing an anterior and left lateral fields with alternating 45° and 60° wedges was used.

controlled by a dose of 4500 to 5000 rad, whereas epithelial tumors require 7000 rad or more to achieve a reasonable level of control.

2.   Size: Small lesions are more radiocurable than large ones. The response of small tumors is better and repair of normal tissue is more complete after completion of radiation therapy.

3.   Invasion of soft tissue, bone, or cartilage: When these structures are invaded, response to radiation is diminished and healing is delayed. The delayed healing can result in deformity, which can ultimately affect the quality of the patient's survival.

4.   Physical factors, e.g., poor oxygenation: Large necrotic tumors have poorly vascularized components. These tumors are less responsive to radiation therapy and require a higher dose to achieve control. However, giving a high dose can result in a severe reaction of normal tissue. The clinical use of hypoxic cell sensitizers and hyperthermia is an attempt to improve results.

Figure 10.12 shows the treatment plan for a patient with recurrent squamous cell carcinoma in the neck. The CT scan showed a necrotic area in the tumor. The patient had been treated initially with a combination of preoperative radiation therapy to the neck followed by a left neck dissection. The primary tumor in the epiglottis had received 7000 rad, and there was no evidence of recurrence. The neck node was deep and fixed, ruling out surgery. The patient refused chemotherapy; therefore, the only treatment available was radiation therapy.

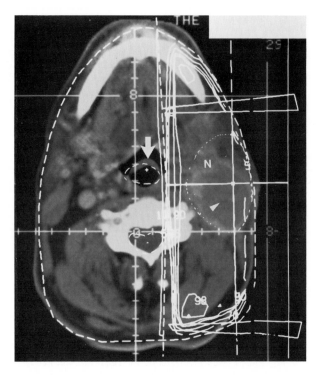

FIG. 10.12. Treatment plan for a patient with recurrent squamous cell carcinoma in the left neck. A treatment plan that would spare the epiglottis (arrow) and other laryngeal structures was utilized. The node (N) extends deep in the neck close to the transverse process and contains a large necrotic area (arrowhead). A pair of anterior and posterior opposed wedged fields was used in treating the patient, and because of the large necrotic area demonstrated by CT, hyperthermia was used in combination with irradiation.

Because this patient was being treated again after previous high-dose irradiation, the treated volume had to be restricted. The larynx was spared in order to prevent necrosis and laryngeal edema. The CT was useful to determine the extent of disease in the choice of a treatment regimen that would spare the larynx and the spinal cord. It also gave important information that would not otherwise have been available, namely, the presence of a large necrotic area within the node. The decision was made to utilize hyperthermia in conjunction with radiation therapy.

Normal Tissue Tolerance Factors

The tolerance of normal tissue to radiation is dose- and volume dependent. Small volumes can tolerate high doses, whereas treating large volumes to a high dose will result in unacceptably high complications. To minimize normal tissue injury, the technique of "shrinking fields" is utilized, i.e., a moderately high dose is delivered to a field that covers the gross tumor and the areas of potential microscopic extension. Following this the field is made smaller and a final boost is given to the gross disease to bring the tumor volume itself to a high dose. To minimize normal tissue injury, this boost can be given by interstitial implants, e.g., radium, cesium, iridium, or radioactive gold seed implants for accessible sites. Electron beam treatment can also be used for boost when deeper structures need to be spared.

Methods of Improving Therapeutic Ratio

The goal in treating patients with head and neck cancer is to control their tumor while maintaining good function and good quality of life. Because of the location of these tumors, radical surgery cannot be carried out without leaving the patient with considerable functional and cosmetic impairment. Radiation therapy has limitations imposed by normal tissue tolerance. In order to improve the results of treatment, methods of improving the therapeutic ratio must be sought. These include

1. Recognition of prognostic factors: The most important prognostic factor in head and neck cancer is the presence of lymph node metastases. Also important is invasion of soft tissue, bone, and cartilage. Invasion of these structures adversely affects the response to radiation therapy. Therefore, where possible, alternate treatment—either surgery or a combination of surgery and radiation therapy—should be employed. CT scan has been very useful in giving details of soft tissue, bone, and cartilage invasion by tumors,[1,16] thereby aiding in the selection of cases for surgery or combined treatment with radiation therapy and surgery.

2. Delivery of more effective treatment: This requires adequate coverage of the tumor by the most efficient radiation fields. The radiotherapist must use adequate treatment volume and must employ techniques that will result in a homogeneous dose to the target volume while sparing as much normal tissue as possible. In order to adequately cover the tumor with radiation treatment fields, the true extent of the disease must be known. Certain sites are relatively inaccessible clinically for adequate determination of tumor extent. In this situation CT scan provides information on the extent of disease and is valuable in planning treatment.

3. Early detection of persistence or recurrence: The use of CT scan to study inaccessible sites in the head and neck region can lead to early recognition of tumor persistence or recurrence so that salvage therapy can be offered when it is most likely to be effective. This can potentially result in a higher rate of tumor control.[30] CT should be done 2 to 4 months after completion of therapy in order to ensure a good baseline. This makes it possible to detect early recurrent disease.

CONCLUSIONS

Cancer of the head and neck is predominantly a local and regional disease, since only about 15 percent of the patients will develop distant metastases.[24] However, 65 percent of the patients die of their disease and in 90 percent of these patients the local disease is uncontrolled. This is a very significant problem, considering the impact of local failure on the quality of life of these patients.

Management of head and neck cancer requires a multidisciplinary approach. Most patients require radiation therapy either as the sole treatment modality or in combination with surgery. There are limitations to radical surgery because of functional and cosmetic considerations. Constraints are imposed on the dose of irradiation that can be delivered by the tolerance of critical dose-limiting structures in the head and neck area. The prognostic factors have been recognized. These include the presence of lymph node metastases, size of the tumor, and tumor invasion of soft tissue, cartilage, and bone. The adequacy of treatment is also an important prognostic factor. To provide adequate treatment, the radiotherapist should be able to determine the extent of the lesion, appreciate the natural history of the disease, and adapt the technique of treatment both to the needs of the patient and to the volume of the tumor. Case selection is very important in order to improve the result of treatment and minimize complications. Thus it is recognized that for advanced disease radiation therapy is less effective. The response to radiation therapy is poor when soft tissue and cartilage or bone are involved. In this situation, the use of surgery combined with irradiation improves the result.

By providing information on the true extent of the tumor and by demonstrating involvement of pharyngeal spaces and invasion of soft tissue, bone, and cartilage, the CT scan aids in selecting treatment and ensures adequate coverage of the tumor volume by the radiation therapist. There is the potential that the use of CT in treating and evaluating head and neck tumors will result in improving local control. This improvement should lead to improved survival.[30]

ACKNOWLEDGEMENTS

We gratefully acknowledge the assistance of Miss Donna Rolli, Mrs. Terry Peters, and Mrs. Barbara Billings in the preparation of this manuscript.

REFERENCES

1. Carter BL, Karmody CS: Computerized Tomography of the Face and Neck, Sem Roentgenol 13:257–266, 1978.
2. Silverberg E, Lubera J: A review of American Cancer Society estimates of cancer cases and deaths, CA 33 (1), 1983.
3. Manual for Staging of Cancer, 1978, American Joint Committee on cancer staging and end results reporting, Chicago, Ill, 1978.
4. Greenberg BE: Cervical lymph node metastasis from unknown primary sites; an unresolved problem in management. Cancer 19:1091–1095, 1966.

5. Creely JJ, Lyons GD Jr, and Trail ML: Cancer of the nasopharynx, a review of 114 cases. S Med J 66:405–409, 1973.

6. Moss WT, Brand WN and Battifora H (eds): Rationale, technique, results. Ch. 6. In Radiation Oncology. CV Mosby, St Louis, 1979.

7. Ohngren LG: Malignant tumors of the maxillo-ethmoidal region, Acta Laryngol (Suppl) 10:1–476, 1933.

8. Cheng VST, Wang CC: Carcinomas of the paranasal sinuses. Cancer 40:3038–3041, 1972.

9. Lewis JS, Castro EB: Cancer of the nasal cavity and paranasal sinuses. J Laryngol Otol 86:255–262, 1972.

10. Shecter GL, Ogura JH: Maxillary sinus malignancy. Laryngoscope 82:796–806, 1972.

11. Jeans WD, Gilani S, Bullimore J: The effect of CT scanning on staging tumors of the paranasal sinuses. Clin Radiol 33:173–179, 1982.

12. Forbes WS, Fawcitt RA, Isherwood I, et al: Computed tomography in the diagnosis of the paranasal sinuses. Clin Radiol 29:501–511, 1978.

13. Parsons C, Hodson N: Computed tomography of paranasal sinus tumors. Radiology 132:641–645, 1979.

14. Lederman M: Cancer of the base of tongue: treatment by radiotherapy. J Laryngol Otol 73:279–288, 1959.

15. Montana G, Hellman S, Von Essen CF, et al: Carcinoma of the tongue and floor of mouth: results of radical radiotherapy. Cancer 23:1284–1289, 1969.

16. Carter BL: Computed tomographic scanning in head and neck tumors Otolaryngol Clin North Am 13:449, 1980.

17. Mancuso AA, Hanafee WN, Juilliard JF, et al: The role of computed tomography in the management of cancer of the larynx. Radiology 124:243–244, 1977.

18. Feuerback S, Conllota U, Schmeisser KJ: Computed tomography of pharyngolaryngeal carcinoma. Eur J Radiol 2:105–108, 1982.

19. Baclesse F: Carcinoma of the larynx. Br J Radiol (Suppl) 3:1–61, 1949.

20. Lindberg RD, Jesse RH: Integrated approach to management of cancer of the larynx and hypopharynx. Ch. 1. In: Oncology 1970, Proceedings of the Tenth International Cancer Congress, Chicago, 1971. Year Book Medical Publishers, Inc.

21. Wang CC, Shulz MD, Miller D: Combined radiation therapy and surgery for carcinomas of the supraglottic larynx and pyriform sinus. Am J Surg 124:551–554, 1972.

22. Lederman M: Cancer of the laryngopharynx. J Laryngol 68:333–369, 1954.

23. McGravran MH, Bauer WC, Ogura JH: The incidence of cervical node metastasis from epidermoid carcinoma of the larynx and their relationship to certain characteristics of the primary tumor. Cancer 14:55–66, 1961.

24. Lanlane GM, Cachin T, Julliard G, Lefur R: Telecobalt therapy for carcinoma of the laryngopharynx. Am J Roetgenol 111:78–84, 1971.

25. Lederman M: Cancer of the pharynx. J Laryngol 81:151–172, 1967.

26. Vandenbronck C,: Results of a randomised clinical trial of preoperative irradiation versus postoperative in treatment of tumors of the hypopharynx. Cancer 39:1445–1449, 1977.

27. Sojker H, Olofson J: Computed tomography in carcinoma of the larynx and pyriform sinus. Clin Otolaryngol 6:335–343, 1981.

28. Mendenhall WM, Million RR, Cassisi NJ: Elective neck irradiation in squamous cell carcinoma of the head and neck. Head Neck Surg 3:15–20, 1980.

29. Merino OR, Lindberg RD, Fletcher GH: An analysis of distant metastases from squamous cell carcinoma of the upper respiratory and digestive tracts. Cancer 40:145–151, 1977.

30. Suit HD: Potential for improving survival rates for the cancer patient by increasing the efficacy of treatment of the primary lesion. Cancer 50:1227–1234, 1982.

11 Comparison of CT and MR of the Head and Neck

ROBERT B. LUFKIN
WILLIAM N. HANAFEE

When comparing computed tomography and magnetic resonance (MR) as imaging modalities in the head and neck region, certain considerations must be kept in mind.

First of all, the two technologies are at very different stages in their development. CT scanning has been in clinical use for more than 10 years. It has evolved through a series of product generations and engineering advances into a stable, essentially industry-standard imaging device found in virtually every major medical center.

MR, on the other hand, has been in limited clinical use only a fraction of that time. It is undergoing an exponential phase of its development, with different manufacturers employing sometimes radically different techniques to create the MR images. New advances are made in system design every few weeks. Although part of the knowledge acquired in CT development such as certain reconstruction algorithms, display software, and the axial tomographic approach to anatomy are similar, the two systems are for the most part completely different in the way the signal is produced to create the image and in the information that that image contains. Therefore in discussing situations where MR scanning is now considered to be inferior to CT, one must add the caveat that the limitation is only for the present and may not be true as MR technology rapidly changes over the next months.

The second consideration is the point of view held by certain proponents of MR. These groups maintain that the real strength of MR does not lie in producing images that compare favorably with the spatial and contrast resolution of CT scanning images but rather rests in the full utilization of the capability of MR to obtain biochemical and physiological data. This may involve the use of coils tuned to atoms other than to protons, such as phosphorus, sodium, and fluorine, and the use of images and spectroscopy based on chemical shift data. They would perhaps argue that a comparison of CT with proton MR imaging overlooks the greatest potential of MR in its ability to detect chemistry in vivo. Because much of the nonproton imaging and chemical shift work with MR is speculative or at best experimental at this time, the remainder of this chapter will consider only proton imaging, which is by far the most common type of MR imaging work done today.

OVERVIEW OF MR

CT has become the "gold standard" in head and neck imaging.[1] CT and other x-ray images are based on a single factor. The x-ray beam is attenuated by the tissue present according to its electron density. This is excellent for imaging bones and for certain industrial applications, but much information about a living organism is contained in regions of soft tissue. The use of intravenous contrast material improves the situation with vascular structures and enhancing lesions. The increased contrast sensitivity available in CT over a conventional x-ray also improves the visualization of soft tissue within the limits of x-ray technology. The problem is that soft tissue structures often have similar x-ray density while varying greatly in chemical composition and biological function.

Unlike CT, the information contained in an MR image is based on a complex relationship of five factors: proton density, flow, T_1 and T_2 relaxation times, and chemical shift information. The proton density (other nuclei will not be considered here) reflects the relative abundance of free protons in the tissue studied. This is somewhat analogous to electron density of x-ray images. In fact, MR images obtained with emphasis on this parameter are similar in appearance to CT images. Flow is an important factor in the MR image and can act as a natural contrast agent. The T_1 and T_2 relaxation times are important MR properties, which reflect the biochemical environment of the tissue. Chemical shift is an effect used in spectroscopy that will not be discussed here. These five factors combine to form the MR image, which allows exquisite delineation of soft tissue detail.

A second well-known advantage in imaging living organisms is that MR produces its images without using ionizing radiation. Finally, as we shall see later, the physics of MR imaging allows scans to be performed in any plane and without any moving parts (such as rotating detectors and an angled gantry).[2]

The first requirement for MR imaging is protons. All protons possess spin, a charge, and, therefore, a small magnetic moment. When placed in a uniform magnetic field, a percentage of the free protons in a patient align themselves with this field. They also wobble (or precess) about the axis of the field at a frequency that is proportional to the applied magnetic field (Larmor frequency). Next, a small amount of energy is added in the form of radiowaves tuned to the Larmor frequency. This causes some of the protons to flip away from the main magnetic field. The radiowaves are then turned off and the protons gradually relax back into alignment with the main field. As this occurs, radiowaves that can be detected by listening coils are emitted from the relaxing protons. These emitted radiowaves are the MR signal. The T_1 and T_2 relaxation times are derived relaxation coefficients reflecting the rate at which the protons reorient with the main magnetic field (T_1) and become out of phase with each other (T_2). These times vary depending on the immediate chemical environment of the protons.

From this discussion, the importance of proton density and T_1 and T_2 relaxation times in forming the MR signal should be apparent. A simplistic explanation of the dependence on flow is that if a stimulated proton is moving rapidly enough, it will move out of the section before its emitted signal can be detected. In practice the effect is not quite so straightforward, but this explanation should suffice for our purposes.[3]

The previous discussion describes how the MR signal is produced. To create an image it is necessary to spatially encode the information in some way. This is accomplished through the use of applied gradients to the main magnetic field. The gradients cause different regions of tissue to be subjected to slightly different magnetic field strengths. Recall that the Larmor frequency of the precessing protons (and therefore their selective radiofrequency) is a function of the applied magnetic field. Therefore, the position of a region of tissue is determined by the frequency of its emitted radio signal. A mathematical tool known as a Fourier transform is performed to easily decode this information from the emitted signals. Once the strength of the signal is known for each region of the tissue being examined, it may be represented as a level of brightness to form the image. The result is that a tomographic image is formed with brightness-reflecting signal intensity.

One of the advantages of MR imaging over CT scanning is the ability of MR to change the appearance of the image (and therefore the information it contains) by changing the relative contributions of flow and relaxation times. This is accomplished by the use of pulse sequences. A pulse sequence is merely a description of how and when the radiowaves are applied to stimulate the protons. Several types of pulse sequences are available but the one most commonly used today is known as the spin-echo (SE) sequence. It is characterized by two parameters TR and TE. (Fig. 11.1). The amount of time from the beginning of one stimulation and listening sequence to the beginning of the next stimulation is the repetition time or TR. The amount of time from the beginning of a sequence until the signal is heard from the protons is known as the echo time or TE. A given spin echo pulse sequence may be described as SE/TR/TE with TR and TE in milliseconds (e.g., SE/670/48). The relationship between the overall intensity (I) of an image element and these factors may be expressed as follows:

$$I = Hf(v)(1 - e^{-TR/T_2})e^{-TE/T_2}$$

H represents proton density and $f(v)$ is the flow function. Although there are certain limitations, from this formula it is possible to see how manipulations of TR and TE will influence the relative contributions of T_1 and T_2 to the image brightness. The flow function is also dependent on the pulse sequence chosen.

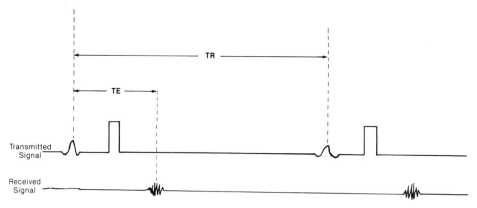

FIG. 11.1 Diagram of the spin-echo pulse sequence illustrating the repetition time (TR) and echo time (TE). The transmitted signals are the RF pulses to stimulate the tissue. The received signal is the emitted MR signal of the tissue.

With the present state of technology a given MR image will differ from a CT image of the same area in the following respects:

Increased Soft Tissue Sensitivity

As mentioned above, because of the various imaging parameters MR may be able to differentiate soft tissue structures that have the same CT density. This is done through selection of the pulse sequence parameters that will maximize the image contrast between the tissues. By the same token, it has been well documented that a given pathology may be rendered inapparent or invisible by selection of the *wrong* pulse sequence parameters.

Another approach to obtaining more information from the tissue is to derive actual T_1 or T_2 values. Derivation may be by direct measurement or by computation. Direct measurement is suitable for small areas but too slow for an entire scan. Calculating the values may be done for an entire image but at the expense of spatial resolution of the resulting data.

Excellent Visualization of Flowing Blood

Although CT can often show vascular structures if intravenous contrast is used, MR always shows rapidly flowing blood without any added contrast agents. This is because of the "flow void" phenomenon mentioned above. At slower velocities or where turbulence is present, the effect is more complicated. A vessel may appear bright or as a void. Until the causes of signal alterations are sorted out, the definitive diagnosis of plaques and mural thrombi requires careful scrutiny.

In the head and neck the ability to visualize flow is very useful in defining the relationship of tumors to major vessels. It is also useful for recognizing structures that may be confused with blood vessels on CT, such as lymph nodes. On MR the nodes show as regions of intermediate signal, which are easily distinguished from large flowing vessels with no signal.

Ease of Scanning in Any Plane

The MR imaging process is achieved by using magnetic fields with gradient coils and radio transmitter and receiver antennae. By electronically adjusting the frequencies and gradients, it is possible to obtain tomographic sections in any plane without moving the patient. This is a great advantage over CT scanning, where the patient (or gantry) must be physically moved in order to align the x-ray tube–detector axis with the plane of section for each scan. Also, because of the physical limitations of the CT gantry bore, certain scanning planes are not possible in the living patient. Although with CT reformatted images may be constructed in any plane from a large number of scans, the spatial resolution is poorer than that from MR. This is because the pixel size is determined by the slice thickness, and even the thinnest CT slice is greater than most current MR image pixel sizes. The second major drawback to reformatted CT images is that they are extremely sensitive to motion, because of the long data acquisition times.

Artifacts from Ferromagnetic Materials Only

CT scanning is very susceptible to artifacts from metallic substances. In the head and neck dental amalgam produces streak artifacts that may completely degrade an image. These streaks occur because materials of high electron density, such as metals, affect the readings on the CT detectors. This effect is propagated throughout the image during the reconstruction process.

With MR not all metals cause artifacts. Only the subset with ferromagnetic properties distort the image. For example, dental amalgam produces no MR artifacts. A homogeneous magnetic field must be present for MR imaging. If a piece of ferromagnetic material is present, a small distortion is created in the otherwise uniform field and will show up on the image. Unlike CT, the effect is not propagated throughout the image and is usually limited to the immediate area of the offending material.

Low Signal from Calcium and Air

Proton density is very important for MR image formation. The protons emit the radiowaves that make up the MR signal. All protons do not take part in this effect but only a subset of them known as free protons. Certain biological materials such as air, calcification, and cortical bone contain few free protons. Therefore, no matter how they are stimulated, or which pulse sequence is used, very little signal is produced, because few free protons are there to produce it.

Fortunately, cortical bone is often adjacent to soft tissues and fat-containing marrow, which have many free protons and emit a high signal. Tissue calcifications are also often surrounded by higher signal soft tissues that allow them to be detected; however, small calcifications are definitely better seen with CT.

The problem in head and neck MR is that certain regions contain areas of bone in close proximity to air. For the study of the middle ear and paranasal sinuses CT continues to have definite advantages over MR. There is also an advantage to having little signal emitted from calcifications and bone in certain situations. Fine details of the cerebellopontine angles and low neck may be obscured on CT scanning by the "beam hardening" artifact caused by the adjacent dense petrous bones and shoulder structures. This does not occur with MR and represents an advantage over CT scanning of these areas.

Long Image Formation Time

The amount of time necessary to obtain an MR image for a given system and image matrix depends on the pulse sequence chosen and the number of signal averages that is necessary to give a sufficient signal-to-noise performance. This translates into image acquisition times on the order of several minutes for current MR scanners versus several seconds for modern CT scanners. For the purposes of estimating patient throughput, the times are not directly comparable. Because of the nature of the MR process it is possible to obtain many images simultaneously. Current MR systems collect 16 or 32 images at the same time whereas CT scanning must obtain each slice separately.

Unfortunately, because each MR slice is acquired over the whole time period, it is susceptible to motion artifact. If the motion is periodic, such as respiration or cardiac, the MR scanning may be gated to the motion. For random movements or swallowing, there is no solution at present.

Acquisition time in MR may be shortened by improving the signal-to-noise performance. Researchers are now trying this through the use of different types of high performance radio coils.

Relatively Thick Image Sections

To keep acquisition times reasonable most MR scanners obtain sections 8-10 mm thick. If thinner sections are desired, longer acquisition times, with increasing susceptibility to motion artifact, are necessary. The use of specialized radio coils to improve the signal and allow thinner sections is also under investigation.

For the present the thick sections of MR images suffer from the same partial volume effects that plagued CT scanning early in its development.

MATERIALS AND METHODS

Unless otherwise mentioned, the cases presented are part of the clinical trials conducted by the Fonar Corporation for their premarketing approval by the Food and Drug Administration. The patients were referred from several medical centers in the New York area. The majority of patients came from Long Island Jewish Hospital, Nassau County Hospital, Beth Israel Hospital, and several private practitioner offices.

Scans were performed on a Fonar Beta 3000 permanent magnet imaging system operating at 0.3 T. The pulse sequences are specified for each image with timing parameters in milliseconds.

APPLICATIONS TO SPECIFIC REGIONS OF HEAD AND NECK

Nasopharynx

The nasopharynx is one of the more promising areas in the head and neck for MR imaging. Its relative lack of motion and abundance of fascial planes and soft tissue anatomy make it ideal for MR study.[4,5]

The anatomy of the region is dominated by the pharyngobasilar fascia. This tough fascia is attached to the skull base and fits inside the superior pharyngeal constrictors much like the segments of a telescope. Inferiorly the fascia ends at the soft palate. It serves as a support to keep the nasopharyngeal airway open during inspiration.

Adjacent to this fascial plane is a capillary bed that is easily visible as an area of low signal on MR imaging. It may also be seen on CT scanning following intravenous contrast infusion. This is a useful CT and MR landmark, because the tough fascia restrains benign disease and is crossed only by aggressive inflammatory processes or malignancies (Fig. 11.2).[6]

Lateral to the pharyngobasilar fascia and superior constrictors are areas of loose areolar tissue that make up the paranasopharyngeal space. The area is well visualized on MR because of the strong signal produced by the lipid-containing spaces. This provides excellent contrast with most masses, which are usually of a lower signal strength. Malignancies of the nasopharynx invade this region after crossing the pharyngobasilar fascia. (Fig. 11.3).

Lying posterolaterally are the carotid arteries and jugular veins. The flowing blood in them reliably appears as areas of low signal intensity on MR. Displacement of these vessels by nasopharyngeal masses may provide useful information about the site of origin of the masses (Fig. 11.4).

Because of the ease of showing flow with MR, this technique should also provide information about tumor invasion of the vessel itself.

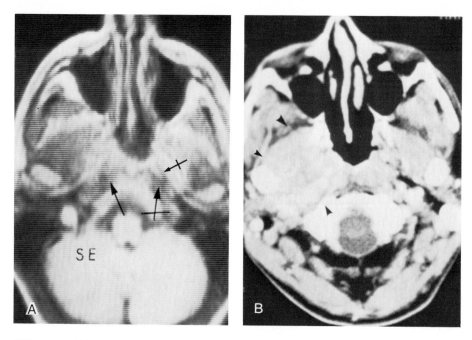

FIG. 11.2 (A) Axial MR (SE/670/48) scan through the high nasopharynx shows a region of low signal on the left (slashed arrow) representing normal pharyngobasilar fascia. Squamous carcinoma has crossed this boundary on the right (arrow). (B) CT through the same level shows obliteration of fascial planes on the involved side (arrowheads).

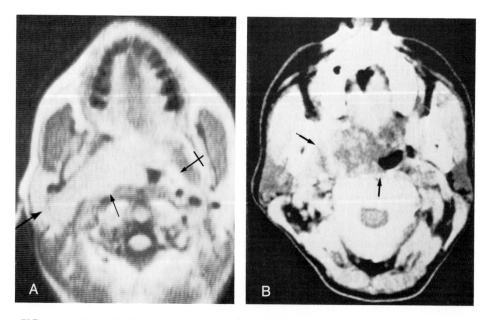

FIG. 11.3 (A) MR (SE/670/48) scan through the low nasopharynx shows carcinoma displacing the airway and spreading to the paranasopharyngeal space on the involved side. The mass is easily differentiated from the surrounding soft tissues and parotid gland (arrow). The contralateral paranasopharyngeal space is intact (slashed arrow). (B) CT scan through the same level again demonstrates the mass effect (arrow).

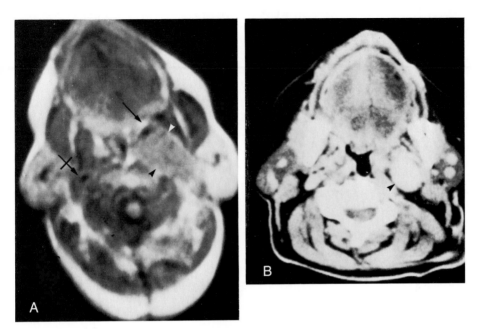

FIG. 11.4 (A) MR (SE/670/48) scan of a patient with a glomus vagale shows a mass (arrowheads) that has displaced the carotid artery anteriorly (arrow). The carotid artery on the uninvolved side is in normal position (slashed arrow). (B) CT scan also shows the enhancing mass (arrowhead). The position of the adjacent vessels is less apparent.

When examining the nasopharynx, it is important to be able to image the skull base because of the propensity of malignancies to spread to this region. The problems of MR imaging of calcium and air have been mentioned. However, most tumors have a higher signal strength than cortical bone so that destruction of the bone by tumor is shown by a region of increased signal (Figs. 11.5–11.7).

Paranasal Sinuses

Unlike the nasopharynx, the arrangement of tissues and anatomy of the paranasal sinuses is far from ideal for MR scanning. Both air and cortical bone produce little signal no matter which pulse sequences are used. The proximity of these structures to each other makes recognition of subtle bony changes (which are so useful on CT scanning) difficult to appreciate on the MR image. Once the sinuses are full of fluid or soft tissue, this proximity is less of a problem and the bony margins are seen better.

A second problem area is the nasal cavity. The mucous membranes covering the nasal passages and turbinates all produce a relatively strong signal on MR that is similar to the effect of malignant disease in the same region. With the use of different pulse sequences or proton chemical shift imaging, this effect may someday be overcome, but it is a problem at present.

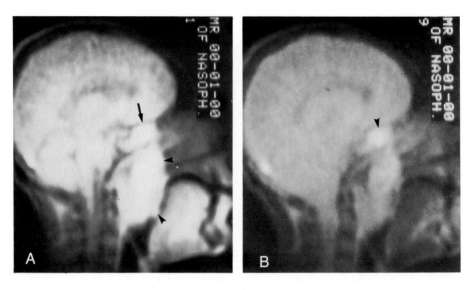

FIG. 11.5 (A) Midsagittal MR scans demonstrate a large carcinoma (arrowheads) of the high nasopharynx. Increased signal from the fluid-filled sphenoid sinus and tumor mass outline the regions of low signal from the intact cortical bone (arrow). (B) The second scan with a different pulse sequence shows high signal coming from the fluid-filled sphenoid sinus (arrowhead), compared with the lower signal from adjacent tumor and brain. (Scans courtesy of R. Nick Bryan, M.D., Baylor University, Houston, Texas)

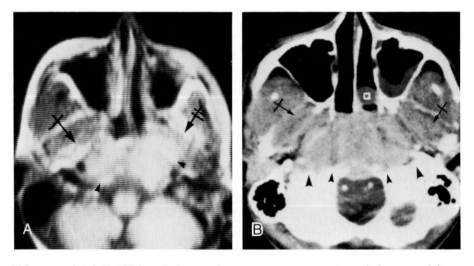

FIG. 11.6 (A) MR (SE/670/48) scan demonstrates interruption of the normal low-signal petrous bone by squamous carcinoma that has invaded the skull base (arrowheads). The right lateral pterygoid muscle remains surrounded by high-signal fibrofatty fascial planes and is free of tumor (slashed arrow). The left pterygoid muscle has been invaded by the mass (double-slashed arrow). (B) CT scan of the same patient a few weeks earlier shows the normal pterygoid muscles (slashed arrows) anteriorly and invasion of the skull base (arrowheads) posteriorly.

312

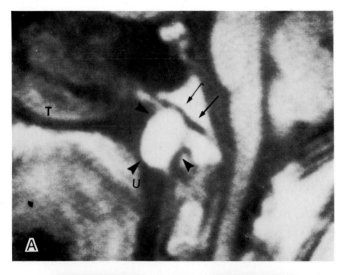

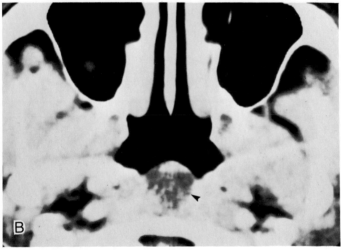

FIG. 11.7 (A) Sagittal MR (SE/1280/110) scan shows a region of high signal caused by fluid-filled mass (arrowheads) in the high nasopharynx. The turbinates (T), uvula (U), and adjacent cortical bone (arrows) are not involved. (B) CT scan of the same region shows a similar finding of a circumscribed area of low density that is characteristic of a Thornwaldt cyst (arrowhead).

A frequent route of spread of antral malignancies is posterior to the infratemporal fossa. The strong signal from the retroantral fat pad and well-demarcated fascial planes of the fossa allow excellent recognition of spread to these areas with MR. Spread to the orbit is also well seen on MR for similar reasons.

Fluid in obstructed sinuses or retention cysts has a characteristically long

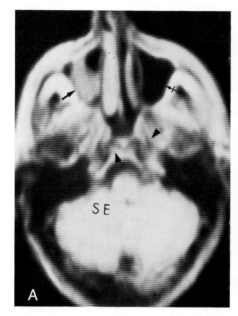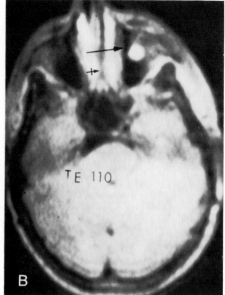

FIG. 11.8 (A) MR (SE/670/48) image shows combined air–bone interface of the normal maxillary sinuses (slashed arrow) seen as an area of low signal. Scan also shows the opposite sinus, with decreased aeration secondary to inflammatory changes, and demonstrates the cortical bone of the posterolateral wall of the antrum (arrow). The normal pharyngobasilar fascia (arrowheads) is also seen. (B) Late echo (SE/1280/110) image of a patient with a retention cyst (arrow) shows high signal from this structure as well as the normal turbinates (slashed arrow).

T_2 that allows easy differentiation from surrounding soft tissues (Figs. 11.8, 11.9). This condition may be recognized with CT scanning after contrast infusion as a region of low density material within the obstructed sinus.

Temporal Bone

The inability of NMR to detect a signal from dense bone is a virtue in the study of cerebellopontine angle masses. With CT scanning, the dense petrous bones attenuate the x-ray beam and result in a beam-hardening artifact that may obscure the posterior fossa and porus acousticus region. MR shows this area clearly (Fig. 11.10) and the MR appearance of a variety of masses found here has been described.[7] For the same reasons, MR shows the intracanalicular portions of the facial and auditory nerves with detail that is not possible with modern CT scanning. It appears that high-resolution thin-section MR will be the study of choice for evaluating possible intracanalicular tumors because it eliminates the need for lumbar puncture and limited air studies.

The middle ear and mastoids have the same close relationship of air and

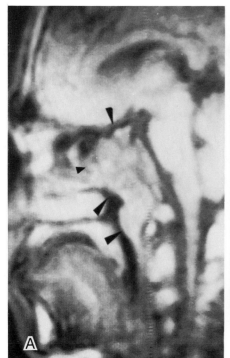
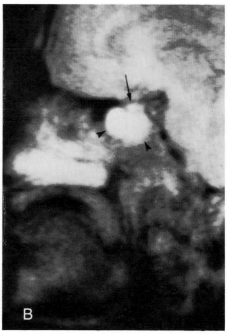

FIG. 11.9   (A) Midsagittal MR (SE/670/48) scan shows a mass of intermediate signal arising from the high nasopharynx and apparently filling the sphenoid sinus (arrowheads). (B) Late echo (SE/1280/110) image shows strong signal from what is actually a fluid-filled sphenoid sinus (arrowheads). The pituitary gland also shows strong signal (arrow).

cortical bone that hinders the effectiveness of MR imaging of the paranasal sinuses. The detection of bony ossicles in a well-aerated epitympanic recess is currently beyond the capabilities of MR scanning. Although soft tissue masses and postobstructive fluid (Fig. 11.11) are easily resolved with MR, it appears that CT scanning will probably continue to dominate the imaging of middle ear disease unless significant improvements are made with MR.

Orbit

The orbital contents are purely soft tissue structures ideally suited for MR imaging. The globes, extraocular muscles, and optic nerves are all well visualized on MR contrasted with the strong signal of the retrobulbar fat. Even the bony walls of the orbit are well demarcated because of the surrounding soft tissues

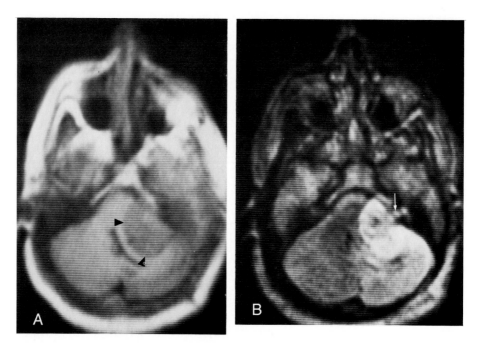

FIG. 11.10 (A) Axial MR (SE/670/48) scan in a patient with an acoustic neuroma shows a low-signal CP angle mass displacing the brainstem and cerebellum (B) The late echo (SE/1280/110) image at a slightly different level again shows the mass as well as a small intracanalicular component (arrow).

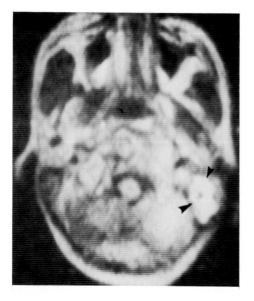

FIG. 11.11 MR (SE/1280/110) scan of a patient with serous otitis media secondary to eustachian tube obstruction shows an area of high signal from the fluid in the mastoid antrum (arrowheads).

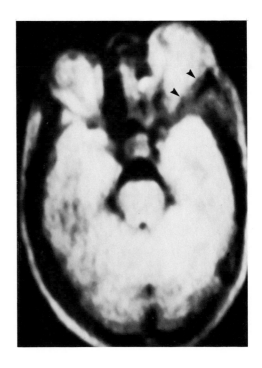

FIG. 11.12 MR (SE/670/48) scan of a patient with meningioma shows bony thickening of the lateral orbital wall (arrowheads) and proptosis.

(Fig. 11.12). However, it is likely that small calcifications or small dense foreign bodies may be better seen with CT scanning than with MR. Orbital tumors are well visualized with MR, with similar detail as in CT scanning.[8] Because reformatted images are so frequently needed in CT of the orbit, the coronal and sagittal plane of MR will be exceedingly useful.

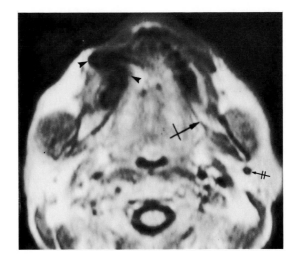

FIG. 11.13 MR (SE/670/48) scan at the level of the oropharynx shows linear region of low signal (slashed arrow) corresponding to Wharton's duct. Local artifacts are present from ferromagnetic dental hardware (arrowheads). The retromandibular vein (double-slashed arrow) is prominent on the left and easily distinguished from the surrounding parotid parenchyma.

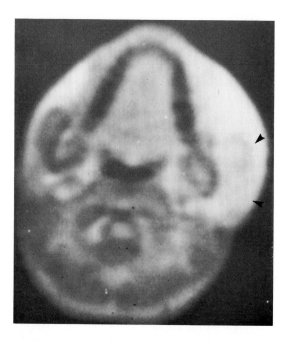

FIG. 11.14 Axial MR scan shows soft tissue swelling and overall increase in signal in the parotid bed (arrowhead) in this patient with a parotid abscess. (Scan courtesy of R. Nick Bryan, M.D., Baylor University, Houston, Texas)

High-resolution thin-section MR scanning of the orbit through the use of surface coils should prove useful because of the superficial location of these structures.

Salivary Glands

The salivary glands appear on MR as regions of intermediate signal strength contrasted to the surrounding high signal fat and lower signal muscle groups. Wharton's ducts are linear regions of low signal intensity coursing from the gland parenchyma to the oral cavity (Fig. 11.13). The retromandibular vein is represented by a region of low signal clearly distinguishable from surrounding gland, lymph nodes, or masses. Small calcifications or calculi within the gland or ducts may be better seen with CT scanning. Otherwise, similar information may be obtained from MR or CT at this stage of development of the technology (Fig. 11.14).

Oropharynx and Tongue

Superb anatomic detail may be obtained regarding the muscle boundaries and fascial planes of the tongue with MR. In a cooperative patient muscle boundaries of this organ are visualized by MR that are not seen with CT scanning. This is the result of a number of responsible factors. MR has inherently better soft tissue discrimination than CT. The use of direct sagittal and coronal scan

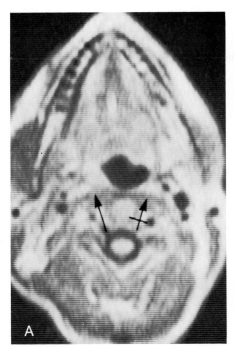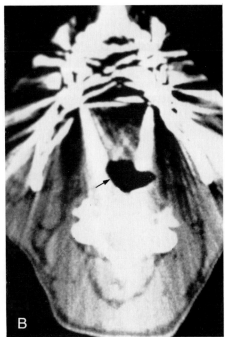

FIG. 11.15   (A) Scan (SE/670/48) of a patient with a carcinoma of the nasopharynx shows tumor indenting the airway (arrow). The opposite side in uninvolved (slashed arrow). The tongue musculature is well visualized in spite of the presence of dental amalgam. (B) CT scan of the same patient shows asymmetry of the airway (arrow), but the marked streak artifacts from the dental amalgam degrade the image.

planes with MR produces images of higher spatial resolution than the comparable CT reformatted image. Finally, the frequently present dental amalgam, which degrades CT images in this region, does not produce any artifact on MR (Fig. 11.15).

The extrinsic muscles of the tongue (genioglossus, hyoglossus, and styloglossus) are clearly visible on both CT and MR. The intrinsic musculature is not definable on CT; however, all four muscle bundles are visible with high-resolution MR. These are the superior longitudinal, inferior longitudinal, transverse, and vertical intrinsic muscle bundles. They are best demonstrated on the sagittal MR scan (Fig. 11.16).

The superior longitudinal intrinsic bundle runs from the tongue base to the tip of the tongue, just below the surface at the midline. A low intensity plane separates this structure from the deeper transverse musculature. The transverse group originates from the fibrous lingual septum 2 to 3 cm posterior to the tip and continues as a thin plate of muscle to the tongue base. The inferior longitudinal musculature lies adjacent to the genioglossus bundles and medial to the interdigitation of the styloglossus and hyoglossus muscles. The

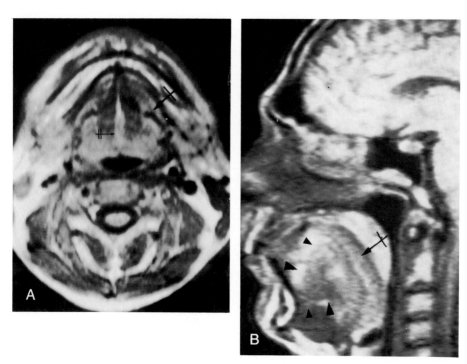

FIG. 11.16 (A) Axial (SE/670/48) image shows the normal lingual artery (slashed arrow) coursing deep in the interdigitation of the styloglossus and hyoglossus muscles. High signal is present in the midline fibrous lingual septum (double-slashed arrow) separating the genioglossus muscles. (B) Sagittal scan (SE/670/48) shows the fibers of the genioglossus muscle radiating outward from the genu of the mandible (arrowheads). The superior longitudinal bundles of the intrinsic musculature (slashed arrow) extend from the tongue base to its tip below the surface. Immediately inferior to this group are the transverse intrinsic bundles seen en face.

vertical intrinsic fibers arise from the surface of the tongue and radiate downward.

This detail is valuable in detecting early malignancies of the tongue manifested as a disruption of these fascial planes. Many of these masses show as regions of high signal on the late spin-echo images (Fig. 11.17). More experience is necessary to determine if this strong signal is from tumor alone or also from the affected surrounding tissues.

On the other hand, areas of muscle atrophy and fatty infiltration appear as regions of increased signal on the early spin-echo images (Fig. 11.18). Lymphoid tissue around the tongue base and oropharynx may show up on CT scanning as soft tissue, which is easily mistaken for tumor. Early experience with MR has shown that lymphoid tissue in these regions is manifested as

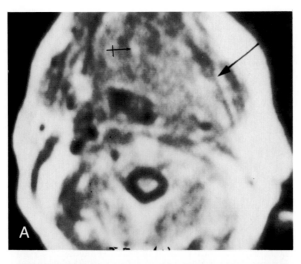

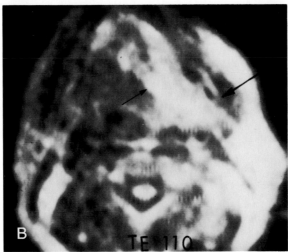

FIG. 11.17   (A) An MR (SE/670/48) scan of a patient with a carcinoma of the tongue base (arrow). The high signal fibrous lingual septum is intact (slashed arrow). (B) Late echo (SE/1280/110) image shows increased contrast definition in the region of the tumor (arrows).

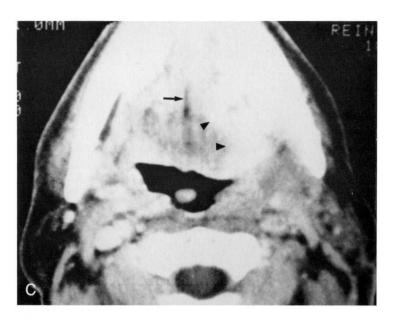

FIG. 11.17 (*Cont.*).   (C) CT scan demonstrates a mass of the left tongue (arrowheads). The midline septum is intact (arrow).

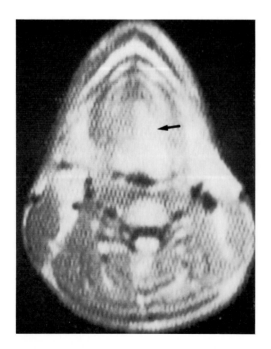

FIG. 11.18 Early spin-echo (SE/670/48) image shows increased signal from a region of fatty infiltration of the tongue (arrow) in patient with unilateral hypoglossal nerve damage.

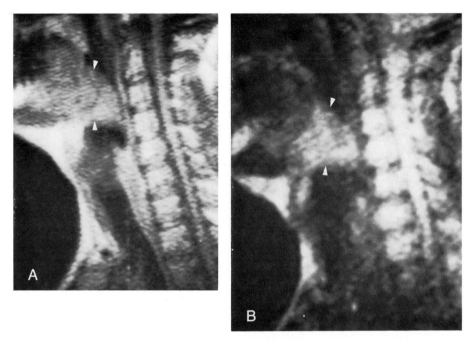

FIG. 11.19   (A) Sagittal (SE/670/48) scan in a patient with lymphoid hyperplasia shows a soft tissue mass at the tongue base and extending into the airway (arrowheads). (B) Late echo image (SE/1280/110) shows increased signal from the region of the lymphoid tissue (arrowheads) separate from the tongue base.

an area of high signal on late spin-echo images. (Fig. 11.19). Again, more experience is necessary to determine if this effect can be differentiated from the similar late spin echo signal enhancement of malignancies in the same region.

Larynx and Hypopharynx

Like the nasopharynx and orbit, the larynx and hypopharynx have ideal anatomy for MR imaging.[9] They are primarily made up of cartilage and soft tissue surrounding an air-filled lumen with very little cortical bone. The cartilage produces a strong signal, which should facilitate the detection of subtle tumor infiltrations and early cartilage destruction. The soft tissues are also well visualized. The loose areolar tissue of the pre-epiglottic space and paralaryngeal spaces also provides a strong MR signal that should be very sensitive to the effects of tumor invasion (Fig. 11.20).

Unfortunately, the usefulness of MR in the larynx and hypopharynx is limited by the currently available technology. Because of relatively long scan times, even moderate respiratory motion will degrade the image (Fig. 11.20A). The 8- to 10-mm thick sections that are currently available are inadequate

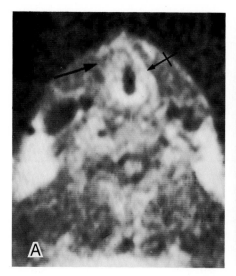 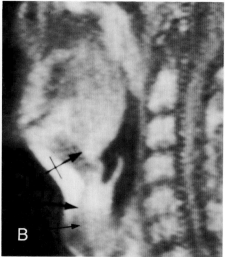

FIG. 11.20 (A) Axial (SE/670/48) scan of a patient with supraglottic carcinoma shows tumor involvement of the paralaryngeal space (arrow). The contralateral side is intact (slashed arrow). Considerable motion artifact is present, manifested by the image degradation and "ghosting" anteriorly. (B) Sagittal (SE/670/48) scan shows the normal geniohyoid muscle (slashed arrow). The strong signal of the pre-epiglottic space is interrupted by the tumor invasion (arrow).

to provide the degree of image resolution free from volume averaging that is necessary for meaningful information about deep spread of malignant tumors.

At the present time the use of dedicated neck coils and surface coils to study the larynx and hypopharynx is being investigated. These produce much better signal-to-noise performance, which allows the acquisition of higher resolution images, thinner sections, and faster scan times. The possibility of respiratory gating is also being considered to overcome some of these problems.

Neck, Thyroid, and Parathyroid

MR imaging of the neck, thyroid, and parathyroid suffers from similar drawbacks as MR of the larynx; however, it does offer advantages over CT scanning in certain situations.

The low neck is well visualized on MR without the problem of the beam-hardening artifact that is present with CT because of the location of the shoulders (Fig. 11.21). The major arteries and veins of the neck are all clearly visible on MR without the use of intravenous contrast materials (Fig. 11.22). The fascial planes of the neck are surrounded by loose areolar tissue, which produces a strong MR signal sensitive to tumor invasion. Lymph nodes are easily differentiated from flowing blood vessels on MR.

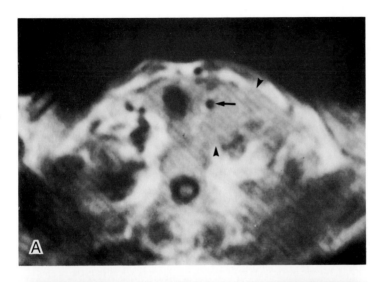

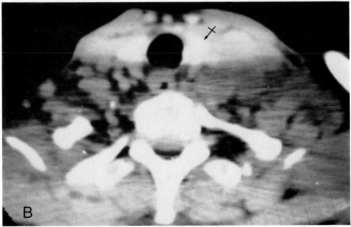

FIG. 11.21 (A) MR (SE/670/48) image in a patient with lymphoma shows adenopathy (arrowheads) separated from the thyroid gland by the carotid artery (arrow) and surrounded by high signal fat. (B) CT scan is degraded by the beam-hardening artifact from the shoulders. The adenopathy is clearly differentiated from the enhancing thyroid tissue (slashed arrow); however, the vascular structures and muscle groups are not as clearly seen as with MR.

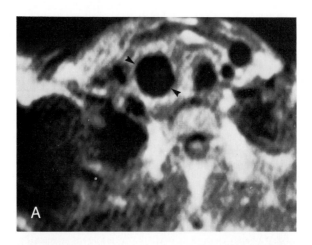

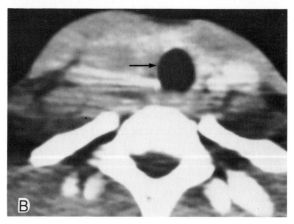

FIG. 11.22   (A) MR (SE/670/48) scan shows aneurysmal dilatation of the innominate artery (arrowhead)
with displacement of the trachea and surrounding
structures. (B) CT scan with contrast enhancement
shows the tracheal displacement (arrow) and contralateral enhancement of the normal jugular vein and
carotid artery. The true vascular nature of the mass
is not apparent from this study.

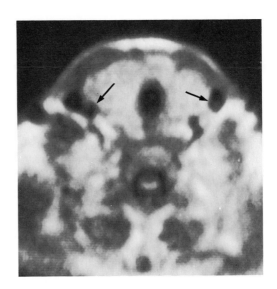

FIG. 11.23 Axial (SE/670/48) shows posterolateral displacement of the normal carotid arteries and jugular veins (arrows) in patient with a goiter.

More experience is necessary with MR imaging of pathology of the thyroid and parathyroid glands (Fig. 11.23). Colloid cysts can be differentiated from surrounding tissue because of the long T_2 of the fluid.

Finally, the ease of obtaining direct axial, coronal, and sagittal images allows more accurate determination of tumor volume for precision radiation therapy in this and other regions of the head and neck.

REFERENCES

1. Mancuso A, Hanafee W: CT of the Head and Neck. Williams & Wilkins, Baltimore, 1982.
2. Young IR, Burl M, Clarke GJ, et al.: Magnetic resonance properties of hydrogen. AJR 137:895–901, 1981.
3. Crooks LE, Mills CM, Davis PL, et al.: Visualization of cerebral and vascular abnormalities by NMR imaging. The effects of imaging parameters on contrast. Radiology 144:843–852, 1982.
4. Lufkin R, Ward P, Yang W, et al.: NMR imaging in malignancies of the upper aerodigestive tract. Radiology (RSNA abs) 149(P):68, 1983.
5. Dillon WP, Mills CM, Brant-Zawadzki M, et al.: NMR imaging of head and neck pathology. Radiology (RSNA abs) 149(P):68, 1983.
6. Mancuso A, Bohman L, Hanafee W, Maxwell D: CT of the nasopharynx: normal and variants of normal. Radiology 137:113–123, 1980.
7. Young IR, Budder GM, Hall AS, et al.: The role of NMR imaging in the diagnosis and management of acoustic neuroma. AJNR 4:223–224, 1983.
8. Hawkes RC, Holland GN, Moore WS, et al.: NMR imaging in the evaluation of orbital tumors. AJNR 4:254–256, 1983.
9. Lufkin R, Larsson S, Hanafee W: NMR anatomy of the larynx and tongue base. Radiology 148:173–175, 1983.

CASE NO. 1 — Charles J. Schatz

Evaluation of a Young Man for Possible Acoustic Neuroma

This 19-year-old man initially complained to his family physician of light-headedness and transient "blackouts" increasing in frequency for about 2 years. Other than a history of multiple allergies, he had no other history of illness. The physical examination was negative. The patient was then sent to an otologist for further evaluation.

The results of the otologist's examination and audiogram were within normal limits. But electronystagmography for vestibular function revealed definite diminution of peripheral responses on the left side. Plain films of the temporal bones were performed, which revealed very large internal auditory canals measuring 13 mm in vertical diameter. Because of the history, suspicious electronystagmography, and the very large internal auditory canals, the otologist proceeded to evaluate the patient for an acoustic neuroma.

A CT scan with additional sections of the posterior fossa was performed. Intravenous contrast material was used. The CT scan confirmed the presence of large (13 mm) symmetrical internal auditory canals (Fig. 1) but a cerebellopontine angle neoplasm was not present. Therefore, gas cisternography of the cerebellopontine angles was done to evaluate the possibility of a intracanalicular acoustic neuroma (Fig. 2A,B). The gas (oxygen) was introduced into the spinal subarachnoid space via a lumbar puncture.

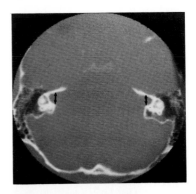

FIGURE 1   Axial CT scan at bone window settings. Large internal auditory canals demonstrated (double arrowheads).

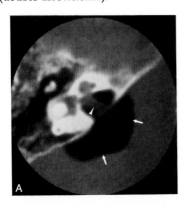
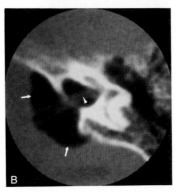

FIGURE 2   (A) Left side. (B) Right side. Gas cisternogram showing gas (oxygen) in cerebellar pontine angles (arrows) with the neurovascular bundle (arrowheads) in the gas-filled internal auditory canals.

DISCUSSION

The technique of gas cisternography has been described many times since 1979.[1-4] This examination is used in the evaluation of small acoustic neuromas after a negative contrast-enhanced CT scan. It can also be used after a negative nonenhanced scan in a person allergic to iodinated contrast material. In the report of Solti-Bohman et al.,[4] 214 gas cisternograms were reviewed. The presence or absence of a tumor was clearly shown in 98 percent of the cases. Only 2 percent had equivocal findings that required Pantopaque studies of the internal auditory canals or further clinical follow-up.

In our patient, the internal auditory canals were unusually large, but symmetrical. However, small tumors can be found with almost identical frequency in symmetrical as in asymmetrical canals.[4] Also, the neurovascular bundle was visualized bilaterally without any particular "bulge." Therefore, this examination must be considered negative. Presumably an "early" acoustic neuroma that has not enlarged the nerve could be present. But with the present CT technology the diagnosis of such an acoustic neuroma cannot be made on the initial study. It can, however, be diagnosed preoperatively with a follow-up gas cisternogram that does show a "bulge" of the neurovascular bundle.

REFERENCES   1. Sortland O: Computed tomography combined with gas cisternography for the diagnosis of expanding lesions of the cerebellopontine angle. Neuroradiology 18:19–22, 1979.

2. Kricheff II, Pinto RS, Bergeron RT, Cohen N: Air-CT cisternography and canalography for small acoustic neuromas. AJNR 1:57–63, 1980.

3. Pinto RS, Kricheff II, Bergeron RT, Cohen N: Small acoustic neuromas: detection by high resolution gas CT cisternography. AJNR 3:283–286, 1982.

4. Solti-Bohman LG, Magaram DL, Lo WWM et al: Gas-CT cisternography for detection of small acoustic nerve tumors. Radiology 150:403–407, 1984.

CASE NO. 2   Charles J. Schatz

Elderly Male with Decreasing Vision of the Left Eye

This 84-year-old man presented to an ophthalmologist in 1981 with a history of recurrent swelling of the left lower eyelid. The clinical examination at that time revealed that the vision in the left eye was not correctable to better than 20/40. No proptosis was noted at that time. On a return visit 5 months later, the vision was not correctable to better than 20/100 in the left eye. Also, on the left side, there was some "paresis" of the medial rectus muscle, a suggestion of mild proptosis, and the lower lid was edematous.

A contrast-enhanced orbital CT examination was then performed in the axial plane. The patient could not assume positioning for a coronal scan. Some orbital plain films were then obtained. The studies demonstrate marked hyperostosis about the left orbit (Figs. 1,2) involving the sphenoidal wings, orbital roof, posterior ethmoid sinus cells and sphenoid sinus. The hyperostosis extends across the mid-line into the right sphenoid sinus (Fig. 2). A large intracranial soft-tissue component was not demonstrated; but a small enhanced mass was found along the anterior aspect of the middle fossa on the left side (Fig. 3).

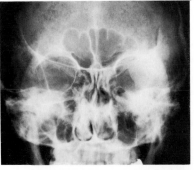

FIGURE 1   Plain film of the orbits, PA view, demonstrating hyperostosis about the left orbit.

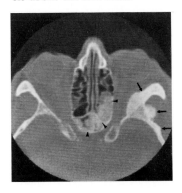

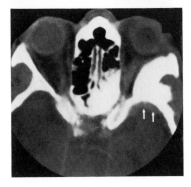

FIGURE 2   Axial CT scan through the orbits with bone window settings. Hyperostosis of the left sphenoid (arrows) and left posterior ethmoid and both sides of the sphenoid sinuses (arrowheads).

FIGURE 3   Contrast enhanced axial CT scan through the orbits. Enhancing soft tissue mass representing the en plaque meningioma is demonstrated at the anterior limit of the middle cranial fossa (arrows).

DISCUSSION

New,[1] in a National Cancer Institute study, found 37 of 164 intracranial meningiomas to be in the sphenoidal-parasellar site. In a meningioma involving the bony orbit, exophthalmos, rather than visual disturbance, is a predominant symptom.[2] Our patient, however, had decreased visual acuity before the exophthalmos was noted by his ophthalmologist. The majority of meningiomas are diagnosed in the 6th and 7th decades of life[1] and there is a 2.4 to 1 ratio of female to male patients.[1]

With nonenhanced and enhanced CT scanning, the diagnosis of "certain or probable meningioma" can be made in 90.5 percent of meningiomas.[1] En plaque meningiomas are differentiated from globular meningiomas by the size and type of intracranial tumor presentations. The globular type has an intracranial tumor mass that is large, frequently broad-based, and has little hyperostosis. The en plaque meningiomas are "carpet-like"[3] and small with subdural spread paralleling the plane of the dura with a disproportionately large degree of hyperostosis. It is this bony change that causes the clinical symptoms. The exact mechanism of the hyperostosis has not been established and a discussion of the various theories is beyond the scope of this case presentation.

In the differential diagnosis of sclerotic lesions of the skull, one must consider fibrous dysplasia, blastic metastases, osteomas, and meningiomas. The former three lesions have no intracranial soft-tissue component adjacent to the hyperostosis. Finding the soft-tissue mass in en plaque meningiomas may be impossible but it has become easier with CT scanning than with older modalities. Seeing this intracranial portion of the lesion is essential in making the preoperative diagnosis of meningioma. However, an additional sign has been described in some en plaque meningiomas by Kim et al.[4] called "the dural lucent line." This is a thin lucent line seen on high-resolution CT scanning or thin section tomography separating the hyperostotic calvarium from an ossified subdural plaque containing meningioma cells. This line may be characteristic of en plaque meningiomas but its absence does not exclude this diagnosis.

The patient had a biopsy of the lesion. The pathological report was "benign meningioma." Because of the patient's age, complete surgical removal was not done; however, because of the change in vision and exophthalmus that occurred in 5 months, radiation therapy was performed.[5] A follow-up CT scan performed 18 months postradiation therapy revealed no change in the size of the meningioma or hyperostosis. The patient remains clinically stable 24 months following therapy.

REFERENCES   1. New PFJ, Aronow S, Hesselink, JR: National Cancer Institute study: Evaluation of computed tomography in the diagnosis of intracranial neoplasms IV. Meningiomas. Radiology 136:665–675, 1980.

2. Pompili A, Caroli F, Cattoni F, Iachetti, M: Intradiploic meningioma of the orbital roof. Neurosurgery 12:565–568, 1983.

3. Rosenbaum AE, Rosenbloom SB: Meningiomas revisited. Seminars in Roentgenology. 19:8–26, 1984.

4. Kim KS, Rogers LF, Lee C: The dural lucent line: characteristic sign of hyperostosing meningioma en plaque. AJNR 4:1101–1105, 1983.

5. Carella, RJ, Ransohoff J, Newall J: Role of radiation therapy in the management of meningioma. Neurosurgery 10:332–339, 1982.

CASE NO. 3   Charles J. Schatz

Elderly Male with Progressive Hearing Loss

This 70-year-old man presented with a progressive hearing loss in the left ear for about 10 years. There had been left-sided tinnitus for a few years, but the patient denied vertigo. The physical examination revealed a decreased corneal reflex on the left. There was no papilledema. The audiogram revealed a bilateral sensorineural hearing loss, which was more severe on the left than on the right with very poor discrimination on the left consistent with a retrocochlear lesion. The patient was sent for a CT scan of the brain. A preliminary nonenhanced scan was followed by a contrast-enhanced scan. The scan showed enlarged lateral ventricles consistent with hydrocephalus (Fig. 1). The nonenhanced scan demonstrated an area of increased attentuation adjacent to the left petrous bone associated with amorphous calcifications along the medial edge of this area (Fig. 2). The enhanced scan demonstrated uniform enhancement of a mass at this same site (Fig. 3A,B). The mass had a broad base of attachment to the petrous ridge and tentorium and covered the medial end of the left internal auditory canal (Fig. 3A). A pre-operative diagnosis of a large "globular type" cerebellopontine angle meningioma was made.

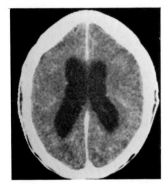

FIGURE 1   Enlarged lateral ventricles with no sulci visualized consistent with hydrocephalus.

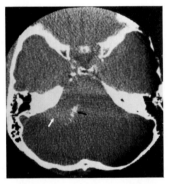

FIGURE 2   Non-enhanced axial CT scan through the posterior fossa demonstrating an area of increased attenuation (white arrow) and psammomatous calcification (black arrow).

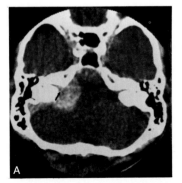

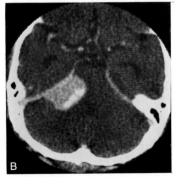

FIGURE 3   (A,B) Enhanced axial CT scan through the posterior fossa demonstrating a homogeneously enhancing, large tumor with a broad attachment to the temporal bone and tentorium. The tumor covers the medial end of the internal auditory canal (arrow).

DISCUSSION

New[1] reported in the National Cancer Institute study that 25 out of 164 intracranial meningiomas were in an infratentorial site. None of these cases demonstrated hyperostosis on plain films or CT but 53 percent had psammomatous calcification. On nonenhanced CT scans, there is some degree of increased density in 91 percent of posterior fossa meningiomas, whereas 9 percent are isodense.[2] Also, 3 percent may show bone erosion.[3] The diagnosis of a posterior fossa meningioma is made by the extra-axial location of the mass suggested by well-demarcated edges, a higher attentuation number than adjacent brain, psammomatous calcifications, and homogeneous enhancement and little or no cerebral edema.[3] Cerebellopontine angle meningiomas generally extend considerably beyond the limits of the internal auditory canal along the posterior aspect of the petrous bone[1,2] giving these tumors a broad base of attachment.

Once the extra-axial origin of the tumor is determined, the main differential diagnostic considerations are an acoustic neuroma or meningoma. An acoustic neuroma is usually excluded because these tumors generally are isodense on nonenhanced scans, enhanced nonuniformly, do not have a broad base of attachment to the petrous bone, lack calcification, and generally do not extend beyond the limits of the internal auditory canal along the posterior aspect of the petrous bone.

Preoperatively, our patient had few symptoms despite the presence of a large tumor. Hirsh[4] described four patients with "giant" meningiomas of the posterior fossa who also had few symptoms or signs of a large tumor. Hirsh feels that the characteristic slow growth of meningiomas allows time for the central nervous system to adjust to a slowly increasing tumor mass. In addition, since only one-third of infratentortial meningiomas have edema,[1] there is usually no additional mass effect secondary to edema. A nonspecific CT sign of meningioma is evidence that the brain accommodates to the presence of a longstanding mass since there is less mass effect than anticipated for the size of the tumor.[5]

A surgical removal of the tumor was made. The pathological report was meningioma. The patient had a stormy postoperative course and died approximately 6 weeks later.

ACKNOWLEDGMENTS

The author wishes to thank Alice Brewer for secretarial assistance and photographer Stephen Y. Shapiro for his expertise in preparing the preceding case presentations.

REFERENCES   1. New PFJ, Aronow S, Hesselink, JR: National Cancer Institute study: Evaluation of computed tomography in the diagnosis of intracranial neoplasms-IV. meningiomas. Radiology 136:665–675, 1980.

2. Thomson JLG: Computerized axial tomography in posterior fossa lesions. Clin Radiol 29:233–250, 1978.

3. Pullicino P, Kendall BE, Jakubowski J: Difficulties in diagnosis of intracranial meningiomas by computed tomography. J Neurol Neurosurg Psych 43:1022–1029, 1980.

4. Hirsh LF, Mancall EL: Giant meningiomas of the posterior fossa. JAMA 240:1626–1627, 1978.

5. Rosenbaum AE, Rosenbloom SB: Meningiomas revisited. Semin Roentgenol 19:8–26, 1984.

Index

Page numbers followed by f represent figures; page numbers followed by t represent tables.

Aberrant thyroid tissue, 43, 44f
Abscess
  vs. cellulitis in children, 261
  cerebellar, in mastoiditis, 188f
  lingual, 94–95
  orbital subperiosteal, 154f, 154
  of salivary glands, 231, 233, 234f
Acinetobacter anitratum, involvement in meningitis, 262f–263f
Acoustic neuroma, 196–199, 197f, 198f, 199f, 200f
  case study of, 329–330, 329f
Adenocystic carcinoma, 76, 77f, 81f, 123, 124f, 287f
  of lacrimal gland, 146, 146f
  and salivary gland mass, 228–229, 228f
Adenoma
  parathyroid, *see* Parathyroid adenoma
  pleomorphic, *see* Pleomorphic adenoma
Air-fluid levels, in nasal cavity, causes of, 116
Allergic disease, of nasal cavity, 114–121
Ameloblastoma, 124
Aneurysm, of the ophthalmic artery, 139–140, 141f
Angiofibroma, 125, 126f
Angiography, for parapharyngeal space lesions, 74
Ann Arbor Clinical Staging Classification, for lymphoma, 244
Anterior triangle of the neck, 33
Antrochoanal polyps, 70, 71f, 118, 118f
Apert's syndrome, in children, 270
Arteriovenous (AV) malformation, of the orbit, 151
Aryepiglottic fold, 5f, 9, 9f
Aryepiglottic fold carcinoma, 19, 20f
  without palpable neck masses, 23f
Arytenoid cartilages, 6, 7f, 8f
Atresia, of right external auditory canal, 180f, 181f
Attico-antral disease, 186, 188f, 189f

Bacterial inflammatory disease, of the orbit, 153, 153f, 154f, 154

Bacterial sinusitis, 114, 115f
  air-fluid levels in, 116
Basal cell nevus syndrome, 270, 271f
Bone erosion, 125
Bone remodeling, malignancies of nasal cavity and, 124
Bony orbit, anatomy of, 135
Branchial cleft cyst, 222–223, 224f
  in children, 274
Buccal cavity, tumors of
  pattern of spread of, 287–288
  staging for, 281t
Buphthalmos, 142

Calculi, in salivary glands, 231, 232f
Capillary hemangioma, 221–222, 223f
Carcinoma
  adenocystic, 76, 77f, 123, 124f, 287f
  of aryepiglottic folds, *see* Aryepiglottic fold carcinoma
  epiglottic, *see* Epiglottic carcinoma
  glottic, 292
  of the hypopharynx, 73, 74f
  metastatic, of lungs to mandible, 77–78, 78f
  nasopharyngeal, 65–67, 65f, 66f, 67f, 68f
    in children, 245, 246f, 247f
  oat cell, metastatic to orbit, 143, 144f
  of piriform sinus, 20, 21f
  and radiotherapy planning, *see* Radiotherapy planning
  of right ear, 201
  squamous cell, *see* Squamous cell carcinoma
  supraglottic, 292
  of the thyroid, 51f
  of tongue base, 95, 96t, 96f, 97, 97f, 99
  transglottic, 20, 22f–23f
  of true vocal cords, 14–15, 15f, 16f, 17, 17f
Carotid-cavernous sinus fistula (CCF), 151, 152f, 153
Carotid sheath structures, 39f, 40
  migration following thyroidectomy, 50, 50f
Carotid triangle, of the neck, 33
Cartilage
  arytenoid, 6, 7f, 8f
  epiglottic, calcification of, 6f

Cartilage—*Cont.*
  cricoid, *see* Cricoid cartilage
  thyroid, *see* Thyroid cartilage
  and trauma to the larynx, 25, 27f, 27
Cellulitis
  postseptal, 261
  preseptal, *see* Preseptal cellulitis
Cerebellar abscess, in mastoiditis, 188f
Cerebellopontine pneumocisternogram
  for acoustic neuroma, 199f, 200f
  normal, 199f
Chemodectoma, 73
Choanal atresia, in children, 269–270, 269f
Cholesteatoma
  density of, 176
  of middle ear and mastoid, 187, 189f, 190–
    191, 190f, 191f, 192f
Chondrosarcoma, 78, 79f
Chordoma, 78–79
Choroidal osteoma, of the eye, 162–163, 163f
Chronic laryngeal stenosis, 29f, 29
Cocaine abuse, 120
Cochlear otosclerosis, 203f, 203–204, 205f
Computed tomography
  for head and neck trauma in children, 256,
    257f, 258, 259f, 260f
  of laryngeal anatomy, 1–2
  and MR, compared, 303–304
  for nasopharynx, infratemporal fossa, and
    skull base, 64
  for neck, 40–41
  for orbit, 131–133
  for paranasal sinuses, 102, 103f
    contrast in, 104
    coronal scan in, 102, 103f
    window settings in, 104
  in pediatric use, 237–238
  and pneumocisternography, for acoustic neu-
    roma, 196–199
  for salivary glands, 208–209, 209f
  of temporal bone
    dosimetric analysis in, 174–175
    enhancement study in, 177
    prerequisite for, 171–173, 172f, 173f, 174f
    projections used, 179t
  for tongue base, 85–86
Computed tomography sialography
  of the parotid, 71, 72f
  of the salivary glands, 216–217
Congenital lesions, in children, 266–267, 268f,
    269, 269f, 270, 271f, 272f–273f, 273–276
Coronal scans, of paranasal sinuses, 102, 103f
Craniofacial malformations, in children, 267
Craniometaphyseal dysplasia, in children, 272f–
    273f, 273
Craniosynostosis, in children, 270
Cricoid cartilage, 6, 8f, 9, 38f, 38
  fracture of, 27, 28f
Crista galli, 108, 109f
Cylindroma, 123, 124f

Cyst
  dermoid, in children, 256
  epidermoid, of petrous bone, 191, 192f
  epidermoid-dermoid, of the orbit, 147, 148f
  mucus retention, 116–118, 117f
Cystic hygroma, in children, 274

Dermoid cysts, in children, 256
Distant metastases, classification of, 282t

Ectopic thyroid tissue, adenoma in, 45–46, 46f
Embryonal rhabdomyosarcoma, 123–124
Encephalocele, 70
Enhancement, in CT of temporal bone, 177
Epidermoid cyst, of petrous bone, 191, 192f
Epidermoid-dermoid cysts, of the orbit, 147,
    148f
Epiglottic carcinoma, 18f, 19, 19f
  with lymph node metastases, 24f
Epiglottis, 2, 4f–5f
  calcification of, 6f
Esthesioneuroblastoma, 123
Eustachian tube, and nasopharyngeal carci-
    noma, 66f, 66–67
Extraocular muscles, anatomy of, 135
Eye, lesions of, 159–163, 160f, 161f, 162f, 163f,
    164f

Facial nerve, anomalies of, 180, 182
Facial paralysis, 183–184
False vocal cords, 7f, 10–11, 10f
Fascial planes, 63–64, 63f
  infection of, 80
Fenestral otosclerosis, 202–203, 202f
Fibrous dysplasia, 120f, 121
  in children, 250, 252, 253f
Fonar Corporation, 309
Foramen cecum, 42
Foreign bodies, in soft tissue, 258, 260f
Fracture
  pediatric evaluation of, 257f, 258
  of temporal bone, 183–184, 184f, 185f
Frontal sinus, 104–106, 105f, 106f

Gas cisternography, in case study of acoustic
    neuroma, 329–330, 329f
Giant cell lesions, in children, 252
Glioma, of the optic nerve, 138, 140f, 158–159
Globe, metastatic disease of, 142–143, 143f
Glomus complex tumors
  jugulare, 73, 193, 193f, 194f, 194, 195f–196f,
    196
  in children, 250, 251f
  tympanicum, 192f, 193
Glottic carcinoma, 292
Glottic tumors, 14–19
Goiter
  intrathoracic, *see* Intrathoracic goiter
  multinodular, 46f, 47, 47f
  substernal, 48, 49f, 50f

Gorham's disease, in children, 252, 254f, 254
Granulation tissue, density of, 176
Granulomatous disease, of the nasal cavity, 118–
    120, 119f
  inflammatory, 120–121, 120f
Grave's disease, 154–155, 155f
Grisel's syndrome, 259f

Hearing loss, progressive, case study of, 333–
    334, 333f
Hemangioma
  in children, 275
  of the orbit, 150
Hemangiopericytoma
  in children, 256
  of the orbit, 151
Hematogenous metastatic disease
  of the mandible, 77–78, 78f
  of skull base, 79
Hemimandibulectomy, 81–82, 82f
Hemophilus influenzae meningitis, 262f, 263f
Histiocytic lymphoma, of left maxillary sinus,
    286f
Histiocytosis X, in children, 249–250
Hodgkin's lymphoma, in children, 244
Hyoid bone, 2, 4f–5f
  CT anatomy of, 34, 35f
Hyperostosis, case study of, 331–332, 331f
Hypopharynx
  carcinoma of, 73, 74f
  MR imaging of, 323–324, 324f
  tumor staging for, 282t
Hypoplasia, of maxillary antrum, in children,
    276
Hypothyroidism, 41, 42f

Infection, of nasal cavity, 114–121
Inferior-orbito-meatal (IOM) scans, of parana-
    sal sinuses, 102, 103f
Inflammatory lesions, in children, 260–261,
    262f, 263f, 264, 264f, 265f, 265, 266f
Inflammatory lesions
Infratemporal fossa
  anatomy of, 62, 63f
  pathology of, 74–78, 75f, 76f, 77f, 78f
Inner ear, anomalies of, 180, 182f
Intergroup Rhabdomyosarcoma Study and stag-
    ing groups, 239
Intrathoracic goiter, 48, 48f
  CT findings in, 48–49
Inverting papilloma, 122–123, 123f

Juvenile angiofibroma, 69–70, 70f

Lacrimal gland, 145
  adenocystic carcinoma of, 146, 146f
  anatomy of, 136
  benign mixed tumors of, 145
  epithelial tumors of, 145
  inflammatory lesions and, 146–147
  pleomorphic adenoma of, 145–146, 145f
Laryngeal airway, 11–12

Laryngeal anatomy
  CT technique in, 1–2
  normal, 2–12
  vascular, 12f, 12, 13f
Laryngeal skeleton, 2, 3f, 4–6, 4f, 5f, 6f, 7f, 8f
Laryngeal soft tissues, 9–11, 9f, 10f, 11f
Laryngeal stenosis, chronic, 29f, 29
Laryngeal ventricle, saccule of, 11f, 11
Laryngocele, CT findings in, 24, 25f, 26f
Laryngopharynx, pattern of tumor spread in,
    291–293, 293f
Laryngoscopy, 12
  and false laryngeal mass, 28, 29f
Larynx
  airway of, 11–12
  anatomy of, *see* Laryngeal anatomy
  benign masses of, 24, 25f, 26f
  deep soft tissue spaces of, 5f, 9f, 11
  MR imaging of, 323–324, 324f
  neoplasms of, 12–24
  postoperative, 20
  skeleton, 2, 3f, 4–6, 4f, 5f, 6f, 7f, 8f
  soft tissues of, 9–11, 9f, 10f, 11f
  trauma to, 25, 27f, 27–28, 28f, 29f
  tumor staging for, 282t
Lingual abscess, 94–95
Lingual thyroid gland, 93, 93f
Lingual thyroid tissue, 43–44, 45f
Lingual tonsil, 91f, 91
Lipoma, in children, 250
Lymphangioma, of the orbit, 150
Lymph nodes
  enlarged, 20, 23f, 24f
  infection of in children, 265, 266f
  involvement in nasopharynx, 67, 68f
  involvement in salivary gland tumors, 227
Lymphocytic lymphoma, 149f
Lymphoma
  in children, 244–245, 244f
  lymphocytic, 149f
  and salivary gland involvement, 229–230

Macroglossia, 93–94, 94f
Magnetic resonance, 304–306
  calcium and air signals in, 307–308
  and CT, compared, 303–304
  ferromagnetic distortions in, 307
  image formation time in, 308
  image section thickness in, 308–309
  increased soft tissue sensitivity in, 306
  of larynx and hypopharynx, 323–324, 324f
  of nasopharynx, 309, 310f, 311f, 311, 312f–
    313f
  of neck, thyroid and parathyroid, 324, 325f–
    327f, 327
  of orbit, 315, 317f, 317–318
  of oropharynx and tongue, 318–320, 319f,
    320f, 321f–323f, 323
  of paranasal sinuses, 311, 313–314, 314f, 315f
  of salivary glands, 317f, 318f, 318
  scanning in any plane in, 307

Magnetic resonance—*Cont.*
  spin-echo pulse sequence in, 305, 306f
  of temporal bone, 314–315, 316f
  visualization of flowing blood in, 306–307
Malignant melanoma, of the eye, 161, 161f
Malleus, dislocation of, 183
Mandible, metastatic carcinoma to, 77–78, 78f
Mandibulofacial dysostosis, 267
Mastoid, cholesteatomas of, 187, 189f, 190–191,
    190f, 191f, 192f
Maxillary antrum, hypoplasia of, in children,
    276
Maxillary sinus, 110–111, 110f
  histiocytic lymphoma of, 286f
  odontogenic malignancies in, 124
  postoperative, 126f, 127f, 127, 128f
  and pterygopalatine fossa, 111f, 111–112
  tumor staging for, 281t
Maxillectomy, CT evaluation following, 126–
    127, 126f, 127f, 128f
Melanoma, malignant, of the eye, 161, 161f
Meningioma, 73
  case study of, 331–332, 331f
  cerebellopontine angle, case study of, 333–
    334, 333f
  involving infratemporal fossa, 75–76, 76f
  of the orbit, *see* Orbital meningioma
Meningitis, in children, 262f–263f, 264, 264f
Meningoencephalocele, in children, 267, 268f,
    269
Metastatic disease
  in children, 245, 248f
  of eye and orbit, 142–143, 143f, 144f
  from salivary gland tumors, 228
Metastatic hypernephroma, 125
Metastatic papillary carcinoma, of the thyroid,
    51f
Metastasis
  distant, classification of, 282t
  to paranasal sinuses, 124–125
  and salivary gland tumors, 230–231, 230f
Middle ear, cholesteatomas of, 187, 189f, 190–
    191, 190f, 191f, 192f
Mondini anomaly, of inner ear, 180, 182f
Mucocele, 118, 119f
Mucormycosis, 119f
Mucus retention cyst, 116–118, 117f
Multinodular goiter, 46f, 47, 47f
Multiplanar diagnostic imaging center (MPDI),
    173
  and reformatted images of temporal bone,
    177f, 178f
Muscle
  extraocular, anatomy of, 135
  mylohyoid, 31, 32f
  omohyoid, 37, 37f
  pterygoid, 81–82, 82f
  sternocleidomastoid, 36, 37f
Muscle triangle, of the neck, 33
Mylohyoid muscle, 31, 32f
  CT anatomy of, 34, 35f

Nasal polyposis, and allergic disease, 116, 116f
Nasopharyngeal angiofibroma, in children, 246,
    249f, 249
Nasopharyngeal carcinoma, in children, 245,
    246f, 247f
Nasopharynx
  anatomy of, 59–60, 60f, 61f, 62, 63f
  benign lesions of, 69–70, 70f
  and lymph node involvement, 67, 68f
  MR imaging of, 309, 310f, 311f, 311, 312f–
    313f
  other malignancies of, 69
  secondary involvement of, 69, 69f
  squamous cell carcinoma of, 65–67, 65f, 66f,
    67f, 68f
  tumors of
    spread pattern of, 283–284, 283f, 284f
    staging for, 281t
Neck
  CT technique for, 40–41
  gross anatomy of, 31–34
  MR imaging of, 324, 325f–327f, 327
  normal anatomy of, 34–40
Neuroblastoma, in children, 245, 248f
Neurofibromatosis, 98f, 99
  in children, 255
  of orbital-facial region, 140–142, 142f
Neuroma, in poststyloid parapharyngeal space,
    73, 73f
Nodes, classification of, 282t
Nuclear magnetic resonance (NMR), and orbit
    evaluation, 131–132

Oat cell carcinoma, metastatic to orbit, 143, 144f
Ocular coloboma, in children, 273–274
Odontogenic malignancies, in maxillary sinus,
    124
Omohyoid muscle, 37, 37f
Ophthalmic artery, aneurysms of, 139–140, 141f
Optic nerve
  anatomy of, 135–136
  optic neuritis/papilledema of, 159
Optic nerve drusen, 162, 162f
Optic nerve glioma, 138, 140f, 158–159
Optic nerve sheath meningioma, 138, 139f
Optic neuritis, of the optic nerve, 159
Orbit
  anatomy of, 133, 133f, 134f, 135–136
  in children
    inflammatory lesions of, 260–261
    tumors of, 254–256
  CT evaluation of, coronal sections and, 164–
    165
  CT technique for, 131–133
  embryonal rhabdomyosarcoma of, 147
  epidermal-dermoid cysts of, 147, 148f
  infection of, and its cerebral complications,
    153–158
  intracranial lesions extending into, 137–142
  lymphoid tumors of, 147–148, 149f, 150
  metastatic disease of, 142–143, 143f, 144f

Orbit—*Cont.*
MR imaging of, 315, 317f, 317–318
secondary tumors in, 143–144
vascular neoplasms of, 150–151, 152f, 153
Orbital fascia, anatomy of, 135–136
Orbital meningioma, 137
CT appearance of, 137–138, 138f
Orbital osseous dysplasia, 142
Orbital pseudotumor, 156–158, 156f, 157f
Orbital teratoma, in children, 273–274
Orbital vessels, anatomy of, 136
Oropharynx
MR imaging of, 318–320, 319f, 320f
tumors of
spread pattern in, 288–289, 289f, 290f, 290–291, 291f
staging for, 281t
Ossicular chain, traumatic disruption of, 183
Osteoma
in children, 255
choroidal, 162–163, 163f
Otitis, malignant external, 80–81
Otitis media, 189f
Otomastoiditis
acute, 185–186, 186f, 187f, 188f
chronic, 186, 188f, 189f
Otosclerosis, 202
cochlear, 203f, 203–204, 205f
fenestral, 202–203, 202f

Papillary cystadenoma lymphomatosum, 217–218
Papilledema, of the optic nerve, 159
Paraganglioma, 73
Paranasal sinuses
anatomy of, 104–106, 105f, 106f, 107f, 108, 108f, 109f
in children, inflammatory lesions of, 261, 262f–263f, 264, 264f, 265f, 265, 266f
CT scanning protocol for, 102, 103f, 104
malignancies of, 121–128
MR imaging of, 311, 313–314, 314f, 315f
as source of secondary tumors to orbit, 143–144
tumors of
spread pattern of, 284–285, 286f, 287f, 287
staging for, 281t
Parapharyngeal space, pathology of, 70–71, 72f, 73–74, 73f, 74f
Parathyroid, MR imaging of, 324, 325f–327f, 327
Parathyroid adenoma
bilateral subcapsular, 53, 55f
CT evaluation of, 53, 55
left, 54, 55f
radiographic evaluation of, 52–53
right, 54, 55f
ultrasound evaluation of, 53, 55
Parathyroid glands, 52–53, 53f, 54f, 55
Parotid gland
anatomy of, 209–210, 210f, 211f–212f, 213

Parotid gland—*Cont.*
branchial cleft cysts of, 222–223, 224f
and lymphoma, 229–230
mass densities in, 216, 217f, 218f
and parapharyngeal space, tumor origin differentiation of, 218–219, 220f, 221f
recurrent pleomorphic adenoma in, 229, 229f
tumor vs. lipoma in, 221, 222f
Warthin's tumor in, 217–218, 219f
Petrous bone, epidermoid cyst or cholesteatoma of, 191, 192f
Pharyngeal space, and parotid gland, tumor orgin differentiation of, 219, 220f, 221f
Phthisis bulbi, of the eye, 163, 164f
Piriform sinuses, 5f, 9, 9f
carcinoma of, 20, 21f
tumors of, 292–293, 293f
Pituitary tumor, 79
Plasmacytoma, 124, 125f
Pleomorphic adenoma, 72f
of lacrimal gland, 145–146, 145f
of the parotid gland, 214, 216, 217, 223, 225f
recurrent, 229, 229f
recurrence of, 219, 221f
of submandibular and sublingual gland, 217
Plexiform neurofibroma, 141, 142f
Pneumocisternography, and CT, for acoustic neuroma, 196–199
Polyp, antrochoanal, 118, 118f
Postseptal cellulitis, in children, 261
Preseptal cellulitis
in children, 261
of the orbit, 153, 153f
Prestyloid lesions, 70–71, 72f
Pseudomonas aeruginosa, and carcinoma of the ear, 201
Pseudotumor, orbital, 156–158, 156f, 157f
Pterygoid muscle, pseudoenlargement of, 81–82, 82f
Pterygopalatine fossa, 111f, 111–112
and angiofibroma, 125, 126f

Radiation, in pediatric practice, 238
Radiation dosimetry, in CT evaluation of orbit, 133
Radical neck dissection, for salivary gland tumors, 227
Radiotherapy management, 295
dose-related factors in, 295–298, 298f
and methods of improving therapeutic ratio, 299
normal tissue tolerance factors in, 298–299
Radiotherapy planning
for buccal cavity, 287–288
epidemiology of cancer and, 279
for laryngopharynx, 291–293, 293f
for nasopharynx, 283–284, 283f, 284f
for oropharynx, 288–289, 289f, 290f, 290–291, 291f
for paranasal sinuses, 284–285, 286f, 287f, 287
for salivary gland tumors, 293–294, 294f

Radiotherapy planning—*Cont.*
for skin cancer, 294–295, 296f–297f
and tumor anatomic groupings, 280
and tumor pathology, 280
and tumor staging, 280, 281t–282t
Rathke's pouch tumor, 79
Recurrent papillary carcinoma, of the thyroid, 51f
Retinoblastoma, 159–161, 160f
in children, 255
Rhabdomyosarcoma, 69
in children
CT findings of, 239, 240f, 241f, 242
lymphatic spread in, 242, 243f
meningeal involvement in, 242–243
metastatic spread of, 242
staging of, 239
of the orbit, 147
Rotary subluxation, of C-1 on C-2, 258, 259f

Sialography, *see* Computed tomography sialography
Salivary glands
anatomic relationships of, 209–210, 210f, 211f, 212f, 213–214, 213f
CT sialography of, 216–217
CT scanning methods for, 208–209, 209f
histology of, 214
and lymphoma, 229–230
MR imaging of, 317f, 318f, 318
other diseases of, 231, 232f, 233–235, 234f, 235f
Salivary gland tumors, 71, 123, 124f
benign, 216–223
classification of, 214, 215t
cystic lesions and, 222–223, 224f
enhancement by contrast medium, 221–222, 223f
incidence of, 214, 216
malignant, 223–231
and lymph node involvement, 227
metastasis and, 228, 230–231, 230f
treatment modalities for, 225
in nasal cavity, 123, 124f
radiotherapy planning for, 293–294, 294f
W.H.O. classification of, 214, 216t
Sarcoidosis, of salivary glands, 233–234
Sarcoma, synovial, 74, 75f
Sialadenitis, chronic, 233
Sinus
ethmoid, 106, 107f, 108, 108f, 109f
frontal, 104–106, 105f, 106f
maxillary, *see* Maxillary sinus
paranasal, *see* Paranasal sinuses
piriform, *see* Piriform sinuses
sphenoid, 112, 112f, 113f, 114f, 114
supraorbital ethmoid, 106, 107f
Sinus opacification, 114, 115f
Sjögren's syndrome, 230, 235f
and chronic sialadenitis, 233

Skin cancer, radiotherapy planning for, 294–295, 296f–297f
Skull base
anatomy of, 62–63
and infection, 80–81, 80f
pathology of, 78–79, 79f
Sound conducting system, anomalies of, 179, 180f, 181f
Sphenoid sinus, 112, 112f, 113f, 114f, 114
Spin-echo pulse sequence, in MR, 305, 306f
Squamous cell carcinoma
of nasal cavity and paranasal sinuses, 122, 122f
of salivary glands, 225, 226f–227f
of skin, 296f–297f
treatment plan for, 297–298, 298f
Staphyloma, of the eye, 163, 164f
Sternocleidomastoid muscle, CT anatomy of, 36, 37f
Subclavian artery and vein, 40f, 40
Sublingual gland, anatomy of, 214
Submandibular gland
anatomy of, 212f–213f, 213–214
and contrast medium for imaging of, 209f
and lymphoma, 229–230
mass density in, 216–217
Submandibular triangle, of the neck, 33
Submental triangle, of the neck, 33
Subperiosteal abscess, of the orbit, 154f, 154
Substernal goiter, 48, 49f, 50f
Supraglottic carcinoma, 292
Synovial sarcoma, 74, 75f

Temporal bone
and common tissues densities, 176
congenital anomalies of, 178–180, 180f, 181f, 182f, 182
CT prerequisites for study of, 171–173, 172f, 173f, 174f
and fibrous dysplasia in children, 250, 252, 253f
MR imaging of, 314–315, 316f
primary malignant neoplasms of, 201, 201f
reformatted images of, 177f, 178f
trauma to, 183–184, 184f, 185f
Therapeutic ratio, methods for improving, 299
Thoracic inlet, 34
and subclavian artery and vein, 40f, 40
Thyroglossal duct, 42
Thyroglossal duct cyst, 42–43, 43f
in children, 275
of tongue base, 92–93, 92f
Thyroid cancer, metastatic to base of tongue, 98f, 99
Thyroid cartilage, 4–6, 7f
destruction of, 15, 16f, 17f
fracture of, 27, 28f
inferior cornu of, 38f, 39
superior cornu of, 36, 36f
and thyroid notch, 36, 37f

Thyroidectomy, and postoperative scans, 50, 50f, 51f, 52
Thyroid gland
  anatomy of, 39f, 40
  embryology of, 42
  hypothyroidism and, 41, 42f
  imaging modalities for, 41
  lingual, 93, 93f
  MR imaging of, 324, 325f, 327f, 327
  normal tissue of, 41, 41f
  pathology of, 42–52
Thyroid notch, 36, 37f
Tongue, base of
  arteries and veins of, 88f, 89f, 90
  carcinoma of, 95, 96t, 96f, 97, 97f, 99
  congenital lesions of, 91–94
  CT technique in, 85–86
  lymphatic drainage of, 90–91, 91f
  miscellaneous tumors of, 98f, 99
  muscle anatomy of, 86, 87f–89f, 90
  MR imaging of, 318–320, 319f, 320f, 321f–323f, 323
Tonsil, lingual, 91f, 91
Tornwaldt's cyst, 70
Transglottic carcinoma, 20, 22f–23f
Trauma
  to head and neck, in children, 256–260
  to the larynx, 25, 27f, 27–28, 28f, 29f
  to temporal bone, 183–184, 184f, 185f
Triangles, of the neck, 31, 32f
  anterior, 33
  posterior, 34
True vocal cords, 7f, 9–10, 10f
  carcinoma of, CT role in, 14–15, 15f, 16f, 17, 17f
Tubotympanic disease, 186
Tumor
  anatomic groupings of, 280
  of buccal cavity, *see* Buccal cavity, tumors of

Tumor—*Cont.*
  glomus complex, *see* Glomus complex tumors
  glottic, 14–19
  of lacrimal glands, 144–147
  of middle ear and mastoid, density of, 176
  of the nasopharynx, 64–65
  orbital lymphoid, 147–148, 149f, 150
  of parapharyngeal space, 70–71, 72f, 73–74, 73f, 74f
  pathology of, 280
  pattern of spread of, 280
  of salivary glands, *see* Salivary gland tumors
  secondary, in the orbit, 143–144
  staging of, 280, 281t–282t
  supraglottic, 18f, 19–20, 19f, 20f, 21f
  transglottic, 20, 22f–23f
  Warthin's, 72f, 217–218
Tympanosclerosis, density of, 176

Ultrasound, evaluation of parathyroid adenoma, 53, 55

Vascular anatomy, of the larynx, 12f, 12, 13f
Vascular anomalies, of temporal bone, 182
Vascular neoplasms, of the orbit, 150–151, 152f, 153
Vision, decrease in, case study of, 331–332, 331f
Vocal cord fixation, 17–19

Vocal cords
  carcinoma of, 14–17
  false, 7f, 10–11, 10f
  true, 7f, 9–10, 10f

Warthin's tumor, 217–218
  cystic, 72f
World Health Organization, classification of salivary gland tumors by, 214, 216t
Wyburn-Mason syndrome, 151